W9-CKJ-403

BOTTOM LINE'S

Treasury of Natural Remedies

Over **1,000** Ways to Halt, Heal or Prevent Common Ailments

Bottom Line Books

www.BottomLinePublications.com

Contents

■ Contents ■

Preface

We are proud to bring you *Bottom Line's Treasury of Natural Remedies*. We trust that you'll find the best natural healing techniques and money-saving solutions to your health concerns.

Whether it's advice about herbs and supplements or cutting-edge nutrition, our editors talk to the people—from doctors and healers to consumer health advocates—who understand time-tested health wisdom and the latest research.

How do we find all these top-notch medical experts? Over the past three decades, we have built a network of literally thousands of leading physicians in alternative and conventional medicine. They are affiliated with the premier medical institutions and the best universities throughout the world. We read the important medical journals and follow the latest research that is reported at medical conferences. And we regularly talk to our advisors in major teaching hospitals, private practices and government health agencies.

Bottom Line's Treasury of Natural Remedies is a result of our ongoing research and contact with these experts, and is a distillation of their latest thinking and advice. We trust that you will enjoy the presentation and glean new, helpful and affordable information about the health topics that concern you and your family.

As a reader of a Bottom Line Book, please be assured that you are receiving reliable and well-researched information from a trusted source.

But, please use prudence in health matters. Always speak to your physician before taking vitamins, supplements or over-the-counter medication…changing your diet…or beginning an exercise program. If you experience side effects from any regimen, contact your doctor immediately.

The Editors, Bottom Line Books, Stamford, Connecticut.

1

Healthy Food Remedies

Had Enough Salmon and Blueberries?

By now, we all can name plenty of "superfoods," and chances are that salmon, blueberries and spinach are at the top of your list. But what if you would like to add some variety to your diet—or never liked the taste of these highly publicized, nutritionally rich foods in the first place?

Good news: There are plenty of other nutritional superstars that you can try with or instead of the more well-known ones.

If you can't find any of the foods mentioned below at your local grocery store, try a specialty food store, such as Trader Joe's or Whole Foods, or an online food retailer, such as *www. lotusfoods.com* (866-972-6879)…or *www.eden foods.com* (888-424-3336).

Tasty, underrated superfoods that are worth trying…

•**Instead of salmon…try red quinoa.** Pronounced "KEEN-wah," this hearty whole grain offers a colorful alternative to popular sources of protein, such as fish and meat.

Nutritional benefits: Quinoa is one of the few grains that, like salmon, is considered a "complete protein"—that is, it contains all eight essential amino acids that the body needs. For this reason, quinoa is an excellent alternative for vegetarians or others who may want a tasty substitute for protein-rich salmon. One cup of cooked quinoa contains 8 g of protein—and modest amounts of a plant-based form of the heart-healthy omega-3 fats that are found in salmon.

Quinoa is also a good source of zinc (important for immunity) as well as magnesium and potassium (both of which help reduce blood pressure). What's more, quinoa is rich in fiber—one cup of the cooked grain delivers 5 g.

Susan Mitchell, PhD, RD, registered dietitian based in Winter Park, Florida. She has coauthored three books, including *Fat Is Not Your Fate* (Simon & Schuster), and is the host of "Straight Talk About Eating Smart," a podcast on WDBO.com (AM 580 WDBO is a central Florida news/talk radio station).

Tasty options: Stir fluffy cooked quinoa into soups and stews...sprinkle over salads... or use in chili in place of ground beef or turkey.

• **Instead of brown rice...try black rice.** According to ancient Chinese legend, only the ruling emperor was allowed to indulge in this extra-dark, nutty-flavored grain—that's why it's often called the "forbidden rice."

Nutritional benefits: Like brown rice, black rice is rich in fiber. However, black rice is also a good source of antioxidants called anthocyanins, which are found in blue/purple superfoods, such as blueberries, grapes and eggplant. These antioxidants are responsible for the deep-purple hue that develops when black rice is cooked.

Important scientific finding: A spoonful of cooked black rice packs the same amount of anthocyanins as a spoonful of fresh blueberries, but with less sugar and more fiber and vitamin E, according to research recently presented at a meeting of the American Chemical Society.

Tasty options: For a delicious stir-fry, top black rice with mushrooms (button or portobello, for example), red pepper and pineapple.

• **Instead of blueberries...try cherries.** Compared with blueberries, these dark red gems are definitely underrated.

Nutritional benefits: Cherries are loaded with healthful compounds that are believed to help prevent inflammation and possibly even some types of cancer, including colon cancer.

Cherries also are a good source of the sleep hormone melatonin, which helps fight insomnia and jet lag.

Research shows that tart cherry juice eases postexercise muscle soreness—members of the New York Rangers hockey team drink it for this reason.

Important scientific finding: In a study reported in the *Journal of Nutrition*, 18 healthy men and women who supplemented their daily diets with just over two cups of Bing cherries daily for 28 days reduced their levels of C-reactive protein, an inflammatory marker in the blood that can signal plaque formation, by 25%.

Tasty options: Sprinkle dried cherries on top of yogurt, stir them into oatmeal or make a superfood trail mix with granola, dried cherries, almonds and dark chocolate. Unsweetened frozen or dried cherries are available at Trader Joe's.

As a postexercise treat, drink five ounces of tart cherry juice with seltzer or blended into a smoothie.

• **Instead of spinach...try kale.** Many people are wary of this cruciferous vegetable—it's big and bushy and often has a bitter smell. But when cooked, kale has a mild taste.

Nutritional benefits: Kale is packed with fiber, calcium, iron and vitamins A, C and K. (For this reason, anyone who is taking a blood thinner should avoid kale—its vitamin K content can reduce the drug's effect.) Kale also contains a chemical called sulforaphane, which has been linked to reduced cancer risk in numerous studies.

Delicious cooked kale: Wash and thoroughly dry kale, remove the center stalk and tough ends, cutting the leaves on each side into bite-size pieces. Add olive oil, chopped scallions, garlic and/or fresh pepper, if you like. Cook in a sauté pan until the kale is tender. For even more flavor, sauté in chicken or vegetable broth.

• **Instead of sweet potatoes...try plantains.** Plantains look like bananas, but they're not eaten straight from the peel unless they're extremely ripe (when their peel turns completely black).

Nutritional benefits: Plantains are a rich source of potassium and vitamins A and C. One cup of cooked plantains also contains an impressive 3.5 g of fiber. What's really exciting about these fruits is their potential to help people with Crohn's disease, a chronic inflammatory disorder of the digestive tract.

Recent study finding: The fiber in plantains may help reduce symptoms of Crohn's disease, such as diarrhea and bleeding, according to preliminary research published in the journal *Gut*.

Tasty options: Popular in Latin American cooking, plantains are often fried. However, lightly broiling or grilling them will help you avoid most of the excess fat and calories of frying. Grilling or broiling ripe plantains also brings out the natural sugar. Use them as a delicious, healthful topping for vanilla frozen yogurt.

Fresh Garlic Better Than Bottled Garlic

Garlic contains allicin, which is a pungent compound that may help fight infection, prevent food poisoning, and protect against blood clots and certain cancers. Bottling interferes with enzymes needed to activate allicin.

Best: Stick to fresh cloves to get the most from garlic's immune-boosting properties.

Toyohiko Ariga, PhD, professor, department of applied life sciences, Nihon University Graduate School of Bioresource Sciences, Japan, and leader of a study published in *Journal of Agricultural and Food Chemistry*.

Dry, Wrinkled Fruit... Strong Bones

Bahram H. Arjmandi, PhD, RD, Margaret A. Sitton Professor and chair, Nutrition, Food, and Exercise Sciences, College of Human Sciences, The Florida State University, Tallahassee, Florida.

Prunes...it's not a particularly pleasant word nor a particularly pretty food, but I think these dark, wrinkly dried fruits are in the process of getting a facelift. Not only are marketers trying to make prunes more appealing by rebranding them as "dried plums" (which is what they are, of course), but the US Department of Agriculture (USDA) has funded some impressive research that puts muscle behind the makeover, cataloging a long enough list of nutritional benefits that prunes now can be considered a real "superfood." The newest study, from Florida State University, finds that including prunes in your daily diet offers powerful protection against both osteoporosis and bone fracture.

SWEET PROTECTION FOR YOUR BONES

Prunes are amazingly good at strengthening bones, said the study's lead author, Bahram H. Arjmandi, PhD, RD, chairman of Florida State's department of nutrition, food and exercise sciences in its College of Human Sciences. Having studied how various fruits, including figs, raisins and strawberries, affect bone health, Dr. Arjmandi said that prunes are uniquely helpful in preventing and/or reversing osteoporosis. That's because they contain compounds that help suppress the natural process of bone breakdown more technically known as resorption—which is a big issue for older people since bone breakdown tends to exceed the rate of new bone growth as people age.

"Yes, you can take medication to make your bones stronger," Dr. Arjmandi said, "but I don't think you can compete with nature in producing anything that is as effective in promoting bone health, while also being healthy in other ways, as prunes are."

This is some pretty dramatic talk—so let's look closely at the study. It spanned one year and involved 236 women who were one to 10 years postmenopausal, either nonsmokers or who smoked 20 cigarettes per day or less, did not have any metabolic diseases and were not taking hormone replacement medication or any other medication that could influence bone health. For the study, half of the women ate 100 grams of prunes (about 10 prunes) each day, while the control group ate 75 grams of dried apple (equal to about two fresh apples, and comparable to the amount of calories, carbohydrates, fat and fiber in 100 grams of prunes). Participants' diets remained the same as normal otherwise. Additionally, everyone in the study took daily doses of calcium (500 milligrams) and vitamin D (400 international units), as do many women.

After a year, a standard bone density x-ray of the ulna (one of two long bones in the forearm) and spine showed that, on average, the women who had been eating the prunes...er, dried plums...had significantly increased bone mineral density compared with their measured levels before eating prunes. The women who had been eating dried apples, on the other hand, did not lose any bone density during the

3

year of the study, as would have been expected, and their bones showed a slight increase in bone density—indicating that apples are also slightly bone protective, but not to the extent that prunes are. Other bones were measured, but the most dramatic changes were in the ulna and spine—which is gratifying because the ulna and spine are the two major fracture sites linked to osteoporosis.

LEARN TO LOVE PRUNES

So, what is it about prunes that helps bones? First, they are unusually high in several types of phytonutrients including the antioxidants neochlorogenic acid and chlorogenic acid, which have been shown to prevent bone loss. Prunes contain larger amounts of boron than most other fruits, and boron helps preserve bone mineral density by modulating bone and calcium metabolism. Prunes also contain iron and potassium, important for blood and heart health.

The women in the study were asked to eat 10 prunes a day, which may be difficult for someone unaccustomed to eating prunes. But Dr. Arjmandi reckons that eating as few as three prunes a day will have important health benefits. I wondered whether all the sugar in prunes caused any problems—he told me that the glycemic index of prunes is about 27, among the lowest of all fruits, and that none of the women gained any weight during the study (which, he said, could be because prunes contain so much fiber). He added that prunes (unlike other dried fruits) don't contain sulfites—good news for the many folks who are allergic to this common preservative. To prevent mold and yeast spoilage, the preservative potassium sorbate, which is generally regarded as safe and is unlikely to cause allergic reactions, is used. But anyone who wants to avoid it can find prunes that are preservative-free in health-food stores and online.

And what about the laxative effect so often attributed to prunes? They have lots of fiber, including insoluble fiber, which Dr. Arjmandi said makes them exceptionally good at helping to keep the gastrointestinal (GI) system healthy. "Forgetting about the bones for a minute," he said, "prunes are really great for digestive health. It's something people may not want to hear about so much, but the truth

is, the health of the entire body depends on the health of the GI system." While drinking prune juice certainly can make the bowels move—quickly—Dr. Arjmandi said that eating dried prunes doesn't have the same effect.

Personally, I like prunes—they're chewy and sweet but not overwhelmingly sweet like dates, and they have an earthy tartness that I enjoy. I snack on them straight from the box, and I also like them chopped up and mixed with nuts or chopped into salads. There are also some really tasty main courses, such as chicken Marbella, that are made with prunes… you can get some unique and delicious recipes by looking online at *http://www.california driedplums.org/recipes*.

Supercharge Your Meals

Joy Bauer, RD, CDN, author of several nutrition books, including *Your Inner Brain: 4 Steps to Thin Forever* (William Morrow) and *Joy Bauer's Food Cures* (Rodale). Bauer is the nutrition expert for the *Today* show. *www.joybauer.com*

Until recently, most nutrition research has focused on the health benefits of individual nutrients. For example, it's well-established that vitamin A is good for the eyes…calcium builds stronger bones… and zinc boosts immunity.

Now there is strong scientific evidence that nutrition is much more complex than that. When certain foods are combined, their nutritional value is much greater than when the foods are eaten individually.

That's why dietitians recommend eating a varied diet with plenty of fruits, vegetables, whole grains and low-fat proteins—the greater the variety, the better your chances of maximizing the health benefits of your food.

Latest development: Scientists are beginning to understand exactly which specific food combinations are the most effective in helping the body fight common ailments.

For example…

TO FIGHT ARTHRITIS

• **Combine Carotenes and spices.** Carotenes are a group of powerful antioxidants that attack toxic, cell-damaging molecules known as free radicals.

In addition to the widely known beta-carotene, there are other carotenes, including beta-cryptoxanthin, which has been shown to fight rheumatoid arthritis and osteoarthritis.

Good sources of both beta-carotene and beta-cryptoxanthin: Winter squash (especially butternut), pumpkin, red bell peppers and carrots...apricots and watermelon.

The spices turmeric (with its antioxidant oil curcumin) and ginger contain phytochemicals that help suppress inflammatory reactions that can lead to arthritis. Turmeric is the bright yellow, dried spice found in curry powder. Ginger is available in powdered form as a spice and also as a fresh root.

My favorite arthritis-fighting combos: Curried butternut squash soup...pumpkin-ginger muffins...Asian ginger stir-fry with red bell peppers...and curried carrots.

TO FIGHT HEART PROBLEMS

• **Combine lycopene and monounsaturated fats.** Lycopene is a fat-soluble antioxidant that has been shown to reduce the risk for heart disease, perhaps by stopping the process that leads to atherosclerosis (fatty buildup in the arteries).

Good sources of lycopene: Tomatoes, red and pink grapefruit, watermelon and guava.

Helpful: Eat cooked tomatoes—they contain three to four times more lycopene than raw tomatoes.

Monounsaturated fats are believed to protect against heart disease and have a number of cardiovascular benefits. These healthful fats help the body absorb all fat-soluble nutrients, including lycopene.

Good sources of monounsaturated fats: Olive oil and canola oil...avocado...almonds, walnuts, peanuts and cashews.

My favorite heart-healthy combos: Roasted tomatoes with a touch of olive oil...any meal made with homemade or store-bought tomato sauce that contains olive oil...a salad of grapefruit and avocado...and turkey, avocado and tomato sandwiches.

TO FIGHT MEMORY LOSS

• **Combine folic acid and anthocyanins.** One of the B vitamins, folic acid (also known as folate) helps lower blood levels of the amino acid homocysteine—a process that research suggests may promote blood flow to the brain. Folic acid also enhances communication between brain chemicals known as neurotransmitters.

Good sources of folic acid: Fortified whole-grain breakfast cereals and oatmeal...green, leafy vegetables, bok choy and broccoli...oranges (or orange juice) and berries (such as strawberries and blackberries).

Anthocyanins are antioxidant phytochemicals that have been shown to not only help prevent memory loss but also improve failing memory.

Good sources of anthocyanins: Berries (especially blueberries—their antioxidant flavonols help protect against brain degeneration), red or black grapes...red or purple cabbage, beets, red onions and eggplant.

My favorite memory-enhancing combos: Folic acid–fortified breakfast cereal with berries...coleslaw with red cabbage and bok choy...chicken-vegetable stir-fry with red onions and broccoli...and fruit salad with oranges and blueberries.

TO FIGHT FATIGUE

• **Combine iron and vitamin C.** Iron helps red blood cells carry oxygen throughout the body. Without enough iron, your cells can become starved for oxygen. This can lead to anemia, which causes listlessness, headache, irritability and general lack of energy.

Good sources of iron: Lean beef, turkey, chicken, lamb and pork...clams, oysters and shrimp...soybeans, chickpeas and lentils...spinach, asparagus and green, leafy vegetables.

Vitamin C is a powerful antioxidant, but most people don't realize that it can help fight fatigue by enhancing the body's ability to absorb iron. By adding a food that contains significant amounts of vitamin C to a meal with an iron-rich food, your body will absorb up to three times more iron.

This is especially important for vegetarians, premenopausal women (who lose iron through menstruation) and people with a genetic predisposition to anemia (determined through blood tests).

Caution: People with hemochromatosis, a dangerous disorder that causes iron to build up in the blood, should not combine foods high in iron and vitamin C.

Good sources of vitamin C: Bell and hot chili peppers, broccoli and kale…tomatoes, mangoes, oranges (or orange juice), strawberries and pineapple.

My favorite fatigue-fighting combos: Spinach salad with mandarin oranges…bean chili (such as kidney, pinto or black bean) with crushed tomatoes…steak with sautéed broccoli…and chicken cacciatore with tomatoes and peppers.

TO FIGHT MOOD SWINGS

• **Combine soluble fiber and protein.** Mood swings often are caused by fluctuations in blood sugar (glucose).

Low-quality carbohydrates, such as white rice, white bread, cakes and soft drinks, cause blood sugar spikes that usually lead to a sluggish, depressed feeling when they begin to plummet about one hour after consumption of such foods.

High-quality carbohydrates, such as vegetables, fruits and whole grains, contain soluble fiber that causes a slower, less dramatic rise in glucose.

Good sources of soluble fiber: Oatmeal…barley, lentils, beans (such as kidney, lima and black) and peas…apples (all types), raisins, oranges and bananas…cauliflower and sweet potatoes.

Protein is another natural blood sugar stabilizer—it helps slow the absorption of carbohydrates in your diet. Pairing protein with soluble fiber at every meal will help keep your blood sugar as steady as possible.

Good sources of lean protein: Turkey or chicken breast…fish (all types)…pork tenderloin…lean beef…egg whites…yogurt (low-fat or fat-free)…milk (low-fat or fat-free)…and beans (such as pinto and black).

My favorite mood-stabilizing combos: Three-bean turkey chili with pinto, black and kidney beans…plain, low-fat or fat-free yogurt with fresh fruit (such as berries or peaches)…pork

tenderloin with sweet potatoes and cauliflower… hard-boiled eggs with turkey bacon and fruit… and oatmeal with a hard-boiled egg.

Vitamin C for Healthier Hips

In a four-year study of 606 men and women, researchers found that men with the highest intake of vitamin C (314 mg daily) from food and supplements had the lowest levels of bone loss in the hip. Vitamin C is required for the formation of collagen, the main protein in bone. There was no similar finding in women, possibly because they already had adequate vitamin C levels.

For strong bones: Strive to eat five to nine servings daily of vitamin C–rich fruits and vegetables (such as strawberries and red peppers).

Katherine L. Tucker, PhD, director, Dietary Assessment and Epidemiology Research Program, Human Nutrition Research Center on Aging, Tufts University, Boston.

Six Ways to Liven Up Your Heart-Healthy Diet

Janet Bond Brill, PhD, RD, expert in nutrition and cardiovascular disease prevention based in Valley Forge, Pennsylvania. She is director of nutrition for Fitness Together, a franchise company of almost 500 personal fitness-training studios, has served as a nutrition consultant for several corporations and is the author of *Prevent a Second Heart Attack* (Three Rivers). *www.drjanet.com*

Just about everyone knows that a Mediterranean-style diet can help prevent heart disease. Even if you've already had a heart attack, this style of eating—emphasizing such foods as fish and vegetables—can reduce the risk for a second heart attack by up to 70%.

Problem: About 80% of patients with heart disease quit following dietary advice within one year after their initial diagnosis. That's often because they want more choices but aren't sure which foods have been proven to work.

Solution: Whether you already have heart disease or want to prevent it, you can liven up your diet by trying foods that usually don't get much attention for their heart-protective benefits…

Secret 1: Popcorn. It's more than just a snack. It's a whole grain that's high in cholesterol-lowering fiber. Surprisingly, popcorn contains more fiber, per ounce, than whole-wheat bread or brown rice.

Scientific evidence: Data from the National Health and Nutrition Examination Survey found that people who eat popcorn daily get 22% more fiber than those who don't eat it.

Important: Eat "natural" popcorn, preferably air-popped or microwaved in a brown paper bag, without added oil. The commercially prepared popcorn packets generally contain too much salt, butter and other additives. Three cups of popped popcorn, which contain almost 6 g of fiber and 90 calories, is considered a serving of whole grains. Studies have shown that at least three servings of whole grains a day (other choices include oatmeal and brown rice) may help reduce the risk for heart disease, high cholesterol and obesity.

Secret 2: Chia seeds. You're probably familiar with Chia pets —those terra-cotta figures that sprout thick layers of grassy "fur." The same seeds, native to Mexico and Guatemala, are increasingly available in health-food stores. I consider them a superfood because they have a nutrient profile that rivals heart-healthy flaxseed.

In fact, chia seeds contain more omega-3 fatty acids than flaxseed. Omega-3s increase the body's production of anti-inflammatory eicosanoids, hormonelike substances that help prevent "adhesion molecules" from causing plaque buildup and increasing atherosclerosis.

Scientific evidence: A study published in the *Journal of the American College of Cardiology*, which looked at nearly 40,000 participants, found that an omega-3 rich diet can prevent and even reverse existing cardiovascular disease.

Other benefits: One ounce of chia seeds has 10 g of fiber, 5 g of alpha-linolenic acid and 18% of the Recommended Dietary Allowance for calcium for adults ages 19 to 50.

Chia seeds look and taste something like poppy seeds. You can add them to baked goods, such as muffins, or sprinkle them on salads and oatmeal or other cereals.

Secret 3: Figs. They're extraordinarily rich in antioxidants with an oxygen radical absorbance capacity (ORAC) score of 3,383. Scientists use this ORAC scale to determine the antioxidant capacity of various foods. An orange, by comparison, scores only about 1,819. Fresh figs are among the best sources of beta-carotene and other heart-healthy carotenoids.

Scientific evidence: In a study published in the *Journal of the American College of Nutrition*, two groups of participants were "challenged" with sugary soft drinks, which are known to increase arterial oxidation. Oxidation in the arteries triggers atherosclerosis, a main risk factor for heart disease. Those who were given only soda had a drop in healthful antioxidant activity in the blood…those who were given figs as well as soda had an increase in blood antioxidant levels.

Bonus: Ten dried figs contain 140 mg of calcium. Other compounds in figs, such as quercetin, reduce inflammation and dilate the arteries. Perhaps for these reasons, people who eat figs regularly have much less heart disease than those who don't eat them, according to studies. Most dried figs contain added sulfites, so it's best to buy organic, sulfite-free dried figs.

Secret 4: Soy protein. Tofu, soy milk and other soy foods are "complete proteins"—that is, they supply all of the essential amino acids that your body needs but without the cholesterol and large amount of saturated fat found in meat.

Scientific evidence: People who replace dairy or meat protein with soy will have an average drop in LDL "bad" cholesterol of 2% to 7%, according to research from the American Heart Association. Every 1% drop in LDL lowers heart disease risk about 2%.

A one-half cup serving of tofu provides 10 g of protein. An eight-ounce glass of soy milk gives about 7 g. Edamame (steamed or boiled green soybeans) has about 9 g per half cup.

Avoid processed soy products, such as hydrogenated soybean oil (a trans fat), soy isoflavone powders and soy products with excess added sodium.

Secret 5: Lentils. I call these "longevity legumes" because studies have shown that they can literally extend your life.

Best choices: Brown or black lentils.

Scientific evidence: In one study, published in the *Asia Pacific Journal of Clinical Nutrition*, the eating habits of five groups of older adults were compared. For every 20 g (a little less than three-fourths of an ounce) increase in the daily intake of lentils and/or other legumes, there was an 8% reduction in the risk of dying within seven years.

Lentils contain large amounts of fiber, plant protein and antioxidants along with folate, iron and magnesium—all of which are important for cardiovascular health.

Similarly, a Harvard study found that people who ate one serving of cooked beans (one-third cup) a day were 38% less likely to have a heart attack than those who ate beans less than once a month.

Caution: Beans have been shown to cause gout flare-ups in some people.

Important: Lentils cook much faster than other beans. They don't need presoaking. When simmered in water, they're ready in 20 to 30 minutes. You need about one-half cup of cooked lentils, beans or peas each day for heart health.

Secret 6: Pinot Noir and Cabernet Sauvignon. All types of alcohol seem to have some heart-protective properties, but red wine offers the most.

Scientific evidence: People who drink alcohol regularly in moderation (one five-ounce glass of wine daily for women, and no more than two for men) have a 30% to 50% lower risk of dying from a heart attack than those who don't drink, according to research published in *Archives of Internal Medicine*.

Best choices: Pinot Noir, Cabernet Sauvignon and Tannat wines (made from Tannat red grapes). These wines have the highest concentrations of flavonoids, antioxidants that reduce arterial inflammation and inhibit the oxidation of LDL cholesterol. Oxidation is the process that makes cholesterol more likely to accumulate within artery walls.

Bonus: Red wines also contain resveratrol, a type of polyphenol that is thought to increase the synthesis of proteins that slow aging. Red wine has 10 times more polyphenols than white varieties.

In a four-year study of nearly 7,700 men and women nondrinkers, those who began to drink a moderate amount of red wine cut their risk for heart attack by 38% compared with nondrinkers.

If you are a nondrinker or currently drink less than the amounts described above, talk to your doctor before changing your alcohol intake. If you cannot drink alcohol, pomegranate or purple grape juice is a good alternative.

Can Beets Beat High Blood Pressure?

Amrita Ahluwalia, PhD, professor of vascular pharmacology, Centre for Clinical Pharmacology, William Harvey Research Institute, Queen Mary's School of Medicine & Dentistry, London, UK.

Beyond being a treat for the eyes, with its gorgeous deep red color, beet juice serves up some pretty attractive health benefits—especially for people who need to bring down their blood pressure. Drinking beet juice appears to have a protective effect on blood vessels, which helps keep blood pressure under control, according to researchers from the UK. To learn more about the study and what it means for consumers, we contacted researcher Amrita Ahluwalia, PhD, professor of vascular pharmacology at Queen Mary's School of Medicine & Dentistry in London.

NITRATES IN BEETS PROTECT BLOOD VESSELS

In the study, 14 people with normal blood pressure drank two cups of either pure beet juice (with no additives) or water. Dr. Ahluwalia and her colleagues checked the participants' blood pressure at regular intervals both before and after ingestion. *They found that...*

• **Blood pressure began to drop** in the beet group about 60 minutes after drinking the juice.

• **Blood pressure reached its lowest level** in the beet group two to three hours after drinking the juice (a reduction of approximately 10 mmHg systolic at two and a half hours and 8 mmHg diastolic at three hours).

• **No similar impact was observed in the control group, who drank water.**

Dr. Ahluwalia believes the nitrates in beets are what help control blood pressure by protecting blood vessels. She explained that colonies of bacteria on the back of our tongues chemically change nitrate to nitrite. When we swallow saliva, this nitrite enters the stomach and then crosses into circulation, where it is changed into a very important molecule called nitric oxide (NO). This is a "vasodilator," which means that it opens up blood vessels so blood flows more easily. With less resistance to blood flow, blood pressure comes down.

Results of the study were published in *Hypertension*.

HBP RX: BEETS

"Our hope is that simple dietary interventions—such as including more beets and other fresh produce in the diet—may one day replace some blood pressure medicines," says Dr. Ahluwalia. We're not there yet, however. She advises people with high blood pressure to carefully discuss all treatment options with their doctors before stopping any medication. In the meantime, you can buy fresh beet juice at most health food stores or make it yourself by steaming and juicing several whole beets. If you find beet juice too heavy, lighten it with apple juice. Other excellent sources of nitrates are spinach, lettuce and root vegetables. Two cups of beet juice is a lot, Dr. Ahluwalia notes, so she's currently testing the effect of lesser amounts and will also be studying its effect on people who have high blood pressure.

Smoothies for Health

Pat Crocker, culinary herbalist, author, *The Smoothies Bible* (Robert Rose). She is based in Neustadt, Ontario, Canada.

There is an intriguing study from Germany about smoothies. It highlights a particular health benefit of these favorite warm-weather beverages—one that may surprise you a bit, but read on, as this may help prevent colon cancer! How? By delivering the critical nutrients in apples directly to the colon.

Earlier research has suggested that the antioxidant and anti-inflammatory polyphenols found in apples help prevent colon cancer, but to be useful they must not be absorbed by the small intestine. Instead, they need to get to the colon where they can be effective. This study found that smoothies delivered significantly more polyphenols and quinic acid to the colon than apple juice or cider. That is a valuable bit of information, because these key nutrients protect against colon disease. The researchers speculate that this is because smoothies made with the whole apple (including the skin but not the core) retain much more of the fruit's cell wall components than apple juice, and these likely bind the nutrients, thus protecting them from being digested by the small intestine further up the gastrointestinal (GI) tract.

In truth, you can get the same benefits by just eating an apple—but what's particularly great about smoothies is that they're an easy, efficient and utterly delicious way to boost your intake not only of fruits and vegetables, but also herbs, spices and other nutrients you can add to smoothies to support specific health needs and enhance general well-being.

For more ideas about how smoothies can contribute to health and also to get tips on how to prepare them most healthfully, we spoke with Pat Crocker, culinary herbalist and author of *The Smoothies Bible*.

THE MOST HEALTHFUL SMOOTHIES, STEP BY STEP

Crocker said that smoothie recipes usually begin with about one-half cup of liquid per serving—milk, yogurt, fruit juices (fresh if possible), vegetable juice (generally tomato, carrot or beet), chicken or beef stock, or green and herbal teas. Added to the liquid are two, three or more of a wide variety of fresh or frozen fruits and/or vegetables. Crocker emphasizes the importance of using high-quality organic ingredients of many colors for maximum antioxidant levels. You can add a splash more of antioxidants with such nutrient-rich ingredients as acai berries, pomegranate (including the seeds, which are edible and contain most of the fiber and antioxidants) and blueberries. If you are using fruits high in natural sugars, for example pineapple, mangoes or kiwis, add lower-sugar fruits for balance, such as apples, watermelon or strawberries.

HEALTH & FLAVOR ENHANCERS

Crocker has a long list of spices, herbs and other health promoters that you can add to smoothies, but the following are among those she particularly advises. Many of these are in your supermarket and if not, health-food stores will have them.

Note: Always put these in with the other ingredients before you blend to be sure that they are well mixed.

Here are some suggestions to help improve general healing…

•**Cinnamon promotes digestion and insulin sensitivity and relieves nausea.** Add one-quarter teaspoon per smoothie serving—especially delicious with apples and blueberries.

•**Ginger calms nausea, aids digestion, relieves diarrhea and flatulence and may soothe pain of arthritis.** Try one-quarter teaspoon of powdered ginger per serving or one-half inch of crystallized or peeled fresh ginger, coarsely chopped. (Ginger is not recommended for anyone with a bleeding disorder, gallstones, or who is taking a blood thinner, and it is not recommended for children under age two.) Ginger is a good complement to pears and peaches.

•**Dandelion supports liver, gallbladder and kidney health, helps with high blood pressure and is a mild laxative.** Add one teaspoon of crushed, dried roots to vegetable smoothies.

To boost the immune system…

•**Astragalus boosts the immune system** and alleviates adverse effects of chemotherapy. Use one teaspoon of dried, powdered astragalus per serving. It has little or no taste.

Note: If you are using steroids, you should discuss with your doctor whether it's okay to consume astragalus.

•**Burdock,** a mild laxative (it contains the fiber inulin), has prebiotic properties and is a diuretic. Crush dried roots into a fine powder, and use one to two teaspoons per serving. It has a crisp, slightly sweet taste. Burdock often is used in sushi, so it goes well with sweet or savory smoothies.

•**Cayenne stimulates blood circulation and digestion,** is a diuretic, and has a beneficial effect on the nervous system. Start by adding just one-eighth teaspoon of powdered cayenne per smoothie serving and increase to one-quarter teaspoon if the spicy flavor doesn't bother you. Cayenne can be used in fruit or vegetable smoothies.

•**Cloves have antioxidants and anti-inflammatory properties,** and help relieve nausea, flatulence and diarrhea. If you don't mind the strong taste, add one-eighth teaspoon of ground cloves per serving. Cloves mix well with apples and peaches.

Other healthful candidates…

•**Flaxseed is a good vegetable source of omega-3 fatty acids,** plus it contributes to regularity. Add one tablespoon of ground flaxseeds per serving.

Note: Flaxseed will thicken your smoothie—especially if you leave the smoothie standing awhile before you drink it.

•**Lecithin is an excellent source of choline,** which improves memory. Add the contents of two capsules or one tablespoon of granules to one to two cups of smoothie.

•**Sea vegetables** provide a high concentration of vitamin A, protein, calcium, iron and other minerals. These work as a diuretic and may be an immune enhancer and also reduce risk for cancer. Add one to two tablespoons of powder or crumbled leaves to vegetable smoothies—their salty taste isn't good with fruit. You may want to start with a smaller amount and increase as you get used to the taste.

• **Wheat germ is** a good source of vitamin E and thiamin. Use two tablespoons per smoothie.

• **Blue-green algae,** a type of sea vegetable, is rich in carotenoids and chlorophyll.

Add two tablespoons per serving to vegetable smoothies.

• **Coconut oil improves cholesterol ratio by raising HDL (good cholesterol).**

• **Protein is helpful for satiety and stabilizing blood sugar.** Good choices include one tablespoon of powdered whey or two tablespoons of nuts, such as almonds or cashews.

EASY SMOOTHIE INSTRUCTIONS

Always make smoothies in a blender, not a juicer, to retain fiber and those important cell wall constituents.

Crocker recommends using a blender with numerous speeds, including one for crushing ice.

Here is how to make smoothies easily and quickly…

Put the liquid in first, which will protect the blades of your blender.

Add other ingredients roughly chopped and top with ice (if using).

Start blending on a low setting for 10 to 30 seconds, then increase to high, purify or liquefy settings for another 10 to 30 seconds.

If a smoothie is too sweet, squeeze in a little lemon juice to correct…if too sour, add chopped fruit (banana, grapes, pineapple or dried apricots or dates) in small increments to reach desired sweetness.

Crocker's book includes numerous smoothie recipes, or you can go to many Web sites for ideas.

And cleaning your blender is as easy as pushing a button.

Rinse the container, put in a drop or two of dish detergent, fill halfway with warm water, cover and blend on a low speed for 30 seconds. Rinse and dry.

Now you have no excuse not to add these healthy treats to your day!

Power Breakfast: Root of a Healthy Day

Jonny Bowden, CNS, nationally known expert on weight loss and nutrition, and author of the best-selling *Living the Low Carb Life* (Sterling) and *The 150 Healthiest Foods on Earth* (Fair Winds). *www.jonnybowden.com*

If breakfast really is the most important meal of the day, shouldn't we select what we eat more carefully? And what exactly are the proven benefits of eating breakfast in the first place?

"There's an old saying that goes 'Eat breakfast like a king, lunch like a prince and dinner like a pauper,'" said nutritionist and weight-loss coach Jonny Bowden, CNS. "But most of us do the opposite." According to Bowden, this is exactly the wrong way to eat if we're trying to lose weight. It also works against us if we're trying to keep our energy up during the day and our performance level high. "Remember, you've just completed eight hours without food," he told me. "You're literally breaking a fast. Your body is craving nourishment, and your brain needs glucose to function at its best. Skipping breakfast is one of the worst possible things you can do. You set yourself up for disaster in a number of different ways later in the day."

Indeed, the research points that way. Between 35% and 40% of all Americans skip breakfast, and many kids leave for school without it. The implications are dramatic, both physically and mentally (more on that in a moment). "People who skip breakfast are more than four times as likely to be obese than people who eat something in the morning," Bowden informed me.

Then there's performance. "Numerous studies over the years have shown that skipping breakfast impacts the behavior and mental performance of school kids," Bowden said. "Kids who eat breakfast have better memory, and higher math and reading scores. And kids who are hungry have a large number of behavior problems, including fighting, stealing, having difficulty with teachers and not acknowledging rules."

Additionally, people who eat breakfast are far more likely to get a healthy intake of vitamins and minerals than those who don't. In one study published in the *Journal of the American College of Nutrition*, researchers found that people who ate a hearty breakfast containing more than one-quarter of their daily calories had a higher intake of essential vitamins and minerals and lower serum cholesterol levels to boot. Sounds weird, doesn't it? Getting adequate and sufficient nutrients when your body needs them is the best way to maintain optimal body function.

THE BEST BREAKFAST

So what constitutes a good breakfast? Is it the high-carb, low-fat "Breakfast of Champions" that was so in vogue several decades ago? Or is it a plate piled high with meat and bacon minus the bread and potatoes á la "Robert Atkins"?

"Higher protein breakfasts translate into a more sustained level of energy throughout the morning and possibly the day," Bowden told me. "Protein fills you up longer, and you're less likely to have midmorning cravings. You're also less likely to overeat at lunch." And higher protein at breakfast may increase metabolism, helping you to maintain a healthy weight. "In one study, a high-protein breakfast increased the metabolism of healthy young women by a shocking 100%," Bowden said.

"There are definite advantages to higher protein intakes in the morning," Bowden continued, "but that doesn't mean 10,000 calories of bacon." He recommends that at least one-third of your breakfast come from a lean protein source and the rest from healthy fats and fibrous carbs. "And if you eat eggs, for goodness' sake, don't throw out the yolks," he urged. They're loaded with good nutrition, and may even lower your cholesterol levels, he added.

"Moreover, don't be afraid to think outside the box," Bowden advised. He pointed out that in Asia, the traditional Japanese breakfast consists of a small piece of fish (like salmon), some light vegetables and a tiny portion of rice, accompanied by a small bowl of miso soup. "The health benefits of fish and vegetables in the morning are huge," Bowden reported. "And the omega-3s in salmon are terrific for your skin, plus they help regulate mood." *If salmon's too much of a stretch for you, Bowden has his own list of favorite breakfasts for more Western palates…*

• **Eggs.** "I think eggs are one of nature's perfect food sources," he told me. "They are loaded with protein and other nutrients such as phosphatidyl choline for the brain and heart."

A Bowden breakfast favorite: Scramble some eggs with spinach and sliced apples in some coconut oil, and season with turmeric and lemon pepper. "It's loaded with protein and nutrients for the eyes, like lutein and zeaxanthin," he explained. "Plus the turmeric is one of nature's great anti-inflammatories." (Note: Bowden strongly recommends free-range eggs—from hens that had access to the outdoors where they could run around and eat more natural food, which changes the fat content and nutrition of their meat and eggs.)

• **Yogurt that contains active cultures.** "One of my favorite quick breakfasts is yogurt with nuts and red or purple grapes," Bowden said. "I always use goat's or sheep's milk yogurt because it's less likely to have hormones in it and has a better nutrient balance. Then I sprinkle on some walnuts or almonds or pecans."

• **Peanut butter and banana sandwich.** "If you're someone who can tolerate grains," said Bowden, "buy a good whole-grain bread, preferably sprouted grain, take one slice and make a 'half sandwich' using natural, unsweetened peanut or almond butter, a banana and, if you like, a dollop of yogurt on top."

• **Whey protein shake.** "Whey is my favorite protein powder," Bowden told us, because it raises glutathione, the most important antioxidant in the body, and has shown in one study to lower blood pressure by about 5 mmHg. "You can make a nutritious shake using water, whey protein and frozen berries, with a little cranberry or pomegranate juice. Or almond or rice milk. Throw in a handful of raw oats for texture—it tastes much better than it sounds. Adding a splash of olive oil to the shake will reduce the glycemic index and help the smoothie 'stick' with you a little longer. Experiment. Peanut butter is another great add-in."

• **Homemade muesli or granola.** According to Bowden, "Raw foods have a lot to recommend them. They contain enzymes, they haven't been processed, they tend to have fiber and they're loaded with nutrients."

Bowden's favorite: "Take some raw oats…soak in a little pomegranate juice…add nuts, berries or sliced apples, and flaked coconut. You can sweeten with xylitol if you need to (though it has been found to cause diarrhea in some), but it's delicious without it. You can also use raw cold-pressed honey or blackstrap molasses if you like."

Fabulous Flaxseeds

Mark A. Stengler, NMD, licensed naturopathic medical doctor in private practice, Stengler Center for Integrative Medicine, Encinitas California…adjunct associate clinical professor at the National College of Natural Medicine, Portland, Oregon…author of many books and the *Bottom Line/Natural Healing* newsletter. *www.drstengler.com*

There are many benefits to eating flaxseeds. Here is an explanation of each one.

• **Fiber,** which prevents and treats constipation and reduces blood glucose and cholesterol levels.

• **Lignans,** compounds that convert during digestion into hormonelike substances that may protect against breast and prostate cancers by preventing the cancer-promoting effects of estrogen.

• **Omega-3s,** fatty acids that reduce inflammation and promote heart, brain, joint and skin health.

Flaxseeds also provide copper to protect connective tissues…folate for normal cell division…magnesium to help the heart contract…manganese for joint health…phosphorous to strengthen bones…and vitamin B-6 to aid in liver detoxification. Flaxseed oil offers some but not all of the benefits of the seeds.

How to eat flaxseeds: To be digested properly, flaxseeds must be ground before being eaten. Grind seeds in a coffee grinder until flaky—about five seconds for the recommended daily serving of one to two tablespoons—or buy preground flaxseeds called flax meal. To prevent cramps and constipation, always drink eight to 10 ounces of water when eating flaxseeds. (If you have the digestive disorder diverticulitis, ask your doctor before eating seeds.)

Choose a product in a vacuum-packed, resealable bag to prevent spoilage. Once opened, keep the bag in the refrigerator. Ground flaxseeds are delicious when added to cereals, salads and shakes. When cooking, substitute three tablespoons of ground flaxseeds for one tablespoon of butter…or replace each egg with one tablespoon of ground flaxseeds soaked in three tablespoons of water. Recipes for chicken, rice, baked goods and more can be found at *www.ameriflax.com.*

For a light, nutritious snack, try Organic Flax Crackers from Foods Alive (*www.food salive.com*), sold at health-food stores. They come in seven flavors, including onion/garlic and Mexican harvest.

My favorite: Maple and cinnamon.

Strawberries Join the Fight Against Cancer

Tong Chen, MD, PhD, research assistant professor in medical oncology, The Ohio State University Comprehensive Cancer Center, Columbus.

Strawberries are high on a select list of super-healthy foods that virtually everyone likes. And listen up—now comes news that they are much more important to our health than previously thought. A new study done at The Ohio State University Comprehensive Cancer Center on freeze-dried strawberries and precancerous esophageal lesions found that the berries were extremely effective in slowing the development of those lesions.

Anything that helps the fight against esophageal cancer is very welcome news. Not only have the number of cases been growing, it's also a very deadly cancer.

BERRIES BRING REVERSALS

The research (which was sponsored by the California Strawberry Commission) was done in China, where the incidence of esophageal cancer—the type known as squamous cell carcinoma—is extremely high. Americans more typically suffer from a different type of esophageal cancer, known as adenocarcinoma. Lead researcher Tong Chen, MD, PhD, research assistant professor in medical oncology at Ohio State, told me that strawberries may similarly affect the type of cancer common in the West because they impact some genes common to both types.

The study had 36 participants, average age 54, all of whom had precancerous lesions of the esophagus. Dr. Chen said that such precancerous lesions are graded mild or moderate (severe ones are clinically considered cancer) and that eventually about 25% of patients with mild lesions and 50% of those with moderate lesions progress to cancer. However, in her study, in which each participant ate about two ounces of freeze-dried strawberries a day, 29 of the 36 participants—about 80%—experienced at least some reversal of lesion progress, with some moderate lesions becoming mild and some mild ones reverting to normal. Dr. Chen said, "Our study is important because it shows that strawberries may be an alternative to—or may work together with—chemopreventive drugs to help stop esophageal cancer. But we will need to test this in randomized placebo-controlled trials in the future."

BIG POWER IN A LITTLE BERRY

As a cancer fighter, strawberries have a powerful combination of molecular components, says Dr. Chen. They contain antioxidant polyphenols, of course, and also vitamins A, C and E, folic acid, calcium, selenium and zinc. As she points out, you can buy all of these in supplemental form, but in strawberries there seems to be a synergistic effect among the components that makes them more potent than the individual components are on their own. Freeze-drying the fruit takes it to an even more impressive level as a nutrient powerhouse—this process removes water from the fruit, leaving a much denser nutritional content within. In the case of strawberries, which are 90% water, when freeze-dried, the end product is 10 times more nutritious than the equivalent weight of fresh berries.

Freeze-dried strawberries are widely available now in supermarkets and health-food stores. This is one rare case in which a processed version of a food might be more healthful than the natural version—probably because freeze-drying takes out only water and adds no flavorings or sugar. As to whether eating strawberries can prevent esophageal cancer in people who don't already have lesions, I'd be surprised if studies on that question don't follow—the potential is just too exciting.

Grocery Cart Smarts
What to Buy...and Why

Mark A. Stengler, NMD, licensed naturopathic medical doctor in private practice, Stengler Center for Integrative Medicine, Encinitas California...adjunct associate clinical professor at the National College of Natural Medicine, Portland, Oregon...author of many books and the *Bottom Line/Natural Healing* newsletter. *www.drstengler.com*

Friends sometimes tease my wife, Angela, and me for being health-food fanatics, feigning amazement at our "exotic" meals. But then they ask, in all seriousness, for hands-on instruction in healthful food shopping. Going to the market with our family of five—including Angela (who is also a naturopathic doctor) and our three children, ages nine, six and four—they marvel at how much our kids know about nutrition.

That's why I thought it would be fun to take readers shopping, too. So come along for a tour of the market.

VERY HEALTHFUL VEGGIES

The fresher the food, the more nutritious it generally is, so we shop several times each week. We go to a nearby health-food store for locally grown produce (which hasn't spent days in transit) and organic products (which aren't contaminated with pesticides) and head straight for the vegetables.

•**Eggplant,** is often the first item in our cart. The skin is a rich source of nasunin, a potent anti-oxidant (a substance that neutralizes disease-causing molecules called free radicals). Eggplant provides minerals that promote good circulation and/or strong bones, including potassium, manganese, copper and magnesium…plus B vitamins for heart health, including B-1 (thiamine), B-3 (niacin), B-6 (pyridoxine) and B-9 (folate). This versatile vegetable can be diced and stir-fried…thin-sliced and grilled…or cut in half, oven-baked until tender (about 20 minutes at 350 degrees), then topped with cottage cheese.

Note: Avoid eggplant if its alkaloids (organic compounds) aggravate your arthritis.

• **Beets** help to detoxify the body by raising levels of the antioxidant glutathione in the liver…improve gallbladder function by thinning bile (a digestive fluid)…and provide folate and manganese for joint health. Red beets provide the most betacyanin, a plant pigment that protects against colon cancer. Beets can be combined with carrots and juiced…grated and added to salads…or cut into chunks and roasted.

• **Broccoli** contains the antioxidants sulforaphane and chlorophyl…vitamins A, C and E, which strengthen the immune system…calcium and vitamin K for bone health…folate for normal cell division…and lutein (a plant pigment) for eye health. Cauliflower provides many of the same phytonutrients (beneficial plant chemicals) as broccoli.

• **Carrots** pack easily into lunch boxes. We love baby carrots dipped in salad dressing, so we buy dressings with no unhealthful hydrogenated fat, high-fructose corn syrup or monosodium glutamate (MSG), a salty additive. For carrot juice, we peel large carrots and put them in our Vita-Mix (from $379, 800-848-2649, *www.vitamix.com*), a high-power blender that preserves the fiber-rich pulp of fruits and vegetables.

• **Cabbage** is a super source of vitamin K (for bone health)…vitamin C (for tissue growth and repair)…and organic compounds called indoles (for cancer prevention). Red cabbage has more healthful plant pigments than white. Since its juice has a very mild flavor, Angela adds red cabbage to almost everything we make in the Vita-Mix. Our kids get a kick from the looks on their friends' faces when we add cabbage to a fruit sorbet or fruit smoothie—and it's even more fun when their friends love the taste!

• **Cherry tomatoes,** rich in vitamins A and C, taste great with sliced low-fat mozzarella cheese.

• **Salad greens** we eat daily include romaine, red- or green-leaf lettuce and fresh spinach. They provide vitamin K, as well as fiber for bowel regularity.

FAVORITE FRUITS

We love fresh fruit for snacks and desserts.

Mango, one of my favorites, is rich in fiber, beta-carotene, magnesium, potassium and vitamins B-1, B-2 (riboflavin), B-3 and B-6. Sweet, tangy and juicy, mangoes make a delicious (if messy) snack when peeled and sliced. Mango slices also can be added to green salad and fruit smoothies or baked in pies.

• **Kiwifruit**—fuzzy brown outside, brilliant green inside—is packed with vitamin C. The kiwifruit is a natural blood thinner that reduces blood levels of triglycerides (fats). Peel and slice to eat alone, add to a fruit salad, or blend into a smoothie.

• **Apricots** are rich in vitamin A and healthful plant pigments called carotenoids (such as beta-carotene and lycopene), which aid vision. Lycopene also may fight heart disease and prostate problems.

• **Apples** provide fiber plus heart-healthy quercetin. Slice and spread with almond butter (for protein), or sprinkle with cinnamon (to balance blood sugar).

• **Bananas** are rich in potassium, to maintain normal blood pressure and heart function…and provide B vitamins, which help to balance brain chemicals called neurotransmitters. Our after-dinner snack often consists of bananas with cinnamon or peanut butter.

• **Blueberries** contain purplish pigments called anthocyanins (also found in red grapes and cranberries), which fight urinary tract infections and may protect the brain from oxidative stress, reducing the effects of dementia. Blueberries have vitamin E and other nutrients that strengthen blood vessels.

• **Oranges** have more than 170 phytonutrients and more than 60 flavonoids (healthful plant pigments) that fight inflammation, blood clots and various cancers. Other citrus fruits provide similar benefits.

●**Avocados** are rich in oleic acid, a mono-unsaturated fat that lowers LDL "bad" cholesterol. Peel and slice them into salads, add them to burritos, or mash as a sandwich spread.

BODY-BUILDING PROTEINS

Protein is required for muscle and tissue repair, blood sugar balance and proper immune function.

●**Eggs** we buy are organic (laid by chickens that eat grains free of chemicals and that are not treated with hormones or antibiotics) and enriched with omega-3 fatty acids for cardiovascular health. We each have three to five eggs weekly—boiled, poached or scrambled with cheese.

●**Poultry** (skin removed) is typically lower in saturated fat than red meat and therefore is healthier for the cardiovascular system. We select poultry labeled "free range" (meaning the animals were not constantly caged and were not fed antibiotics). From the deli counter, we buy cooked, sliced turkey and chicken breast for sandwiches, opting for low-sodium, preservative-free brands. Favorite dinner entrées include turkey loaf (ground turkey can be substituted for beef and pork in meat loaf recipes) and pan-fried or broiled turkey burgers. Our favorite baked chicken breasts are seasoned with rosemary, lemon and poultry seasoning. We seldom barbecue meat or poultry because doing so creates cancer-causing compounds called heterocyclic amines (HCAs).

●**Wild ocean salmon** (which we consider to be more healthful than farm-raised) we buy when it is in season, to bake or broil with olive oil and lemon. In addition to being low in calories and saturated fat, salmon is high in protein…omega-3s…vitamins B-3, B-6 and B-12 (cobalamin)…phosphorous… and magnesium. We avoid tuna—including canned—due to concerns about mercury contamination. However, canned ocean salmon packed in water is healthful, as are canned sardines—though I confess that we do not enjoy the taste (or smell) of sardines.

●**Cheeses** we enjoy in moderation include Colby and string cheese for snacks and shredded cheddar on burritos. Along with protein and calcium, cheese provides the amino acid tryptophan, which promotes thyroid function and positive moods.

CANS, CARTONS & JARS

Packaged goods can be healthful, provided they don't have added preservatives, oils, sugars or salt.

●**Beans are a must for Mexican-style tostados.** Their soluble fiber promotes proper cholesterol and blood sugar levels. Black beans are rich in antioxidant anthocyanins. Pinto beans have magnesium, potassium, manganese, copper and molybdenum, which help the liver with detoxification.

●**Almond milk is rich in potassium.** Blue Diamond's unsweetened almond milk tastes great in cereal and scrambled eggs. A sweetened brand called Almond Breeze has 7 grams (g) of sugar per eight-ounce serving. We pour it over hot oatmeal and drink it as a snack. We also buy oat milk and rice milk. (We avoid drinking cow's milk because it can cause allergic and immune reactions and digestive distress.)

●**Peanut butter.** We buy pure peanut butter (in a glass container to avoid chemicals that may leach from plastics) that has no added sugar or partially hydrogenated fat. Peanut butter has heart-healthy monounsaturated fats, vitamin E, niacin, folate, manganese and resveratrol (the same antioxidant found in red wine). We also like almond butter, which is similar in nutrient content.

GREAT GRAINS & OTHER GOODIES

Selecting grains can be complicated for people who—like my youngest son and me—experience nasal congestion, bloating and diarrhea after consuming foods with gluten (a protein complex). Wheat, rye and barley all contain gluten.

●**Gluten-free grains** include corn, amaranth, rice, buckwheat and quinoa. Of the gluten-free breads we have tried, those from Kinnikinnick Foods (877-503-4466, *www.kinnikinnick.com*) taste best. Pastas, cereals, pretzels, corn chips, tortillas and tostado shells also come in gluten-free varieties.

- **Cereals** we select have no more than 3 g of sugar and provide at least 2 g to 3 g of fiber per serving. Favorites include Rice Crunch-Ems from Health Valley…Amazon Frosted Flakes from Nature's Path…and Kix or Cheerios from General Mills. We also get oatmeal—a source of energy-sustaining complex carbohydrates, as well as manganese, selenium and silicon, which promote bone and cartilage health. The slow-cooking kind has the most fiber.

- **Seeds and nuts** are on our list, too. I grind up two tablespoons of flaxseeds each morning, place them on my tongue, and wash them down with water. Flaxseeds provide fiber and essential fatty acids, and may combat cancer. Hemp seeds are high in protein and omega-3s. Almonds and walnuts are rich in antioxidants and omega-3s, respectively. Angela and I eat one-quarter cup daily, and we try to get our kids to eat a few.

- **Chips are big hits,** especially bruschetta chips from Wild Oats (800-494-9453, *www.wildoatsproducts.com*). Made with potatoes, tomatoes, basil and olive oil, they provide protein and fiber but no sugar or saturated fat.

- **Oils** are important to good cooks (like Angela). Extra-virgin olive oil is what we use when cooking fish and chicken or roasting vegetables. Its monounsaturated fats promote cardiovascular health. To scramble eggs, we use organic canola oil, which contains vitamin E and omega-3s. Macadamia nut oil is best for stir-frying because it has a higher smoke point (the temperature at which a cooking oil breaks down and smokes, giving food an unpleasant taste).

Fun foods we enjoy without guilt include Rice Dream Bars (ice cream bars made from rice milk)…Newman's Own brand fig cookies…Ghirardelli semisweet chocolate chips…and SunSpire carob chips.

Eating healthfully comes at a premium. The price of organic foods is about 25% higher than the cost of foods that may have been grown using pesticides or made with unhealthful processing methods. We are happy to pay the price because our family's health is worth it. I suspect you feel the same way.

WHAT WE WON'T BUY

We check labels and stay away from…

- **Artificial sweeteners** (sucralose, aspartame and saccharin), which may cause headaches, rashes and mood changes.

- **High-fructose corn syrup,** which contains many calories but no nutritional benefit.

- **Monosodium glutamate** (MSG), a salty "flavor enhancer" that can cause headaches and/or digestive upset.

- **Partially hydrogenated fats,** also called trans fats, which harm the cardiovascular and immune systems.

- **Sodium nitrate and potassium nitrate,** preservatives that are linked to cancer.

Beans—The Ultimate Health Food

Jo-Ann Heslin, MA, RD, CDN, Douglaston, New York–based registered dietitian. She is author of 28 consumer nutrition books, including *The Healthy Wholefoods Counter* (Pocket), and two college textbooks on nutrition. A former faculty member of the State University of New York, Downstate Medical Center, in New York City, she was the editor of the *Journal of Nutrition for the Elderly* for 23 years.

Ask someone to name the food that is richest in disease-fighting antioxidants, and you're likely to hear "blueberries" or "cranberries." Few people are aware that red beans actually have more antioxidants than these nutritional-powerhouse berries.

WHAT MAKES BEANS SO SPECIAL?

Some foods are rich in protein, while others provide healthful unsaturated fats, vitamins and minerals or fiber.

Beans (in a class of vegetables known as legumes) are all of the above—the ultimate "combination food," providing maximum nutritional value, including about 15 g of protein and about 13 g of fiber per cup cooked. (A typical serving is one-half cup cooked.)

Compelling scientific evidence: In a landmark study of nearly 800 people (ages 70 and over) from Japan, Sweden, Greece and Australia, the risk for death over a seven-year period dropped by 7% to 8% for each 0.7 ounces (about one-quarter cup cooked) of beans consumed daily.

Bonus: It's especially important to eat beans as we grow older. As we age, our metabolism slows, and we tend to eat less—even though we need more vitamins, minerals and other food-based chemicals to support a weakening immune system...fiber to keep digestion functioning smoothly...and protein to offset the age-related loss of muscle tissue. Beans provide all these benefits—and they're economical and easy to eat for those who have difficulty chewing or swallowing.

BEAN STANDOUTS

More than 100 types of beans are grown worldwide and offer similar basic nutritional advantages. *However, some varieties stand out...*

•**Red beans** not only have more antioxidants than blueberries, but also are a good source of iron (5.2 mg iron per cup cooked).

•**Kidney beans** are also rich in antioxidants and are an especially good source of fiber (13 g fiber per cup cooked).

•**Pinto beans** have been shown to reduce markers for heart disease, including total cholesterol, when one-half cup cooked was consumed daily for eight weeks, according to research published in the *Journal of the American College of Nutrition.*

•**Lima beans** are a good source of potassium and have been shown to reduce blood glucose levels.

•**Navy beans,** which also are a rich source of potassium as well as calcium and magnesium, have been linked to reduced risk for high blood pressure and heart attack.

•**Black beans** are another excellent source of antioxidants—one cup cooked offers the same antioxidant levels as a six-ounce glass of red wine.

•**Garbanzo beans** (also known as chickpeas) have been shown to reduce LDL "bad" cholesterol by nearly 5%.

•**Soybeans** have higher-quality protein—it closely matches that of eggs, meat and milk—

and more of it (60% of your daily needs in a single cup) than other types of beans.

Important: Soybeans are the richest source of isoflavones—phytochemicals with estrogen-like properties. Although research findings have been mixed, there is some concern that high intake of isoflavones may promote the growth of precancerous or malignant breast cancer cells. The American Cancer Society recommends that women who are at high risk for breast cancer or with a history of the disease eat no more than moderate amounts of soy foods and avoid isoflavone supplements.

BEST WAYS TO ADD BEANS TO YOUR DIET

Aim for at least three cups of cooked beans (six servings) per week. *For example, you can try...*

•**Garbanzo or kidney beans** in lettuce salads.

•**Navy beans or black beans** in soups.

•**Roasted soybeans** (soy nuts) and edamame (fresh soybeans) as convenient snack foods.

•**Three-bean salad** containing more dried beans (such as chickpeas and kidney beans) than yellow or green string beans.

For even more variety: Try adzuki beans in rice dishes...anasazi beans in Southwestern soups...and fava beans in stews. These varieties are available at health-food stores and most supermarkets.

NO MORE GAS!

Many people avoid beans because they can cause intestinal gas. To minimize gas, add beans to your diet gradually—start with one-quarter cup on top of a salad, for example... and increase your intake to half-cup and full-cup servings over a period of weeks.

Other gas-control secrets: Get dried beans when they're fresh (otherwise, the beans' natural starches degrade and become more difficult to digest). Look for a "best by" date or buy dried beans at a store where business is brisk. Soak them overnight, then rinse them thoroughly before cooking.

SODIUM-REDUCING TRICKS

The high salt content of canned beans (it's added to preserve texture) is a problem if you're on a low-sodium diet. Canned beans typically contain 300 mg of sodium per one-cup serving. By washing the beans, you can lower the sodium content by 40% or more. Rinsing canned beans thoroughly also helps prevent intestinal gas.

When cooking dried beans, it is not necessary to add salt. However, seasonings, including salt (in moderation), can be added once the beans are cooked. For convenience, freeze serving-size portions for later use. Frozen cooked beans also are becoming increasingly available at supermarkets and are nearly sodium-free.

TOP 10 ANTIOXIDANT FOODS

1. Red beans
2. Wild blueberries
3. Red kidney beans
4. Pinto beans
5. Cultivated blueberries
6. Cranberries
7. Artichokes
8. Blackberries
9. Prunes
10. Raspberries

Source: US Department of Agriculture.

Nuts—Now to Prevent Heart Disease

Among women who have type-2 diabetes (which puts them at high risk for heart disease), those who ate five or more servings a week of nuts or peanut butter had a 44% lower risk for heart disease than those who rarely or never ate these foods.

Theory: Monounsaturated fat in nuts reduces cholesterol and inflammation.

Best: At least five times weekly, have one ounce of nuts or one tablespoon of peanut butter.

Frank Hu, MD, PhD, professor of nutrition and epidemiology, Harvard School of Public Health, Boston, and lead author of a 22-year study of 6,309 women.

The New Nordic Diet

Anja Olsen, PhD, researcher, Institute of Cancer Epidemiology, Danish Cancer Society, Copenhagen, Denmark.

Have you heard about the "new" Nordic diet? It turns out that Scandinavians who follow their countrymen's traditional way of eating seem to live longer. But, sorry to tell you, the key is not Danish pastries and Swedish meatballs...they eat a lot of whole-grain rye bread—real rye bread, not the mushy "rye" found alongside white bread in supermarkets—and cabbage. *But there's more to the Nordic diet than that...*

LIVE LIKE A VIKING

Anja Olsen, PhD, a researcher at the Danish Cancer Society, and a team of researchers collected information about the diets and lifestyles of approximately 57,000 Danes ages 50 to 64. Over the 12-year study period, 4,126 died. After accounting for lifestyle differences (such as exercise, weight, smoking, alcohol use and education), the researchers found a strong correlation between eating traditional Nordic foods and length of life. For instance, men who followed the traditional Nordic diet most closely had a nearly 36% lower risk of dying during the 12 years of follow-up. And women who ate the most Nordic staples reduced their risk for death by 25%.

These results appeared in the *Journal of Nutrition*.

Whole-grain rye bread, which most study participants ate daily (the median amount was two-and-a-half slices) appeared to have the strongest protective effect, especially in men.

Adding further to the chance of living longer, both whole-grain rye and cabbage help in the battle against obesity. And cabbage has been related to a decreased risk for both cancer and heart disease.

However, as in other Western countries, many Nordic folk today eat too much processed and/or fatty food, including pasta, french fries, pizza and sugary desserts, and, as a result may suffer from high rates of heart disease, diabetes and cancer.

19

DANISH MODERN...NOT?

To encourage better health, Dr. Olsen recommends that we focus on old-style dietary habits as they've long existed in most traditional cultures, be they Nordic or from other countries. They tend to emphasize natural, whole and often wild foods—in contrast to our modern approach of eating highly refined foods

Luckily, you don't have to be a Dane, Swede or Norwegian to eat like one. *Here are some ways you can enjoy the benefits of the healthy Nordic diet...*

•**Eat real rye bread.** Whole grains such as rye, barley and oats abound in dietary fiber, minerals and antioxidants that protect against heart disease, type 2 diabetes and cancer. In this study, whole-grain rye had the most positive impact on health—but it's important to realize that this is not the rye bread we grew up with in the US. Instead, in this country, you'll most easily find this European-style rye by looking for German whole-grain rye, such as the Mestemacher brand, usually found in the deli section of grocery stores, and also in health-food stores, health-oriented markets such as Whole Foods and even online from Amazon.com.

•**Cut up some cabbage.** Cabbage is packed with fiber and isothiocyanates (the sulphur-containing compounds found in cruciferous vegetables). Enjoy both red and green cabbage shredded raw in salads and slaws or lightly steamed.

•**Root for root vegetables.** Root vegetables, especially carrots, are rich in phytochemicals such as carotenes, which neutralize free radicals that damage cells in your body and may cause cancer. Parsnips and turnips also are good choices.

•**Enjoy apples, pears and wild berries.** Wild berries, which are easily available in Scandinavia, are especially rich sources of substances such as omega-3 fatty acids, essential to normal growth and development, as well as antioxidants and phytoestrogens such as lignans, which help lower cancer risk. But even though wild berries contain many more of these healthful components, the berries you find in US grocery stores—i.e., cultivated ones—are still a good source of these important nutrients.

2

Herbal Remedies and More

Popular Herbs with Unexpected Health Benefits

You may know that the tiny, fiber-rich seeds of the flax plant can be used as a laxative and that ginger helps ease nausea. But can you name any of the other health benefits provided by these plant-derived remedies?

Few people can. However, credible scientific evidence shows that many herbs that are well-known for treating a particular ailment have other important—but little-known—uses.* *For example...*

ARTICHOKE LEAF

Artichoke leaf extract is used by some people with mildly elevated cholesterol levels as an alternative to prescription statin drugs. Exactly how the herb works is unknown, but animal studies suggest that it inhibits HMG CoA-reductase, an enzyme that plays a key role in the liver's production of cholesterol.

In a placebo-controlled, randomized study conducted at the University of Reading in England, adults who took 1,280 mg of artichoke leaf extract daily for three months reduced their cholesterol levels by 4.2%, on average, while levels increased by 1.9%, on average, in those taking a placebo.

What else artichoke leaf can do: Calm indigestion. In a placebo-controlled, randomized study, patients rated their chronic indigestion as significantly improved after taking artichoke leaf extract twice daily for six weeks. Tests on rats suggest that the herb stimulates the gallbladder's production of bile, which helps facilitate the digestion of dietary fat.

*If you use prescription drugs and/or have a chronic medical condition, such as diabetes, cancer or heart disease, speak to your doctor before trying herbal remedies. In some cases, herbs may interfere with medication or cause an undesired effect on a chronic medical problem. Women who are pregnant or breast-feeding also should consult a doctor before taking herbs.

Holly Phaneuf, PhD, expert in medicinal chemistry and author of *Herbs Demystified* (Avalon). She is a member of the American Chemical Society and is conducting research on exercise and herb use.

21

Typical dose: About 320 mg daily of artichoke leaf soothes digestive complaints. This dosage can be taken until the indigestion is no longer a problem.

Caution: Avoid artichoke if you are allergic to plants in the daisy family or if you have gallstones (artichoke appears to make the gallbladder contract).

FLAX

Often used as a gentle laxative, the seed of the flax plant (flaxseed) contains fiber and phytonutrients known as lignans—a combination that helps draw water into the gut to speed digestion. For laxative effects, eat one tablespoon of whole or ground seeds (sprinkled on cereal, for example) daily. Be sure to drink at least eight ounces of water when eating flaxseeds to prevent them from forming a temporary blockage in the intestines.

What else flaxseed can do: Help prevent breast and prostate cancers. Lignans form estrogen-like compounds that inhibit the body's production of the hormone in women and men. This effect is believed to reduce risk for estrogen-dependent malignancies, including some breast and prostate cancers.

Typical initial dose: One to two tablespoons of ground flaxseed daily, which can be increased gradually to as many as five tablespoons daily.

Grinding flaxseed (in a coffee grinder, for example) rather than eating it whole releases more of its cancer-fighting compounds. Also, ground flaxseed is better than flaxseed oil, which lacks the plant's beneficial lignans unless they are replaced during the manufacturing process.

Helpful: Be sure to refrigerate flaxseed to prolong freshness and preserve potency.

Caution: Do not consume flaxseed within two hours of taking an oral medication—flaxseed may interfere with absorption of the drug.

GARLIC

With its powerful blood-thinning effects, garlic is widely used to help prevent artery-blocking blood clots that can lead to a heart attack or stroke. The typical recommendation for this purpose is one clove of fresh garlic or one-half to three-quarters of a teaspoon of garlic powder daily.

What else garlic can do: Help prevent stomach and colorectal cancers. The National Cancer Institute funded an analysis of 23 clinical studies that linked garlic consumption (raw, cooked or from garlic supplements) to a 10% to 50% decrease in risk for these types of cancers. This cancer-fighting effect is believed to result from the antioxidant activity of garlic's sulfur-containing molecules. Garlic also is a popular remedy to stave off the common cold, but research on its virus-fighting properties has shown mixed results.

Recommended: A fresh crushed garlic clove four to seven times a week.

GINGER

Ginger is widely used to treat nausea, including that due to motion sickness (one-quarter to one-half teaspoon of ginger powder)… and chemotherapy (one to two teaspoons daily of ginger powder). Ginger is believed to quell queasiness by stopping intense stomach motions that can interfere with digestion.

What else ginger can do: Relieve arthritis pain. With its aspirin-like effects, ginger inhibits both COX-1 and COX-2 enzymes, two substances that are involved in the production of inflammatory hormones known as prostaglandins.

Typical dose: One-quarter to one-half teaspoon daily of ginger powder.

TURMERIC

In India, turmeric is a popular remedy for indigestion. It contains curcumin, an oily, yellow pigment that appears to prevent gut muscles from contracting and cramping.

What else turmeric can do: Relieve arthritis, morning stiffness and minor sprains. Turmeric reduces levels of an inflammatory, hormone-like substance known as PGE2. In lab studies, researchers also are finding that turmeric helps prevent colorectal and skin cancers, but its cancer-fighting mechanism has not yet been identified.

In addition, turmeric is being studied for its possible role in decreasing risk for Alzheimer's disease. Test tube and animal studies suggest that turmeric interferes with the formation of amyloid plaque, a hallmark of this neurodegenerative disease.

Recommended: Consume turmeric powder regularly by adding it to food, such as Asian dishes.

Caution: Because turmeric can cause gallbladder contractions, people with gallbladder problems should avoid the herb.

Cheers for Chia Seeds

Diana Allen, MS, CNS, certified nutrition specialist and holistic health educator in private practice in Montague, Massachusetts, and author of *Chia Seed* (Woodland). *www.eat2evolve.com*

Chia seeds—which can be black, white or mottled—come from the salvia hispanica plant, a relative of sage. With only about 60 calories per tablespoon, chia seeds are an exceptionally good source of the heart-healthy omega-3 fatty acid alpha linolenic acid as well as fiber, protein, calcium, magnesium, iron and antioxidants. Chia seeds also have been found to soothe the stomach, reduce gut inflammation and help control appetite. They also benefit the heart. One recent study compared the effects of eating about three to four tablespoons per day of chia seeds with the effects of eating an equal amount of wheat bran. After 12 weeks, the chia group showed greater improvements in blood pressure and levels of C-reactive protein (a marker of inflammation). You can find chia seeds online and in many health-food stores. They have a slightly nutty, branlike taste that is mild enough so they won't overpower the flavor of whatever other foods you add them to. Because their outer seed coat is soft and tender, you don't need to grind chia seeds before eating or cooking with them (though for use in baked goods, the seeds are ground). Add chia seeds to…Creamy or pureed soups, using one tablespoon of seeds for each cup of soup. Allen explained that chia seeds are like little sponges, absorbing more than 10 times their weight in water. For this reason, they act as a natural thickener,

giving soups a pleasing velvety texture… and they also are hydrating, helping your body hold moisture. Salads, tossing in one to two teaspoons of seeds for each serving of greens. Smoothies, stirring in one tablespoon of seeds per cup of smoothie. Pancakes and baked goods (muffins, cookies), replacing up to one-fourth of the flour in a recipe with ground chia seeds.

Easy and refreshing beverage: Chia Fresca (a kind of thick lemonade). Mix one tablespoon of chia seeds with one cup of water and the juice of one-half lemon. Sweeten to taste with maple syrup, agave or stevia. Let sit for 30 minutes to thicken. Refrigerate to chill if desired. Makes one serving.

Delicious dessert: Maple-Banana Chia Tapioca. Soak one cup of whole raw almonds, cashews or Brazil nuts in three cups of water for four to eight hours to soften. Drain and rinse nuts, discarding soaking water. In a blender, blend nuts and three cups of fresh water until smooth. Add one banana, two tablespoons of maple syrup, one tablespoon of vanilla extract and a pinch of sea salt. Blend well. Pour mixture into a bowl and briskly stir in one-half cup of chia seeds, combining well. Refrigerate for at least one hour to let the pudding set. Makes four servings.

For more recipes: See Allen's nutrition blog at *www.eat2evolve.blogspot.com.*

Chasteberry for Women

Mark A. Stengler, NMD, licensed naturopathic medical doctor in private practice, Stengler Center for Integrative Medicine, Encinitas, California…adjunct associate clinical professor at the National College of Natural Medicine, Portland, Oregon…author of many books, including *The Natural Physician's Healing Therapies* and coauthor of *Prescription for Natural Cures* (both from Bottom Line Books)…and author of the *Bottom Line/Natural Healing* newsletter. *www.drstengler.com*

If you were to examine some of the many "women's hormone-balancing" products in health food stores and pharmacies, you would most likely see chasteberry (also known as Vitex agnus-castus) listed as an ingredient. It has been recommended for female conditions, including hormone-related acne, fibrocystic breast syndrome, endometriosis, infertility, lactation difficulties, menopausal hot flashes, menstrual disorders, ovarian cysts and uterine fibroids. In other words, it is touted as helping almost all major female conditions.

The herb comes from the berries of the chasteberry tree, actually a shrub found in subtropical climates. The ancient Greeks used chasteberry as a symbol of chastity in young women, hence the name "chasteberry" or "chaste tree."

HOW IT WORKS

Chasteberry does not contain hormones. It acts on the pituitary gland in the brain to increase the production of luteinizing hormone (LH). LH stimulates the ovaries to release eggs, as occurs with ovulation. Ovulation triggers a surge in levels of the hormone progesterone. This release of progesterone is important in maintaining a balance with the other major female hormone, estrogen. Research has shown that some premenopausal women do not ovulate regularly. This sets the stage for what is known as "estrogen dominance"—too much estrogen relative to progesterone. By helping to normalize progesterone levels, chasteberry promotes hormone balance. This is why it is effective for so many female conditions, including premenstrual syndrome and fibrocystic breast disease as well as uterine fibroids in women of all ages, which are in large part caused by estrogen dominance.

Chasteberry also has been shown to lower levels of the hormone prolactin. When elevated, this hormone, which is secreted by the pituitary gland, is associated with premenstrual syndrome, irregular menstrual cycles and infertility.

DOSAGE

For all of these conditions, I commonly recommend 160 mg to 240 mg daily of a 0.6% aucubin or 0.5% agnuside extract (important active ingredients) in capsule form—available from Enzymatic Therapy (800-783-2286, *www.enzymatictherapy.com*) and Natural Factors (sold by Vitacost, 800-381-0759, *www.vitacost.com*). Or I suggest 40 drops of the tincture in four ounces of water, taken once daily.

For best results, chasteberry should be used until the problem is alleviated and then for an additional three months. Women may notice improvements within two menstrual cycles.

Chasteberry often needs to be taken for four to six months or longer for long-standing cases of hormone imbalance that have resulted in infertility, amenorrhea (no menstrual cycles), irregular menstrual cycles or endometriosis.

Mild digestive upset, nausea, headaches and skin rash are infrequent side effects of chasteberry. Stop taking it if they occur.

Chasteberry should not be used by women taking birth control pills or injections. It also should be avoided by those taking drugs that block dopamine receptors, such as the antipsychotic medication *haloperidol* (Haldol).

As with most herbs, chasteberry should be avoided during pregnancy, although it is helpful for lactation in nursing mothers.

The New Supplement That Soothes Sciatica

Gad M. Gilad, PhD, department of physiology and pharmacology, Sackler Faculty of Medicine, Tel Aviv University, and co-author with Varda H. Gilad of more than 90 scientific papers on nerve function, published in the *Journal of Neuroscience Research, Brain Research, Annals of Neurology* and many other leading medical journals.

The longest nerves in your body are the left and right sciatic nerves. Rooted in the lumbar (lower back) area of the spinal cord, they run through the hips and buttocks and down the back of the legs, powering muscles and providing feeling to the thighs, legs, and feet.

Problem: If there's a rupture in one of the fluid-filled, cushioning disks that sit between the bones (vertebrae) of the spinal column, a gel-like substance can leak out and press on a sciatic nerve—causing painful sciatica.

The pain of sciatica ranges from mild tingling to electric agony, and parallels the path of the nerve, shooting from the low back to the buttocks and down the back of (typically) one leg. Other symptoms can include numbness and weakness in the affected leg and foot.

An estimated 3 to 5 million Americans have sciatica, and most get better in a few weeks or a few months. But in the meantime, the nerve pain is very difficult to treat.

Solution: A recent study shows you can soothe sciatica—by taking a nutritional supplement of agmatine, a compound produced when your body breaks down the amino acid arginine, a component of protein found in small amounts in meat, fish and plants.

FOUR TIMES MORE PAIN RELIEF

Sixty-one people who had suffered with sciatica from two to four months took either agmatine or a placebo for two weeks.

The agmatine group had a 28% improvement in pain levels—compared with 7% for the placebo group.

The researchers also used an extensive questionnaire to measure the participants' "general health status." The agmatine group improved by 70%, compared with 20% for the placebo group.

People suffering from sciatica "undergo significant improvement in their symptoms and in general health-related quality of life" after taking agmatine, concluded the researchers in *Pain Medicine*.

How it works: The compound may work to protect and strengthen nerve cells (neurons) in several ways, says Gad Gilad, PhD, a study researcher at Tel Aviv University in Israel. *Agmatine...*

• **Improves the functioning of cellular receptors for neurotransmitters,** the chemicals that send messages from neuron to neuron

• **Blocks the movement of calcium and potassium salts into neurons,** reducing pain-causing activity

• **Increases the production of polyamines,** molecules that protect nerves

• **Decreases the production of matrix metalloproteases,** enzymes that kill nerves and produce nerve pain

• **Helps regulate nitric oxide,** a "messenger molecule" that plays a key role in how neurons function

• **Limits the formation of advanced glycation end products (AGE),** a byproduct of blood sugar metabolism that damages neurons and other cells.

Suggested dosage: "There is no way to eat enough food to ingest the amount of agmatine necessary to protect nerves," says Dr. Gilad. "But taking a supplement of the compound can help a person with sciatica avoid the painful 'pins and needles,' burning and tingling sensations, and numbness and weakness that characterize the problem."

Dr. Gilad recommends Neurofencine, the agmatine supplement used in the study, which contains G-agmatine, a unique form of the compound.

"Start with two capsules twice a day, for four days," he says. "If there is no decrease in symptoms, take three capsules twice a day for as long as needed for reduction of pain and other symptoms—it may take two to three weeks before you see an effect. Once the symptoms are reduced, switch to two capsules, two times a day, for a maintenance dose."

Resource: You can order Neurofencine at *www.fornervehealth.com* or call 888-484-4523. *E-mail: info@fornervehealth.com.*

Ashwagandha—Ancient Remedy for Stress

Mark A. Stengler, NMD, licensed naturopathic medical doctor in private practice, Stengler Center for Integrative Medicine, Encinitas, California...adjunct associate clinical professor at the National College of Natural Medicine, Portland, Oregon...author of many books, including *The Natural Physician's Healing Therapies* and coauthor of *Prescription for Natural Cures* (both from Bottom Line Books)...and author of the *Bottom Line/Natural Healing* newsletter. *www.drstengler.com*

In the ancient tradition of Ayurvedic medicine—as practiced in India for thousands of years—the herb *ashwagandha* (Withania somnifera) has been used to treat conditions such as fatigue, chronic disease, impotence and waning memory. Now, in the twenty-first-century United States, this well-respected herb has a new and even brighter reputation as a much-needed stress reliever.

Sometimes referred to as "Indian Ginseng," "Winter Cherry" or "Withania," ashwagandha herb has many similarities to Chinese ginseng. In Ayurvedic medicine, it may be used to treat a number of other diseases besides those already mentioned—including asthma, bronchitis, psoriasis, arthritis and infertility. Ayurvedic doctors prescribe it in very specific ways that are suited to certain constitutional types. It's often given with the so-called "warming herbs," such as ginger, to increase its tonic effect.

Ashwagandha root differs from Chinese ginseng in having a mild sedative action. This makes it well suited for the Type A person—that is, someone who's always "on the go" at such a high rate that he or she may be headed for burnout.

MULTITONIC

Research shows that this herb is an excellent adaptogen that helps the body cope with physical and mental stress. Studies show that ashwagandha can help people who have exhaustion from chronic stress, weakened immunity (for instance, if they have cancer) and as a tonic for chronic diseases, especially inflammatory disorders.

This herb also has overall benefits for many body systems. Ashwagandha is unique in acting as a tonic to the nervous system, but also has sedative and antiepileptic effects. It mobilizes different components of the immune system to fight invading microbes and has a modulating or balancing effect if you have inflammation.

A number of animal and laboratory studies have shown this herb has antitumor activity. Ashwagandha has also been shown to have antioxidant activity, so it's helpful in protecting brain cells (which could explain why it helps to prevent memory loss). It also stimulates red blood cell production. Ashwagandha is also said to be a rich source of iron, so it's a potential choice for the treatment of iron-deficiency anemia.

Animal studies have shown that it increases thyroid hormone levels.

Over 35 chemical constituents have been identified, extracted and isolated in this plant. These include some groups of chemicals such as alkaloids, steroidal lactones, saponins and withanolides.

Ashwagandha has been used in only a few human studies—far outweighed by the number of animal or test-tube studies that have been done. However, it has remained popular and highly valued through thousands of years of use in Ayurvedic medicine. This is a classic case of an herb that has often been used for successful treatments yet never "proven" by modern scientific research. In my opinion, ashwagandha should be used when indicated. I am sure there will be continued scientific research that will eventually shed light on the reasons why this wonderful plant has proven so helpful to so many people.

Dosage: The standard adult dosage is 1,000 to 3,000 milligrams daily of the root.

What are the side effects?: No side effects or toxicity have been reported with ashwagandha.

Recommendations for…

• **Aging.** For one full year, 3,000 milligrams of purified ashwagandha powder or placebo was given to 101 normal healthy male volunteers, all between the ages of 50 and 59. The herb had some physical effects that slowed the effects of aging for all the men in the study. All men showed significantly increased hemoglobin and red blood cell count. Improvements in nail calcium and cholesterol were also noted. In addition, nearly 72 percent of the men reported improvement in sexual performance.

• **Anemia and slow growth.** Ashwagandha has been shown in two human studies and several animal studies to increase hemoglobin, red blood cell count and serum iron levels. In a scientific trial that continued for 60 days, 58 healthy children between the ages of 8 and 12 were given milk that was treated with fortified ashwagandha (2,000 milligrams a day). The herb improved the health factors that contribute to growth—leading to a significant increase in hemoglobin and albumin. Researchers concluded that ashwagandha can be a growth promoter in children—and they also noted that these children were less likely to have anemia.

• **Arthritis.** Ashwagandha is used in Ayurvedic herbal formulas for the treatment of arthritis and conditions involving inflammation. In a double-blind, placebo-controlled study, 42 people with osteoarthritis were given a formula containing ashwagandha (along with the herbs boswellia, turmeric and zinc) for three months. Their health was compared with a control group that received a placebo.

The herbal formula significantly reduced the severity of pain and the degree of disability. There were no significant changes in the control of inflammation, however. For this reason, ashwagandha is mainly used in formulas where inflammation-controlling substances are also part of the mix.

• **Fatigue.** Ashwagandha has been historically used for the treatment of chronic fatigue, especially a patient who shows signs of nervous exhaustion.

• **Memory problems.** Some holistic practitioners recommend ashwagandha for its benefit to the brain. It helps improve the ability to reason and solve problems as well as improve memory. Practitioners of Ayurvedic medicine, who are familiar with these outcomes, often recommend it for patients who are starting to experience memory loss. Studies on rats have shown that it improves cognitive function.

• **Stress.** Ashwagandha appears to help the body cope with the effects of stress more effectively. I am sure that ashwagandha will become as popular as the ginsengs in helping to deal with this all-too-common problem.

Banaba—Ancient Herb, Modern Success

It's called banaba in the Philippines, banglang in Cambodia, bungor in Malaya and jalal in India. For thousands of years, folk healers in these southeast Asian countries have used the many-named plant to lower blood sugar. Scientists are catching on.

BREAKTHROUGH STUDIES

Japanese researchers in the Department of Diabetes and Clinical Nutrition at Kyoto University gave 31 people with diabetes and other blood sugar problems either corosolic acid (the active ingredient of banaba) or a placebo. Then they gave them a big dose of dietary sugar, in what's called a glucose tolerance test. An hour later...90 minutes later...and 2 hours later...those taking the banaba had much lower blood sugar levels.

In a similar study conducted in the United States, 10 people with diabetes were given banaba for 2 weeks—and their high blood sugar dropped by 30%.

Why it works: Corosolic acid stimulates cells to absorb glucose, say the researchers.

Suggested intake: 32 to 48 mg a day of a banaba extract standardized to 1% corosolic acid (CRA), the active ingredient.

• **The US study used Glucosol,** a soft-gel formulation found in many products, including Glucotrim from NSI, Gluco Trim from NOW Foods and Glucosol/Rx-Blood Sugar from Nature's Plus.

Chinese Club Moss For Better Memory

Every so often, we learn that an ancient medicinal herb has new and astonishing health benefits. So it is with Chinese club moss. Perhaps you have heard of it by another name—huperzia or Qian ceng ta—but most people haven't heard of it at all. Yet as the baby boomer population ages, people will be talking a lot about Chinese club moss and its active ingredient, huperzine A (HupA).

New finding: HupA improves memory and slows age-related cognitive decline—even in early-stage Alzheimer's disease patients. (Neither HupA nor drugs help much in later stages of Alzheimer's.)

Chinese medicine practitioners have used club moss for centuries as a diuretic and an anti-inflammatory. Two decades ago, a Chinese scientist discovered that an alkaloid (an organic compound) in HupA could improve brain function. This sparked many studies, some on-going, including a clinical trial at the National Institutes of Health.

HupA's cognitive benefits are due mainly to its effects on acetylcholine, a neurotransmitter critical for normal thinking, memory and attention. These mental processes falter when acetylcholine production drops or an enzyme called acetylcholinesterase (which normally breaks down unused acetylcholine) is overactive, degrading the much needed acetylcholine.

HupA appears to inhibit activity of acetylcholinesterase, thereby sparing acetylcholine. This also is how pharmaceuticals for Alzheimer's work—but several human clinical trials suggest that HupA may be even more effective than the drugs *donepezil* (Aricept) and *tacrine* (Cognex). Animal studies demonstrate that HupA further supports cognitive function by protecting brain cells from damage caused by free radicals (harmful negatively charged molecules), toxins and/or lack of oxygen (for instance, from poor circulation or stroke)… and by reducing formation of beta-amyloid, a protein that forms lesions in the brain tissue of Alzheimer's patients.

I began prescribing HupA eight years ago for patients with memory problems—and many have been delighted with their improvement. HupA seems to work better than ginkgo biloba, an herb that increases blood flow to the brain. For ability to improve brain function, on a scale of one to 10, I rate ginkgo at six and HupA at nine. And unlike ginkgo, HupA is safe for people who take blood thinners, such as aspirin or *warfarin* (Coumadin).

For intermittent problems with short-term memory, I recommend that adults under age 55 take 50 micrograms (mcg) to 100 mcg of HupA daily…and that those age 55 and older take 100 mcg twice daily. For more severe memory problems, such as in early Alzheimer's, take 200 mcg twice daily.

HupA is generally safe and can be taken indefinitely. Occasional side effects include nausea, diarrhea, dizziness and/or loss of appetite. Before starting HupA, talk to your doctor. Do not take HupA if you have a cardiac condition that affects heart rate, such as bradycardia (slow resting heart rate) or congestive heart failure, because HupA can decrease heart rate and lead to fainting.

If you take medication for Alzheimer's disease, do not use HupA, because it might worsen the drug's side effects (nausea, vomiting and sweating).

If you are dissatisfied with the Alzheimer's drugs you are taking, ask your doctor about discontinuing them and trying HupA instead.

HupA brands I like include Source Naturals (800-815-2333, *www.sourcenaturals.com*), sold at health-food stores and online (for instance, at *www.iherb.com*)…and Ceriva by Metagenics (800-692-9400, *www.metagenics.com*), available from health-care practitioners.

Cost runs about $20 per month at a dose of 100 mcg daily. In my view, that's a small price to pay for improved memory and clearer thinking.

Indian Frankincense May Relieve Asthma

Boswellia, a white resin from the frankincense tree, is a potent anti-inflammatory that may make breathing easier for people with asthma.

Recent finding: Breathing eased and frequency of attacks dropped in 70% of asthma patients who took boswellia daily for six weeks.

Ask your doctor about taking 300 milligrams (mg) to 400 mg of a standardized extract with at least 60% boswellia acids three times a day.

Laurie Steelsmith, ND, naturopathic doctor and acupuncturist in private practice, Honolulu. *www.drsteelsmith.com*

Bee Pollen—Taking the Sting Out of Allergies

Mark A. Stengler, NMD, licensed naturopathic medical doctor in private practice, Stengler Center for Integrative Medicine, Encinitas, California…adjunct associate clinical professor at the National College of Natural Medicine, Portland, Oregon…author of many books, including *The Natural Physician's Healing Therapies* and coauthor of *Prescription for Natural Cures* (both from Bottom Line Books)…and author of the *Bottom Line/Natural Healing* newsletter. *www.drstengler.com*

There's nothing more "made by nature" than bee pollen, the substance that clings to bees as they gather nectar from flowering plants. It is rich in vitamins A, B-complex and C as well as nutrients such as calcium, magnesium and potassium. Bee pollen also contains flavonoids that have been found to reduce inflammation. Bee pollen supplements mainly are used to reduce hay fever symptoms, treat arthritis and fight fatigue. Are they worth taking?

My experience: One spring, I had a terrible bout of hay fever. None of the natural treatments that I had successfully used in the past were of any help. I was miserable. I tried bee pollen supplements. Bee pollen supplements have a homeopathic effect—they help to desensitize the immune system to the allergic reaction. They contain small amounts of the allergen, which help the body build up its defenses against the allergen and prevent future allergic reactions. These supplements helped me when all else failed. Now I recommend them to prevent or treat flare-ups in some of my patients with hay fever.

My advice: If you suffer from hay fever, start taking bee pollen about two months before hay fever season begins. If it is effective at keeping hay fever at bay, continue taking it throughout hay fever season. Although it is not my first choice for alleviating arthritis symptoms and fatigue in patients, it does help some people with these conditions. Dosage: Two to four capsules (500 mg to 1,000 mg) daily. To relieve acute symptoms, four to eight capsules can be taken as long as needed if no side effects are experienced. Do not take bee pollen supplements if you are allergic to bee stings. Even if you have never had an allergic reaction to a bee sting, test a small amount of bee pollen supplement before taking a whole capsule. To do this, open a capsule and place a small amount of the powder on your tongue. If you experience wheezing, a rash or any other reaction, do not take bee pollen supplements. If you experience digestive upset from taking bee pollen, stop taking it.

To ensure that a bee pollen product does not contain contaminants, such as pesticides, buy from companies that manufacture quality bee pollen supplements, such as Nature's Way (800-962-8873, *www.naturesway.com*) or Natural Factors (800-322-8704, *www.naturalfactors.com*).

Eggshells Can Give You a Break from Arthritis Pain

Anne Winkler, MD, PhD, rheumatologist practicing in Missouri.

Why did the chicken cross the road? To provide relief to the arthritis sufferers on the other side.

Well, that could be a new punch line for the old joke—because a recent study shows that a nutritional supplement made from an extract of chicken eggshells can soothe the stiff, painful joints of people with osteoarthritis.

STUDY DETAILS

Sixty people with osteoarthritis of the knee were divided into two groups. One received a daily supplement of 500 milligrams (mg) of Natural Eggshell Membrane (NEM), a hydrolyzed extract of the inner linings of chicken eggshells. (Hydrolysis uses a protein to predigest the membrane, making it easily absorbable by the body.) The other group received a placebo. Researchers evaluated both groups after 10, 30 and 60 days, for pain and stiffness.

After 10 days, the NEM group had 16% less pain and 13% less stiffness than the placebo group. After 60 days, the NEM group had 16% less pain and 27% less stiffness than the placebo group.

"NEM is a safe and effective option for the treatment of pain and stiffness associated with knee osteoarthritis," wrote the researchers, in *Clinical Rheumatology*.

Why it works: In a joint afflicted with arthritis, the cartilage that covers and cushions the ends of bones degenerates, allowing bones to rub together. The result—pain and stiffness.

NEM contains several compounds—including glucosamine, chondroitin sulfate, hyaluronic acid and collagen—that help maintain and restore healthy cartilage. Animal studies also show NEM alleviates inflammation by reducing the number of pro-inflammatory immune factors called cytokines.

A LESS TOXIC THERAPY

Nonsteroidal anti-inflammatory drugs (NSAIDs) for arthritis, such as ibuprofen (Motrin, Advil) and naproxen (Aleve, Naprosyn) relieve symptoms only about 30 to 40% of the time, says Anne Winkler, MD, PhD, a rheumatologist in Missouri, and a study researcher. NSAIDs also cause gastrointestinal bleeding, hospitalizing 200,000 people a year and killing 15,000 to 20,000.

"If a person wants to try a less toxic therapy, NEM is a good choice," says Dr. Winkler. "It works for a majority of people and—if it works for you—it provides significant relief from pain and stiffness in just 10 days. I recommend it to my patients."

Suggested intake: With the approval and supervision of your primary care physician or rheumatologist, take 500 mg of NEM daily, says Dr. Winkler.

Warning: Don't take NEM if you are allergic to eggs.

Resource: You can order JOINThealth, an NEM-containing product, at *www.membrell.com*, or call 800-749-1291. The Web site also includes a "Store Locator"—enter your zip code to find the store nearest you that sells JOINThealth.

The Power of Pickles

Andrew L. Rubman, ND, medical director, Southbury Clinic for Traditional Medicines, Southbury, Connecticut. *www.naturopath.org*

Foods that are pickled (fermented) dish up serious health benefits. Specifically, they are really good for soothing digestive discomfort of all kinds. Counterintuitive as it may be, eating fermented foods—not only pickled cucumbers, but also peppers, tomatoes and sauerkraut—is a simple and tasty way to resolve heartburn, bellyaches and other intestinal distress.

Pickling is an ancient preservation technique with healthful results. British seamen ate sauerkraut to ward off scurvy…Bulgarians were believed to live longer because they drank fermented milk…and Koreans today eat more than 40 pounds per year of kimchi (a blend of cabbage, garlic, chilis and other ingredients) both for taste and to ease digestion.

PICKLING PROMOTES DIGESTION

The fermentation of foods takes place through the breakdown of carbohydrates by live microorganisms such as bacteria (for instance, Lactobacillus acidophilus or Lactobacillus bulgaricus), yeasts and molds. Kimchi, pickles, sauerkraut and the like act as probiotics, encouraging the growth of positive intestinal microbes. These fermented foods promote efficient digestion, support immune function and boost good nutrition overall. They support availability of B vitamins in certain foods and essential amino acids. They also serve to counteract the ill effects of antibiotics.

According to Dr. Rubman, fermented foods are far better than the over-the-counter antacids or the proton pump inhibitors (PPIs) people routinely swallow to relieve heartburn and stomach upset, which end up causing more harm than good. While they may provide temporary relief, use of antacids or PPIs can backfire because you need acid to efficiently digest foods…and insufficient stomach acid can upset the proper environmental balance of intestinal flora. In contrast, fermented foods encourage the growth of good gut flora while also helping to neutralize the small amounts of stomach acid left in the system between meals, which is a common problem for people with gastritis and GERD.

PICK A PECK

Eating fermented foods a few times a week can make a real difference in how well your digestive system functions. It's easy enough to do—you can spice up stews with a dollop of chutney or a ¼ cup of kimchi, enjoy a bowl of miso soup, slice pickled cucumbers or peppers onto sandwiches or spoon yogurt over fresh fruit. To find fermented foods, visit your local health or gourmet store or shop online…

• **Order fermented foods from farms** such as Wills Valley Farm Products (*www.willsvalley.com*) in Lancaster County, Pennsylvania, which offers fermented vegetables including kimchi, red cabbage, red beets and ginger carrots. Other American picklers include Adamah Farm in Falls Village, Connecticut (*www.isabellafreedman.org/adamah/products*) and Alexander Valley Gourmet in Healdsburg, California (*www.alvalgourmet.com*). In New York City, classic Lower East Side vendors Russ & Daughters (*www.russanddaughters.com*) and Pickle Guys (*www.nycpickleguys.com*) are great sources. You can find many more online.

• **Visit food festivals that celebrate pickling,** such as New York City's International Pickle Day (*www.nyfoodmuseum.org*).

• **Go international.** Explore fermented foods from around the world, such as the pickled Asian plums known as umeboshi. In Japan, these have been consumed for thousands of years for their purported ability to counter nausea, stimulate the digestive system and promote the elimination of toxins. Find them in Asian and gourmet markets and on Web sites such as *www.kushistore.com*. To explore the extensive world of Indian chutneys, visit *www.kalustyans.com*.

• **Choose carefully.** Read labels and buy fermented products that are low in sugar and contain live or active cultures. Dr. Rubman warns that most brands of yogurt, in particular, are loaded with sugar and artificial flavoring, but he notes that Stonyfield Farm and Nancy's are two organic brands that contain live bacterial cultures and no artificial ingredients.

In cases of active intestinal disturbances such as irritable bowel syndrome or gastritis, Dr. Rubman sometimes prescribes fermented foods and/or probiotics (supplements that you can take if you don't enjoy the taste of fermented foods), but he does not recommend that you try this on your own. See a qualified and experienced naturopathic physician who can assess your condition and prescribe an appropriate dosage. But if you're in good health, pile pickles on your plate…pucker up…and enjoy.

Gingerroot—Not Just For Cookies

Mark A. Stengler, NMD, licensed naturopathic medical doctor in private practice, Stengler Center for Integrative Medicine, Encinitas, California…adjunct associate clinical professor at the National College of Natural Medicine, Portland, Oregon…author of many books, including *The Natural Physician's Healing Therapies* and coauthor of *Prescription for Natural Cures* (both from Bottom Line Books)…and author of the *Bottom Line/Natural Healing* newsletter. *www.drstengler.com*

For centuries, ginger (*Zingiber officinale*) has been widely valued as a medicinal herb. It is one of the most widely prescribed herbs by practitioners of Ayurvedic and Chinese traditional medicines. The botanical name for ginger is zingiber, which, in Sanskrit, means "shaped like a horn." Technically speaking, the root is actually a rhizome, a stem that runs underneath the surface of the ground.

It's most commonly used to treat digestive disorders and arthritis in all the healing traditions. It is known as a warming herb, especially suited to people with "cold constitutions," and it's said to enhance circulation. Chinese herbalists use fresh ginger to "warm the lung and stomach."

Ginger is prescribed in Chinese medicine for the common cold, flu, coughs, vomiting, nausea and general digestive upset and bleeding. It also reduces the toxicity of other herbs, so it's essentially an antidote to plants that might have side effects. Also, ginger can help protect an intestinal tract that has been ravaged by tainted or toxic food.

To practitioners of traditional Chinese medicine, every form of gingerroot has certain distinct properties. Fresh ginger has a warming effect on the exterior of the body, while the dried ginger is apt to be recommended for warming the middle of the body.

One of the more intriguing Chinese medicine cures is quick-fried ginger, which is made by frying ginger until the surface is slightly blackened. Practitioners say this is the type that's effective for stopping bleeding and treating conditions that affect the lower abdomen.

Today, ginger is used by herbalists and physicians to treat colds, arthritis, digestive conditions, respiratory-tract infections, headaches, motion sickness and cardiovascular disease.

As with many herbs, ginger has many different active constituents. Dried gingerroot contains between 1% and 4% volatile oils, which account for the strong taste and aroma. (The volatile oils include bisabolene, zingiberene and zingiberol.) Two of the pungent principles—gingerol and shogaol—are believed to be responsible for a lot of the medicinal effects.

Ginger also contains proteolytic enzymes that help to digest proteins and reduce inflammation. Many commercial products are standardized to the constituent gingerol.

DIGESTIVE POWER

Ginger has the unique ability to improve many organs that are involved with digestion. Known as an "aromatic bitter," it tonifies the intestinal muscles and stimulates the digestive organs. It also stimulates secretion of bile from the liver and gallbladder, which helps digest fats. Ginger is also a well-known carminative, meaning that it can reduce gas and bloating.

ANTI-INFLAMMATORY

Ginger acts as a natural anti-inflammatory by inhibiting the release of prostaglandins and other chemicals in the body that promote inflammation and pain. Unlike nonsteroidal medications such as aspirin, it does not have the potential to damage the stomach, liver and kidneys. For centuries, people used ginger as an anti-inflammatory without knowing how or why it worked. Modern tests have now proven the herb's anti-inflammatory powers.

CIRCULATION AND CARDIOVASCULAR HEALTH...

Ginger promotes cardiovascular health by making platelets (cells responsible for blood clots) less likely to clump together. This preventive action allows the blood to keep flowing smoothly and helps prevent hardening of the arteries.

Studies have shown that this protective effect is achieved by inhibiting the formation of thromboxanes, substances that promote blood clotting. Other substances in ginger promote the synthesis of prostacyclin, a component that helps prevent platelets from "aggregating" or clumping together.

Animal studies have also shown that ginger improves the pumping ability of the heart.

Dosage: Fresh gingerroot can be made into tea. It's also sold in capsules, tablets, and tinctures. I have found all these forms to work with patients and myself.

The tea is relaxing and works well for digestive upset, as do the capsule and tincture forms. For the treatment of inflammatory conditions, I recommend a standardized capsule to get high levels of the active constituents that reduce inflammation.

The typical capsule dosage is 500 milligrams two to four times daily. If you're taking the tincture, I recommend 20 to 30 drops two to three times daily.

What are the side effects?: Side effects are rare with ginger, though some people (my wife among them!) report heartburn after taking it. In the short term, pregnant women can take ginger for nausea and vomiting related to morning sickness. One to two grams appear to be safe and effective.

Ginger stimulates bile production, so some herbal experts recommend that you should avoid this herb if you have gallstones.

Although I have seen no human studies on drug interactions and ginger, it theoretically may cause a problem with blood-thinning medications such as Coumadin. So check with your physician before using high doses of ginger if you are on a blood-thinning medication.

One last piece of advice you may not find in many books is that gingerroot by itself may aggravate those who are very warm-blooded.

If you are the type of person who gets warm and sweats easily, then long-term use of ginger is not recommended just because it can cause discomfort by making you even warmer.

Recommendations for...

•**Arthritis.** Many herbal medicine experts mention that ginger is effective in treating arthritis, but in day-to-day treatment of patients, I have not found this to be true. Ginger by itself does not usually provide substantial relief. That said, however, it can be helpful to some people as part of a comprehensive herbal formula, such as practitioners of Chinese herbal formulas have created for patients with a "cold constitution."

•**Bloating and flatulence.** Ginger is the remedy par excellence for relieving bloating and flatulence, which is the common result of what I call SAD (Standard American Diet). It reminds me of one lady who came up to me after a talk, looked around to make sure no one else was listening, and asked if there was anything I could recommend for her 36-year-old son who was having trouble with a lot of gas. It turns out this son was newly married, and his mother was worried that his flatulence would cause marital problems.

I recommended she give her son a bottle of ginger capsules to use with meals. Hopefully it rescued the young groom from some embarrassment—or possibly saved the marriage!

•**Cardiovascular disease.** Since ginger is a natural blood thinner, it promotes good circulation and therefore improves cardiovascular health. Animal studies show that it helps with the pumping action of the heart. To me, it is most beneficial as a synergistic herb—one that makes other herbs more effective rather than working by itself.

•**Diarrhea.** There's a specific type of diarrhea, called "cold diarrhea" in Chinese medicine, that ginger seems to help significantly. This is the kind that gives you a case of the chills as well as loose stools. (What's called "hot diarrhea," as you might expect, is the kind where loose stools are accompanied by a feeling of feverishness.)

•**High cholesterol.** In animal studies, ginger has been found to lower cholesterol levels in rats. Unfortunately, it doesn't show exactly the same effect in humans. But if you're taking ginger for other conditions, there is a possibility that it could also help lower your cholesterol.

•**Morning sickness.** Ginger has actually been studied as a relief for severe morning sickness. In 19 of the 27 women who took ginger for nausea and vomiting, both symptoms became less frequent within four days of treatment. The dosage of gingerroot capsules was 250 milligrams taken 4 times daily.

Since publication of the earliest studies, which were done in 1990, many conventional doctors have started to recommend gingerroot for morning sickness. (My wife's obstetrician, for instance, recommends it to her patients.) However, I don't advise that women take more than one gram daily during pregnancy, and there's no reason to continue taking it after the morning sickness passes.

•**Motion sickness.** Ginger has received a lot of attention for its ability to prevent and treat motion sickness. A study in 1982 revealed that ginger was superior to the drug Dramamine for reducing motion sickness. Not every study, since then, has supported this finding, but some excellent research done in 1994—involving 1,741 people—confirmed that ginger was indeed very effective in treating motion sickness.

The 1994 study was done with a group of people who were taking a whale-watching trip. Before boarding the boat, people were asked to take various kinds of motion-sickness remedies, ginger among them. (None of the passengers knew which remedy they were being given.) The study showed that 250 milligrams of ginger was just as powerful as the pharmaceutical medications, but without side effects such as drowsiness.

•**Nausea and vomiting.** Bad food, flu, chemotherapy and surgical treatments are just a few of the possible causes of nausea and vomiting. No matter what the cause, however, ginger has been shown to be an effective remedy.

In two studies, ginger helped reduce nausea and vomiting in patients who had just undergone surgery where they received anesthesia. (Anesthesia makes some people very nauseated.) If you are scheduled to have surgery, talk with your surgeon about taking one gram of ginger before and after surgery.

33

Beets Beat Fatigue

Andrew Jones, research group leader and professor in the Department of Sports and Health Sciences at the University of Exeter.

Nathan Bryan, PhD, assistant professor in the School of Medicine at the University of Texas Health Science Center, co-author of *The Nitric Oxide (NO) Solution* (Neogenis). *www.neogenis.com*

Scientists at the University of Exeter in England conducted a six-day experiment —with results they described as "remarkable" (a word rarely used in the understated world of scientific research).

The study: They divided eight men into two groups. Every day for three days, four men drank two cups of beetroot juice. (Beetroot juice is juice from the beets themselves, not from beet greens.) The other four drank a look-alike, taste-alike placebo juice.

Over the next three days, the eight men engaged in several short bouts of exercise on a stationary bike, at two levels of intensity...

1. Moderate intensity (it is similar to brisk walking)

2. Strenuous intensity, exercising to total exhaustion, when they couldn't exercise anymore.

Results: During the moderate exercise, the men who drank beetroot juice used 19% less oxygen than the men who didn't drink the juice—in other words, they needed less energy to accomplish the same amount of exercise.

During the strenuous exercise, the men who drank beetroot juice exercised 16% longer until total exhaustion than the men who didn't drink the juice—in other words, they had a lot more energy.

Beetroot juice can boost energy levels—a nifty finding, for sure. But what was so "remarkable" about it?

"The oxygen cost of exercise is a fundamental tenet of human physiology," says Andrew Jones, PhD, a professor in the Department of Sports and Health Sciences at the University of Exeter and a study researcher. "It is highly consistent in humans, and it is virtually unchanged by all other interventions, including

long-term endurance training. Therefore, we were very surprised when we saw these remarkable reductions in the oxygen cost of exercise after drinking beetroot juice."

Bottom line: Drinking beetroot juice accomplished what no other training method, drug, food or supplement has ever accomplished—it allowed the body to use less oxygen during exercise!

And this remarkable result is remarkable even if you're not an exerciser—because maybe you're one of the millions of Americans who would be able to function more energetically if only your muscles demanded less oxygen. *For example...*

If you're over 50, you have the "significantly reduced lung capacity" of aging, says Dr. Jones—and could benefit from muscles that used less oxygen.

If you have heart disease, your heart muscle probably receives less oxygen—if it needed less, it wouldn't suffer as much "metabolic stress," says Dr. Jones.

If you have diabetes—which can narrow arteries, reducing blood flow to the heart—you'd also benefit if your heart required less oxygen.

If you have chronic obstructive pulmonary disease (also called emphysema and chronic bronchitis), with frequent breathlessness, you could have a higher activity level if your body demanded less oxygen.

In short, supplementing the diet with beetroot juice can reduce the "oxygen cost" of daily activities and could "enhance functional capacity and the quality of life" for all the above-mentioned groups, says Dr. Jones—and that includes tens of millions of Americans.

Problem: Who wants to drink beetroot juice every day? You'd have to either juice fresh beets (a lot of work) or shop for it (a lot of money—a sixteen-ounce bottle of beetroot juice is a specialty item costing about $5).

Solution: A new study from the same team of UK researchers shows that a specific nutritional compound in the beetroot juice is behind its remarkable oxygen-sparing, energy-boosting effects—a compound that's available in a wide range of vegetables and a new dietary supplement.

THE POWER OF NITRATE

In the first study, the UK researchers theorized that the active ingredient in beetroot juice was nitrate—the men drinking beetroot juice had a 49% increase in blood levels of this nutritional compound, which is found abundantly in beets and in leafy green vegetables.

In the body, nitrate turns into nitric oxide (NO).

NO is a signaling molecule, explains Nathan Bryan, PhD, assistant professor in the School of Medicine at the University of Texas Health Science Center and co-author of *The Nitric Oxide (NO) Solution* (Neogenis). It signals the body to oxygenate muscles. (It also signals the lining of the arteries to relax, lowering blood pressure.)

In the new study, the UK researchers gave nine people either regular beetroot juice, rich in nitrate, or beetroot juice with the nitrate filtered out. Once again, the study participants exercised after drinking the two types of juice.

Results: The beetroot juice with nitrate reduced oxygen requirements and increased time-to-exhaustion—just as in the first study. The beetroot juice without nitrate didn't have those effects.

"A high-nitrate diet may be beneficial for health and performance," Dr. Jones says. "It also has the potential to improve the cardiovascular health of healthy people and of people with high blood pressure."

HOW TO BOOST YOUR NITRATE

"I think the primary take-home message from my research is to eat a diet that contains lots of high-nitrate foods, such as beets and spinach, says Dr. Jones.

One of the best ways to increase nitrate in the diet is with nitrate-rich, NO-creating vegetables, agrees Dr. Bryan.

To guide people to the foods highest in NO-creating nitrate, Dr. Bryan created "The Nitric Oxide Index." It assigns an overall value based on several factors, including the food's total amount of NO-creating nitrate, and its total

amount of antioxidants, which help preserve NO so the body can use it.

FOODS HIGH ON THE NITRIC OXIDE INDEX

Kale
Swiss chard
Arugula
Spinach
Chicory
Wild radish
Bok choy
Beet
Chinese cabbage
Beetroot juice
Lettuce
Cabbage
Mustard greens
Cauliflower
Parsley
Kohlrabi
Carrot
Broccoli

Dr. Bryan has formulated a special beetroot-containing, NO-boosting supplement called NEO40 Daily. It also contains hawthorne (a nitrate-rich herb) and two amino acids (L-arginine and L-citrulline) that help generate NO in the body. The supplement is dissolved in the mouth rather than swallowed, making use of a recently discovered, saliva-based NO-creating mechanism.

In a clinical study conducted at the University of Texas, NEO40 doubled blood levels of a biomarker for increased NO—and 50% of the people taking the supplement said they felt more energetic.

Resource: You can order NEO40 Daily at *www.neogenis.com* or call 855-636-4040.

Be sure to follow the dosage recommendations on the label.

Reishi—A Mushroom that Heals Bronchitis, Altitude Sickness and Liver Disease

You may be surprised to find that sometimes a remedy is very effective at treating several seemingly unrelated conditions. That's the case with the mushroom reishi (*Ganoderma lucidum*) that grows wild in China and Japan. Reishi is well-known in the East for its potent and wide-ranging medicinal properties, but most people in the West have never heard of it. Used in traditional Chinese medicine for more than 4,000 years, reishi promotes longevity. Research has shown that it can stimulate the immune system…support liver function…improve circulation…reduce inflammation…and lower blood sugar and cholesterol. *I recommend it for the following conditions…*

• **Chronic bronchitis.** Studies have shown that reishi helps ease chronic bronchitis symptoms. It inhibits the release of histamine, a compound that causes swelling and inflammation.

• **Altitude sickness.** Because of its ability to thin blood, reishi can help prevent symptoms of altitude sickness, such as nausea, dizziness and light-headedness. It is most effective if taken daily, starting two weeks before needed (whether you are traveling to a high-altitude location or mountain climbing) and then throughout the trip.

• **Liver problems.** Studies show that reishi can help support liver function, especially in people with hepatitis B.

Dosage: Reishi is available in multiple forms, though I generally recommend it in capsule form. For all of the medical conditions described above, you can take two to five 400-milligram (mg) to 500-mg capsules twice daily of a reishi mushroom extract standardized to at least 10% polysaccharides.

Brand to try: Nature's Way Standardized Reishi (800-962-8873, *www.naturesway.com*, for a store locator).

Side effects: Very rarely, reishi initially causes digestive upset. Reduce the dose, and the upset should go away. Then gradually increase the dose. Because reishi has blood-thinning effects, check with your doctor if you take a blood thinner, such as warfarin (Coumadin). If you have diabetes, talk to your doctor about reishi because it lowers blood sugar and you might need a lower dose of your diabetes medication.

Why Seafood Protects The Heart

Researchers from Finland and Sweden looked at the effects of astaxanthin (a red pigment found in salmon, shrimp, crab and lobster) on blood fats. For three months, 40 healthy young men took daily supplements of 8 mg of astaxanthin or a placebo. Blood test results: Astaxanthin users had significantly less oxidation (cell damage from negatively charged molecules) of blood fats.

My view: A powerful antioxidant, astaxanthin is known to protect against retinal disease—and now appears to benefit the heart, too. Fats that become oxidized promote heart disease by contributing to inflammation and plaque-forming LDL cholesterol. People with a family history of heart disease should supplement daily with 8 mg of astaxanthin. It is sold at health-food stores and has no known side effects.

Mark A. Stengler, NMD, licensed naturopathic medical doctor in private practice, Stengler Center for Integrative Medicine, Encinitas, California…adjunct associate clinical professor at the National College of Natural Medicine, Portland, Oregon…author of many books and of the *Bottom Line/Natural Healing* newsletter. *www.drstengler.com*

Mellow Out with Melon Extract

Claire Notin, nutritionist and study researcher, *Nutrition Journal.*

You're weary, irritable and can't concentrate. Your body is peppered with vague aches and pains. Hanging out with your family or friends seems more burdensome than fun. You're having trouble sleeping. And you're tired all the time.

What's wrong?

Maybe you've OD'd—on stress.

You're not alone. Most of us are overdosing on stress these days, as we try (and sometimes fail) to creatively cope with our 24/7 lives.

Well, if you've OD'd, maybe it's time for SOD—*superoxide dismutase*, a super-powerful antioxidant that a recent study shows can ease the symptoms of stress.

LESS STRESS, MORE ENERGY

When cells are barraged by hyperactive molecules called reactive oxygen species (ROS)—the same molecules that spark the inflammation that fuels chronic disease and aging—scientists say your body is under oxidative stress.

New thinking: Scientists have begun to link oxidative stress with perceived stress—the physical, mental and emotional toll from the relentless demands of modern life.

That's why French scientists decided to see if they could lessen perceived stress with a nutritional supplement containing the antioxidant superoxide dismutase (SOD). This enzyme is found in every cell of the body, where it helps prevents the formation of ROS. Scientists discovered it in 1968, dubbing it the "enzyme of life."

The researchers studied 70 healthy people who (like all of us) were doing their best to deal with everyday demands, and divided them into two groups.

At the beginning of the study, the researchers evaluated both groups for the typical symptoms of perceived stress…

- **Negative feelings about life**
- **Pain**
- **Anxiety**
- **Disinterest in socializing**
- **Irritability**
- **Depression**
- **Poor concentration**
- **Fatigue and weariness**
- **Doubt and indecision**

Then one group started taking a daily supplement of 140 international units (IU) of SOD. The other group took a placebo.

One month later, the researchers compared the stress symptoms of both groups. The SOD group had…

- **50% more energy**
- **38% less insomnia**
- **30% less pain**
- **26% less weariness/fatigue**
- **22% more concentration**
- **22% less irritability**
- **18% more interest in socializing**

"Oral supplementation with SOD, which is known to have antioxidant activity on the cellular level, fighting against oxidative stress, could have a positive effect on several signs and symptoms of perceived stress," conclude the researchers, in *Nutrition Journal*.

THE MELON CONNECTION

"SOD is a unique antioxidant that is a natural part of the body's defense system against ROS," says Claire Notin, a nutritionist and study researcher. "I participate in sports—running and volleyball. After starting to take SOD, I find that even after a long, stressful day at work, I still have energy in the evening for training or competition."

Product: The supplement used in the study was *Extramel*, a freeze-dried concentrate of juice from a hybridized cantaloupe rich in SOD.

"Although there are no contraindications for taking a product that contains Extramel, if you have a medical condition you should talk to your doctor before taking it or any nutritional supplement," says Notin.

Extramel is an ingredient in several nutritional supplements sold in the US.

They include…

- **Melonx,** by O-Life
- **Longevity Antioxidants,** by MDR
- **Defenze,** by Enzymedica
- **Body Boost,** by Nature's Code
- **Genesis,** by Symmetry

• **Xyngular Super Fruit Global Blend,** by Xyngular

• **Oriyen E3 Fruit and Vegetable Diet Mix,** by E3

• **Power Repair Spa Vitamins,** by ClariPlex

• **RAW Cleanse,** by Garden of Life

Good news: In a recent animal study, Extramel blocked the formation of artery-clogging plaque by up to 85% in hamsters fed a high-fat diet.

In another recent animal study on weight loss, researchers concluded that taking Extramel regularly "may represent a new alternative to reduce obesity induced by a high-fat diet."

"The widespread applications of this unique antioxidant are just beginning to be discovered," says Notin.

Snack on Popcorn to Boost Fiber

Whole-grain, high-fiber foods may reduce risk for heart disease, some cancers and diabetes.

New study: Compared with people who did not eat popcorn, those who snacked on popcorn consumed, on average, 250% more whole grains…22% more fiber…and 15% less meat.

Bonus: Popcorn has as little as 15 calories per cup and, unlike some highly processed snack foods, does not trigger potentially harmful spikes and dips in blood sugar levels.

Journal of the American Dietetic Association.

3

Natural Cures for Mind and Body

"Take the Waters" for Insomnia, Flu and More

Lots of people take a hot bath to unwind and help release muscle tension. But few people take advantage of the other health benefits provided by bathing. Also known as "balneotherapy," therapeutic bathing has long been used with many forms of water—for example, hot springs, cold pools, tap or pond water. But mineral springs are among the most well-known for their healing powers. In the 1800s, bathing in mineral springs—also known as "taking the waters"—was fashionable, and mineral water was even bottled and sold as a medicinal beverage. Scientific evidence proving that mineral spring therapy is helpful is limited. But scientists seem to agree that balneotherapy is not harmful, and there's no question that it feels good. I know people who swear that regular mineral spring soakings cured their ailments, including arthritis and fibromyalgia.

You can create your own mineral spring soak at home using a simple, inexpensive substance—Epsom salts. In fact, Epsom salts (a four-pound container is available at most drugstores and supermarkets for less than $4) are a mainstay of my home-treatment recommendations for patients suffering from insomnia, arthritis, fibromyalgia, flu, back strain, acute sprains, itchy dermatitis, sunburn and shingles.

Epsom salts contain magnesium sulfate. Magnesium is, of course, essential to human health (particularly heart and muscle function) and acts as a muscle relaxant. Because magnesium is often depleted in the processing of foods, magnesium deficiency is common—it's estimated to affect more than half of Americans—and can contribute to fatigue, muscle spasm, weakness, irritability, insomnia, high blood pressure,

Jamison Starbuck, ND, naturopathic physician in family practice in Missoula, Montana. She is past president of the American Association of Naturopathic Physicians and a contributing editor to *The Alternative Advisor: The Complete Guide to Natural Therapies and Alternative Treatments* (Time-Life).

sugar cravings and anxiety. Magnesium-rich foods, such as nuts, whole grains and black-strap molasses...and magnesium supplements (typical dose: 300 mg daily) are your best options to keep your magnesium levels adequate. But soaking in a hot tub of Epsom salt water also provides some magnesium via absorption through the skin.

To create your own healing bath: Add two cups of Epsom salts to a tub of comfortably hot water, and soak for 20 minutes. At the end of your soak, moisten a washcloth with cool water and rub it all over your arms, legs and trunk for 30 seconds—to prevent chilling and promote blood circulation. Towel off and then relax by lying down for at least 30 minutes. To complete the healing environment of your mineral soak, use low lights and/or candles, drink several ounces of cool water throughout the bath and ask family members to not disturb you.

As described above, Epsom salt soaking is very safe. However, people with high blood pressure or arterial disease should avoid hot mineral soaks—the high temperature of the water can aggravate these conditions. For this reason, pregnant women should consult a doctor before trying a hot mineral bath.

Visualize Your Way to Healing

Mark A. Stengler, NMD, licensed naturopathic medical doctor in private practice, Stengler Center for Integrative Medicine, Encinitas, California...adjunct associate clinical professor at the National College of Natural Medicine, Portland, Oregon...author of many books, including *The Natural Physician's Healing Therapies* and coauthor of *Prescription for Natural Cures* (both from Bottom Line Books)...and author of the *Bottom Line/Natural Healing* newsletter. *www.drstengler.com*

People often are surprised to find out that they can use their imaginations to heal. Whether you're coping with a debilitating disease...chronic aches and pains...or seasonal allergies, visualization, a form of guided imagery in which you use your imagination to gain a greater understanding of yourself, has been proven to help relieve symptoms. To help you use visualization on your own, we spoke to David E. Bresler, PhD, a pioneer in the field of guided imagery techniques. So sit down and get comfortable—and experience the positive effects of this safe and pleasurable mind-body therapy.

Use your mind to ease your symptoms...

We don't know exactly why imagery works, but studies have shown that guided imagery can help patients ease the symptoms of many chronic conditions (such as arthritis and fibromyalgia) and psychological problems (such as depression and anxiety).

Best: Practice visualization for five to 20 minutes once or twice a day. There is no harm in doing it as frequently as you like. Follow these steps...

1. Quiet your breathing. Sitting comfortably in a quiet place, begin to slow down your breathing. Let it become more regular...deeper...quieter. Quieting yourself will enable you to focus your mind's power on any symptoms you are experiencing.

2. Release tension. Imagine a ball of energy that starts in your lower abdomen and rises to your forehead as you inhale. As you exhale, the imaginary ball goes down your spine and your legs and then into the ground. As this "energy sponge" travels around your body, it absorbs and drains away any tension, tightness, pain or discomfort as you breathe.

3. Bring to mind any symptom that is present. Allow an image to form in your mind's eye that represents or symbolizes a symptom (pain, palpitations) or condition (diabetes, cancer, arthritis). Someone with allergies might imagine them as pollen, red or yellow lights, creatures, energy fields, smells or tastes. Examine the image and notice what part seems to be most uncomfortable.

4. Imagine that your body can heal the symptom. Create an inner healing movie in your mind's eye by imagining that your body is using all of its resources to heal what is most uncomfortable.

Example: A woman with peripheral neuropathy viewed the pain as "fire ants chewing on the nerve." With the help of guided imagery, she learned to focus on her breathing and to imagine that, with each breath, the nerve could release its own natural "insecticide," causing the ants to become smaller and fewer in number. This helped to significantly reduce the intensity of her pain.

5. Create an inner adviser. You can base this image on a mentor or teacher who, in the past, provided you with wise advice, encouragement and guidance. You might ask the adviser, "What can I do to speed up healing?" or, "Am I doing anything that is getting in the way of healing?" You might discover that your body needs more sleep or a change in diet, for example. And with your adviser's help and support, you will be more likely to try it—and succeed.

WORK WITH A PRACTITIONER

Many patients benefit from following instructions on guided imagery CDs or audiotapes, which can be purchased online. You also can work with a certified guided imagery professional. To find one in your area, contact the Academy for Guided Imagery (800-726-2070, *www.acadgi.com*).

What Energy Healing Can Do for You

Gary E. Schwartz, PhD, professor of psychology, medicine, neurology, psychiatry and surgery at the University of Arizona and director of the university's Laboratory for Advances in Consciousness and Health, both in Tucson. He is the author of *The Energy Healing Experiments* (Atria). *www.drgaryschwartz.com*

Western medicine has long scoffed at the claims of Eastern philosophies that espouse the healing powers of "energy" or "life force." In China, such forms of energy are known as "qi"...in India, the term is "prana."

Now: Many mainstream American doctors are taking a more open-minded look at so-called energy healing. For example, the National Institutes of Health's National Center for Complementary and Alternative Medicine is actively involved in the scientific investiga-

tion of energy healing. And energy therapies are quietly gaining popularity among Western patients seeking alternatives to conventional medicine.

Gary E. Schwartz, PhD, one of the world's leading experts in the scientific study of energy healing, answered questions about how such therapies are being used in the US.

•**What exactly is energy healing?** To understand energy healing, it's useful to first discuss energy fields, which play a key role in our society. They support the radio-wave technology that allows us to use cell phones, satellite TV, garage-door openers and any number of other wireless technologies. These radio waves, which cannot be seen, are capable of transmitting data, conversations, music and visual images through the air, often over a distance of thousands of miles. Energy fields also are widely used in technology that diagnoses and treats disease. For example, electromagnetic fields are used in magnetic resonance imaging (MRI) scans and cardiac pacemakers.

Energy healing refers to the use of invisible frequencies of energy. Some of these frequencies have been measured via reproducible methods, while others are theorized. Practitioners of energy healing believe that disturbances in the energy fields that flow throughout the human body can result in illness.

There are studies suggesting that one person's energy fields can overlap and interact with another person's energy fields. For example, even when people are not touching each other, the electrical activity of one person's heart can be registered in the other person's electroencephalogram (EEG), a recorded image of the electrical activity in different parts of the brain.

•**How is energy healing now practiced in the US?** There are various forms. The most popular include Healing Touch (developed in the 1980s)...and Reiki (developed in 1922). With each of these therapies, the practitioner seeks to "manipulate" a patient's life force—or energy. The techniques can involve touching the patient or placing one's hands a few inches or feet from the patient's body. With Reiki, at least four 30- to 90-minute sessions are typically recommended. In a study of older adults receiving Healing Touch, pain reduction was reported after an average of 6.4 sessions.

• **How is energy healing believed to work?** I like to use the metaphor of a ladder, with each step providing a higher and wider view. On one step are electromagnetic fields generated by an energy healer's hands—fields that research shows can resonate with and change plant, animal and human cells. The energy of the healer's hands interacts with the energy of the patient and they respond to each other—something akin to two tuning forks resonating with each other.

• **Is there any scientific proof that energy healing is effective?** As a trained scientist, I started out as a skeptic, but after conducting research on energy healing for 10 years, I am certain that energy plays a role in health and healing.

One remarkable experiment that helped convince me that energy healing is real was conducted here at the University of Arizona and published in the *Journal of Alternative and Complementary Medicine.*

In the experiment, rats were subjected to daily stress from noise. One group of rats was treated with Reiki. Another group was "treated" by fake energy healers who stood in front of the animals' cages moving their arms in a way that mimicked the outward actions of the Reiki practitioners but with no intention to heal the rats.

At the end of the study, the rats treated with Reiki had significantly less stress-caused damage to small blood vessels. This study showed quite convincingly that energy healing is real—because with rats, there is no placebo effect.

Dozens of studies on humans have shown that energy healing, in the form of Reiki and Healing Touch, has improved such medical conditions as pain, wound healing and high blood pressure.

• **If the evidence is strong, why is there such widespread skepticism about energy healing?** There are several reasons. Many people tend to think of the world in material terms, as opposed to invisible, energetic terms. These individuals may not have grown up with cell phones and satellite TV or with

the reality that there are unseen energies all around us that convey information. Also, the first energy healers tended to be "New Agers." Some were frauds and made outlandish claims—and people threw out the baby with the bathwater.

There are also powerful economic forces, such as those wielded by the pharmaceutical industry, that have a vested interest in not accepting a nondrug methodology that can reduce and, in some cases, eliminate the need for drugs.

New scientific ideas are always met with resistance, but I believe there will be a paradigm shift in which energy healing is accepted and becomes widely practiced by health professionals.

• **Why do critics of energy healing claim that the evidence is inconclusive?** Most of these critics have not reached their conclusions based on a thorough knowledge of the literature. Some applications of energy healing, such as its use in stress and pain reduction, are well documented, while other applications have not yet undergone rigorous scientific evaluation and are considered inconclusive.

• **Is energy healing particularly effective for certain health conditions?** Positive effects are uniformly reported in pain reduction, wound healing and stress relief. Energy healing also is effective in diseases caused or exacerbated by stress, such as high blood pressure.

• **Are there any risks associated with energy healing?** The risk for adverse effects is very low, particularly when compared with drugs and surgery. In rare cases, people who are particularly sensitive to energy may have an adverse response, such as a flare-up of allergies. But as a rule, energy healing is safe and can have profoundly powerful positive effects.

• **What's the best way to locate a competent energy healer?** Several organizations train and certify energy healers. To find lists of certified healers, go to the Healing Touch Program, 210-497-5529, *www.htpractitioner.com*... or the International Center for Reiki Training, 800-332-8112, *www.reiki.org*. You also can get a recommendation from a holistic physician or other health professional who is open to energy healing. Or talk to a friend who has had a positive experience with an energy healer.

Rejuvenate Your Mind with Acupressure

Applying pressure to certain areas of the body opens energy pathways by increasing blood circulation.

How to do it: Gently place your thumb and middle finger of one hand on your forehead above each eyebrow, making a bridge. Meanwhile, with your other hand, reach around to the back of your head and apply firm pressure just below the base of the skull on either side of the spine. Use light pressure in front and firm pressure in back for three minutes to refresh your mind.

More information: www.acupressure.com.

Michael Reed Gach, PhD, founder, Acupressure Institute, Berkeley, California.

Surprising Benefits of Biofeedback

Celeste De Bease, PhD, the former chair of the Biofeedback Certification Institute of America, has taught biofeedback therapy for many years and practices it in Bala Cynwyd, Pennsylvania.

The 1970s was an era of bizarre fads and funky ideas like the Pet Rock. Those disappeared quickly—but at least one idea that seemed weird then not only had staying power, but also proved visionary.

Mood rings, made with liquid crystal that changes color based on body temperature, were marketed as a tool to gauge state of mind. These novelties were an early form of biofeedback. Biofeedback was being studied in the 1970s, with research continuing even now, and it has become a highly sophisticated therapy for a host of different health challenges. In fact, even the American Cancer Society acknowledges that biofeedback can help im-

prove cancer patients' quality of life and certain associated health conditions.

ARE YOU "OVER-REACTIVE?"

Dr. De Bease explains that ideally the alarm or arousal levels people experience should be appropriate to the situations they encounter, but that's often not what happens. Many people chronically over-respond to stress and others go through daily life on "high alert" even when nothing particularly stressful is happening. Dr. De Bease calls this having a "hyperactive idling speed." Though they may have no clue that this is happening, they pay a high price in stress-related fatigue and illnesses. Through biofeedback, says Dr. De Bease, such people can learn to "uncouple the primitive and physically taxing survival response of fight or flight from situations that do not call for it."

Biofeedback is used for a wide swath of disorders, many associated with some degree of stress, including Raynaud's disease, urinary incontinence, ADHD, fibromyalgia, anxiety, epilepsy, high blood pressure, migraine and other headaches, sleep disorders, IBS and tinnitus. Treatment usually starts with a psycho-physiological stress test in which people are exposed to stress-inducing situations, such as recounting a stressful experience or hearing a sudden loud noise. They are hooked up to equipment that measures the physical responses to determine their individual levels of reactivity and how long it takes them to recover afterward. Machines used in biofeedback therapy measure muscle tension, blood flow, heart rate and skin temperature, as well as sweat gland activity—all are extremely sensitive to thoughts and feelings. Additional equipment identifies brain activity (neurofeedback), which includes alpha waves (calm relaxation), beta (alert), theta (meditation and light sleep) and delta waves (deep sleep).

LEARNING A BETTER WAY THROUGH BIOFEEDBACK

Once problems are identified, the therapist uses various techniques to retrain clients to improve their physiological responses. One area of change centers on releasing muscle tension. This is the easiest biofeedback goal to achieve, says Dr. De Bease, because we control many of our muscles voluntarily. Then the work moves on to learning control of the autonomic

43

nervous system, which affects vasoconstriction. For example, people who have Raynaud's disease often have cold hands, caused by constriction in the blood vessels leading to them. Biofeedback teaches them to focus on learning how to uncouple this subconscious response and pay attention to what triggered it.

Another key diagnostic area centers on heart rate.

To explain: Normally the heart beats faster on inhalation and slows with exhalation (variability), but that pattern can be disrupted in people who are chronically stressed and whose hearts remain at a fast-paced "ready" rate. People can learn to normalize this heartbeat with breathing exercises, which Dr. De Bease explains is "a great bridge for helping people to balance the influences from the two components of autonomic nervous system function—sympathetic (preparing for attack) and parasympathetic (calm and relaxation)." Eventually people learn to consciously make changes that can affect their autonomic responses, including heart rate and perspiration. Rather than becoming inappropriately stressed yet again, you can learn to modify your response to fit the situation.

THE BODY-MIND LINK

Dr. De Bease observes that using the body to calm the mind is exactly the opposite of the usual path in the Western world, where many believe that if you "think it, you can make it so." Biofeedback works in reverse, she says: "Change your body and it will change your mind." It's a tactic that reminds me of being told to smile when upset or angry—however silly you feel with a grin on your angry face, it does seem impossible to stay mad.

Much of the stress in our culture comes from time constraints and attempts to multitask, thinking about several things at once, says Dr. De Bease. When you find yourself overstressing because of commitments or distractions or fear of not getting everything done, slow down and regulate your breathing. Breathing slowly in and out will help balance the function of the parasympathetic and sympathetic nervous system, allowing for a more appropriate autonomic response to external stressful stimuli.

Biofeedback can help all sorts of health problems—and is generally considered safe. You can find a practitioner near you by going to the Web site of the Biofeedback Certification International Alliance (*www.bcia.org*). Most biofeedback sessions run about 45 minutes and cost in the same range as psychotherapy. Insurance generally pays at least part of the cost—sometimes all, depending on your health condition. Don't expect to solve your problems in one visit, however. Most people require a session a week for 20 weeks or so and some may continue even longer.

So Much More Than a Foot Massage!

Bill Flocco, reflexology teacher and researcher, founder and director of the American Academy of Reflexology, based in Los Angeles and author of several books on reflexology, including *Reflexology Research: Anatomy of a Reflexology Research Study* (William Sanford).

Reflexology has long been viewed by many Americans and medical professionals as little more than a foot massage.

Now: Recent scientific studies show that chronic pain, digestive disorders and other common health problems can be relieved through the use of this practice. Reflexology, which was developed by three medical professionals in the early 20th century, involves applying pressure to specific areas—known as "reflex points"—located on the feet, hands and ears.

How it works: When a body part is injured or stops functioning properly due to disease, irritating chemicals accumulate in distant but related nerve endings in the feet, hands and ears. Various studies have repeatedly shown that when certain parts of the feet, hands and ears are worked on with touch techniques, relief results in corresponding parts of the body.

Bonus: You can perform many basic forms of reflexology on yourself or a partner.*

For best results, work on all of the reflex points described in this article for at least five

*To find a certified reflexologist in your area, contact the American Reflexology Certification Board, 303-933-6921, *www.arcb.net*

minutes twice a day, four or more times a week. Relief can be experienced within minutes, but it sometimes takes days or weeks of repeatedly working on the appropriate reflex areas to get results.

Caution: Do not work on bruises, cuts, sores, skin infections or directly on areas where you have damaged a bone or strained a joint during the preceding three to six months. If you've had surgery or suffered a bone fracture, ask your surgeon when it's safe to perform reflexology on these areas.

The main technique used on most parts of the feet and hands, including those points described below, is the "thumb roll."

What to do: Place gentle pressure with the pad of your thumb against the area on which you wish to work. Maintaining this pressure and moving slowly, bend the knuckle in the center of the thumb in an upward direction and roll your thumb from the pad toward the tip, moving it forward. Next, reverse the movement of the knuckle, so that once your thumb is flattened you can do another thumb roll, each time moving forward in the direction the thumb is pointing.

Reflex points that correspond to common complaints…

HEARTBURN

What to do: While sitting in a chair, place your left foot on your right knee. Use your left thumb to locate the "diaphragm line," which separates the ball of your foot and your instep, where the skin color changes between the pad and soft part of the sole. On this line, about an inch from the inner edge of the foot, press gently with the tip of your thumb while squeezing gently with your index finger on top of the foot for five to 10 minutes.

Next, place the tip of your right thumb on the soft part of your left palm at the point between the base of the knuckles below your index and middle fingers. With the fingers of your right hand gently squeezing the back of your left hand, apply gentle pressure with the tip of your right thumb for five to 10 minutes.

HEADACHE

What to do: Start with the hand corresponding to the side of your head where the pain is most noticeable. On the back of that hand, locate a point about an inch below the base knuckle of your index finger in the fleshy web between your index finger and thumb. Place the tip of the thumb of your other hand on this point and the tip of your index finger of the other hand on the palm side of this point, squeezing to find a spot that's slightly thicker and more tender than the surrounding area. While maintaining steady pressure, gently move the tip of your thumb in small circles over this spot. (This movement is different from the thumb roll.) It usually takes about five minutes of work to alleviate a tension headache, and up to an hour to reduce or eliminate a migraine headache.

Caution: This point should not be worked on during the first trimester of pregnancy, as it could have an adverse effect on the fetus. Instead, work only on the related point on the ear, as described in the next column.

After you have completed the hand reflexology, locate the small, hard flap of cartilage at the top of your earlobe, then feel where this flap and the earlobe meet. With the tip of your thumb on the front of the ear and the tip of your index finger behind the ear, gently squeeze this point between your index finger and thumb, feeling for a spot that's slightly thicker and more tender than the surrounding area. Squeeze both ears at once, holding for five to 10 minutes, while resting your elbows on a table or desk.

IRRITABLE BOWEL SYNDROME

What to do: While sitting, place your left foot on your right knee. With the fingers of your left hand, gently grasp the top of the foot. Using the thumb roll technique in repeated overlapping strips, work across from the inner edge to the outer edge of the foot, on all of the soft part of the sole and the entire heel, for 10 minutes. Repeat, using your right thumb on the bottom of your right foot.

After you have completed the foot reflexology, use your right thumb to perform the thumb roll technique on your left palm. Work from the outside to the inside of the palm, starting just below the base of the fingers and progressing toward the wrist. Repeat, using your left thumb to work on the right palm.

NECK PAIN AND STIFF NECK

What to do: Move your finger slightly above the cartilage flap described in the headache section, and find a ridge of cartilage running up and down the ear. Place the tips of your index fingers on the lower inch of this ridge on both ears while resting your elbows on a table or desk. Squeeze gently but firmly between your index fingers and thumbs, with your thumbs behind the ears. Continue for five to 10 minutes.

Meditation for People Who Don't Like to Meditate

Sharon Salzberg, cofounder of the Insight Meditation Society meditation center in Barre, Massachusetts. She has taught meditation since 1974 and written numerous books, including *Real Happiness: The Power of Meditation* (Workman).

Only about 9% of American adults meditate regularly, even though it's been proven in a variety of studies to reduce stress...lower blood pressure...ease depression...relieve chronic pain...and boost immunity, to name just a few of its many health benefits. So why don't more people meditate?

Despite all its virtues, meditation can be seemingly impossible for many people to do. Fortunately, there are simple solutions for virtually all of the reasons that people cite for not being able to meditate.

DO IT YOUR WAY

The most familiar form of meditation involves sitting or lying down for about 30 minutes and focusing on your breathing—how it feels as air enters and leaves your nose or as your chest or abdomen rises and falls. For most people, it takes about 30 minutes to calm their stress-based thinking—I forgot to call so-and-so, etc.—and reach a deeper level of concentration.

It's simple but not easy. It is common to become frustrated with your mind's constant chatter, or you may feel so restless, bored or distracted that you give up.

My solutions for the most common reasons that people don't try meditation—or give it up…

Problem: Feeling too restless to meditate. Some people find it impossible to sit still for an extended period of time.

Solution: Try walking meditation. Find a quiet, unobstructed, flat area where you can take at least 20 steps before turning around. As you walk slowly, let your attention rest on your feet and legs. Be aware of the sensations in each foot as it lifts off the ground, moves through the air, then settles down.

Feel the contact of the ground in your toes and the soles of your feet. Notice how the muscles of each leg tighten and then relax as you walk. Observe the sensations in the foot (and the leg) that is not bearing weight.

Note: Walking meditation is also ideal for people who tend to fall asleep while meditating in a chair or lying down.

Problem: Getting distracted by noise. It's not always easy to find a quiet place to meditate, and some people are very sensitive to noise.

Solution: Make sound the object of your meditation. The distinction between sound and noise is important. "Sound" is a purely physical phenomenon, while "noise" is sound plus a negative judgment. The idea is simply to notice sounds as they arise—beep, rumble, clang, hiss—without speculating about where they come from.

When you become aware that you're reacting to a sound, observe the thoughts you have about the sound. What does the anger or irritation feel like? Then go back to just hearing it.

Problem: The "mind chatter" won't stop. You may hope that meditation will clear your mind of thoughts, but invariably the thoughts keep on coming—a conversation you had last week …what you want to eat for dinner. Your mind just won't shut down.

Solution: Don't fight the thoughts. Just observe them as they pass through your mind.

It's like sitting on the bank of a river and watching the water float by, noticing leaves, twigs, fish, flashes of sunlight and shadow—without being swept up by the current.

If the thoughts persist, gently bring your attention back to the sensations of breathing… or the feeling of your feet on the floor. When more thoughts arise, repeat the process.

Problem: There's no time to meditate. When your schedule is busy, it may not be possible to devote a half hour (or even 20 minutes) to meditation every day.

Solution: Start with 10 minutes. For many people, it's easier to find three 10-minute periods in the course of the day than to arrange a time for a lengthier break. If 10 minutes seem too long, you can even start with five.

How can five or 10 minutes of meditation be enough to benefit you? The reason is that the dailiness of meditation—making it a regular part of your routine—is more important than the amount of time you meditate. And many people find that after several weeks of five-minute meditation periods, it seems natural—and possible—to meditate longer.

MIX AND MATCH

Do you crave variety? If so, you don't have to meditate the same way every time. Choose whichever way fits your current state of mind. Even a household task like washing dishes can be an occasion to meditate—just focus on your body's movements and sensations as you carry out the task. That, too, is meditation.

Get Hypnotized, Get Healthier

Benjamin Kligler, MD, MPH, associate professor of family and social medicine at Albert Einstein College of Medicine, vice chair of the department of integrative medicine at Beth Israel Medical Center and research director of the Continuum Center for Health and Healing, an integrative medicine practice, all in New York City. *www. healthandhealingny.org*. Dr. Kligler, who is certified in Ericksonian hypnotherapy, is author of *Curriculum in Complementary Therapies* (Montefiore Medical Center).

Hear the word "hypnosis" and you may think of a stage show—a guy in a turban dangling a pocket watch and making you cluck like a chicken or behave in some other silly and uncharacteristic way.

This is not at all what modern hypnotherapy is like.

Reality: Ericksonian hypnosis (named after American psychiatrist Milton Erickson, who pioneered the techniques used today) is a collaboration between you and a trained healthcare practitioner that can help you achieve specific health goals.

Hypnotherapy does not use commands, such as, "Now you will do what I say." Instead, the practitioner offers gentle, nonauthoritative suggestions when you are in a highly relaxed state. The idea behind hypnosis is that there is no separation between body and mind—so you can access the healing potential of the unconscious mind to move yourself in a healthful direction. Unlike classical hypnosis, which works on only a small subset of highly suggestible people, Ericksonian hypnosis can help almost anyone—though it is most effective for those who are motivated and accepting of treatment.

HELP FROM HYPNOSIS

Research shows that hypnotherapy helps treat a variety of physical and psychological problems, including…

• **Anxiety**

• **Chronic pain**

• **Insomnia**

• **Irritable bowel syndrome** (recurring bouts of diarrhea and/or constipation)

• **Menopausal hot flashes**

• **Nausea**

• **Overeating**

• **Phobias,** such as claustrophobia or fear of flying

• **Sugar addiction**

• **Tobacco addiction.**

Examples: One study found that a single 15-minute hypnosis session significantly decreased pain and anxiety in women undergoing breast cancer surgery—and, for unknown reasons, also shortened the procedure time in the operating room. In another study, 68% of women with menopausal hot flashes showed reduced symptom severity and frequency, as well as decreased insomnia, after hypnosis.

How it works: Everybody has chatter in the conscious mind that can get in the way of healthful behaviors, such as controlling consumption of sweets or not panicking in an elevator. Hypnosis quiets the conscious mind so your unconscious can come in and say, "Wait a minute, we're trying to be healthier here"— making it easier to turn down that donut or stay calm in the elevator. Hypnosis relieves physical symptoms, such as pain or hot flashes, by reducing stress hormones that contribute to physical ailments.

Hypnosis by itself does not cure the problem —rather, it creates a heightened state of awareness that opens the way for your own willingness to bring about the desired changes. Hypnotherapy can focus on symptom reduction...strategies for coping with stress... resolution of personal problems...and/or personality development.

WHAT TO EXPECT IN TREATMENT

Typically, the first session with a hypnotherapist lasts one hour. During this visit, the practitioner asks questions about your particular problem—when symptoms began, other treatments you have tried, how the issue affects your life and stress level. Because hypnotherapy is highly individualized, this information helps determine the most appropriate treatment for you. Hypnosis may or may not be done during this first session.

A course of hypnotherapy generally ranges from three to eight sessions, with each weekly hypnosis session lasting about 30 to 40 minutes. Sometimes patients return months or years later for a "booster" session.

During a session, you sit on a comfortable chair or couch in a quiet and softly lit room. Usually your eyes are closed, but you can hear everything around you.

Speaking in a soothing voice, the practitioner leads you into an induction, a trancelike state of deep relaxation. One common technique is the body scan. The practitioner asks you to focus on your feet, relaxing the muscles there. Next you focus on feeling the relaxed sensation in your ankles, your calves, your

knees. Over five to 10 minutes, the practitioner guides you to relax your entire body.

While you are in a state of deep relaxation, the practitioner makes therapeutic suggestions, prompting your unconscious mind to deal more effectively with your health issue. The practitioner does not say something like, "You will not be afraid of the airplane," but rather, "You may find yourself feeling much more relaxed on the airplane than you have in the past." Suggestions are tailored to the specific problem and person. The process generally is pleasant and completely safe. You do not reveal personal secrets or do anything that you don't want to do.

After the therapeutic suggestions, the practitioner typically brings you back to your normal state of consciousness by saying, "I'm going to be quiet now, and over the next few minutes, you can gradually bring yourself back to the room." You may or may not consciously remember what was said to you during hypnosis...you may come to the end of a session thinking that it lasted just a few minutes, when in reality it lasted half an hour.

Over the following few days or weeks, you may notice that your symptoms are improving— for instance, you sleep better, feel less nauseous or fearful, or find it easier to resist cravings for cigarettes.

HYPNOTHERAPY HOMEWORK

The practitioner may assign you some simple self-hypnosis techniques to do on your own. For instance, if you are seeking to change a habit, such as compulsive overeating, self-hypnosis helps you handle cravings as they arise. These techniques typically include physical strategies, such as pressing two fingers together as a reminder of how to reach the relaxation state...or taking a series of deep breaths while focusing on a certain calming image or phrase.

For a physical problem, such as irritable bowel syndrome, the practitioner may tape-record an in-office hypnosis session and have you listen to it at home. As you reexperience the state of deep relaxation again and again, not only your mind but your entire body benefits—making your gut less susceptible to digestive upsets.

Finding a practitioner: In addition to being a licensed doctor, psychologist or social worker, a qualified practitioner should have about one year of hypnotherapy training. To ensure that your practitioner has met educational standards and training requirements in clinical hypnosis, you may want to verify that he/she is certified through the American Society of Clinical Hypnosis (630-980-4740, *www. asch.net*).

Hypnotherapy costs about $125 to $300 per session. Although many insurance companies do not cover hypnosis per se, you may be able to collect under a mental-health benefit if your psychotherapist or integrative physician includes hypnosis among the treatments offered.

Yoga Can Help You—But Which Kind Is Best?

Timothy McCall, MD, board-certified internist, medical editor of Yoga Journal and author of *Yoga as Medicine: The Yogic Prescription for Health and Healing* (Bantam). *www.drmccall.com*

Yoga is powerful medicine. It can improve balance, flexibility and posture …strengthen muscles and bones…lower blood pressure, ease pain and boost immune function…heighten sexual functioning…alleviate stress and depression…and bolster spiritual well-being.

Key: Finding a style that fits your abilities, temperament and goals. With your doctor's okay, consider…

•**Anusara.** This playful, warm-hearted and physically challenging style emphasizes body alignment (often with hands-on adjustments from the teacher) and a positive mindset that looks for the good in all people.

Best for: Physically fit people who want to be part of a like-minded community.

•**Ashtanga ("power" yoga).** A vigorous practice, it includes a fixed series of postures that flow rapidly and continuously, accompanied by energizing breathing techniques.

Best for: People who can handle an intense workout, want to build stamina and strength, and enjoy a set routine.

•**Bikram ("hot" yoga).** An invariable sequence of 26 poses is performed in a studio heated to at least 100°F to loosen muscles, tendons and ligaments.

Best for: People in good health who don't mind heat and want improved flexibility. Bikram, like other vigorous styles, may not be appropriate for frail or older students or those with serious illnesses.

•**Integral.** Beginning classes include gentle poses, breathing techniques, meditation and discussions of ancient yoga texts. The principle of selfless service (such as volunteer work) is emphasized. Some centers offer special classes for students with physical limitations or health problems (such as heart disease or cancer).

Best for: People interested in traditional Indian yoga that includes more than just poses.

•**Iyengar.** Emphasizing meticulous body alignment, this style makes use of blocks, straps and other props so students with limited flexibility can safely and comfortably assume poses. Teacher training requirements are among the strictest.

Best for: Anyone new to yoga or especially in need of better body alignment, such as people with arthritis or back pain.

•**Kripalu.** A blend of Western psychology and Eastern philosophy, this practice provides a safe place to explore emotional issues. Meditation and chanting accompany moderately vigorous and sometimes improvised movement.

Best for: People looking for stress relief and emotional release.

•**Kundalini.** This style includes a wide variety of breathing techniques, intense physical movements, chanting and meditation. The focus is on raising energy rather than on precise body alignment.

Best for: People who are seeking to build prana (life force) and who are open to yoga's spiritual dimensions.

•**Viniyoga.** Gentle flowing poses are held only briefly. Safety and breath work are emphasized. Teachers often focus on private one-on-one sessions rather than group classes.

Best for: People who are new to yoga or out of shape or who are looking to use yoga to help alleviate any of a variety of chronic ailments.

To find a class: Yoga Alliance (888-921-9642, *www.yogaalliance.org*) registers teachers who complete a certain number of hours of training in specific styles. If you have a medical condition, contact the teacher to see if a particular class is appropriate for you or to ask about private lessons. Yoga therapy has been shown in studies to be effective for a wide range of conditions, from diabetes and arthritis to cancer and chronic lung disease.

The Essential Guide to Acupuncture

Effie Poy Yew Chow, PhD, RN, founder and president of East West Academy of Healing Arts in San Francisco (*www.eastwestqi.com*). A California-licensed acupuncturist, qigong grandmaster and registered psychiatric nurse, she was appointed by President Clinton to the original 15-member White House Commission on Complementary and Alternative Medicine Policy.

Acupuncture has been practiced in Asia for more than 5,000 years, but only recently has Western medicine begun to acknowledge this ancient healing therapy. Just over a decade ago, the FDA reclassified acupuncture needles from "experimental" status to "medical device." Around the same time, a consensus panel of the National Institutes of Health (NIH) found acupuncture to be an effective treatment for postoperative dental pain, chemotherapy-induced nausea and several other conditions.

Since then, people in the US have increasingly embraced acupuncture as an alternative or complementary therapy for numerous common ailments—and many health insurance companies now cover it. *What acupuncture can do for you...*

HOW IT WORKS

The human body has 12 major energy meridians (pathways), each corresponding to a different organ system. Flowing through this network is the body's qi (pronounced chee), or life force. Health problems result when there is too much or too little qi in specific places.

Example: If qi flow is excessive, a woman may be congested, feverish or unable to sleep. If qi flow is insufficient, she may lack energy, feel chilly or catch a cold.

Acupuncture often eases arthritis, asthma, migraine and many other conditions (see the list at the end of this article). The practitioner inserts very fine needles into the skin at one or more of about 1,000 specific points. This either calms the flow of excessive energy or stimulates the point if the qi is blocked.

Among Western researchers, the most widely accepted theories are that acupuncture triggers the release of pain-relieving brain chemicals called endorphins...helps release substances that transmit nerve impulses to the brain... and/or stimulates the immune system.

To date, one of the largest and most rigorous trials on acupuncture in the US was an NIH study in 2004 involving 570 participants. The study evaluated acupuncture's usefulness in treating osteoarthritis of the knee.

Results: After receiving 23 acupuncture sessions over 26 weeks, participants showed, on average, 40% more improvement in pain plus significantly more improvement in movement and function compared with a control group that received sham acupuncture. (In sham treatments, fine needles are inserted but not in the appropriate points.)

WHAT TO EXPECT

Before seeing an acupuncturist for a health condition, it is best to have a diagnosis from a medical doctor or naturopathic doctor. This helps the acupuncturist provide appropriate complementary treatment. However, even if a doctor has not been able to diagnose your problem, acupuncture still may correct the underlying cause or causes of your symptoms. For instance, I had a patient with severe asthma plus unexplained joint pain and digestive problems. Within two weeks of her first acupuncture session, her symptoms were gone and she was able to discontinue her many medications.

Your acupuncturist also will want as complete a picture of you as possible—including your health history and medications...diet and supplement use…exercise and sleep patterns… relationships, emotional state and stress level. Healing is most complete when a patient takes responsibility for her own health—so getting stuck with needles is only part of the process. You may be advised to adjust your diet and lifestyle, keep a journal of your feelings and/ or take steps to reduce stress.

At the start of every session, the acupuncturist checks the pulse points that correspond with the various meridians and examines your tongue color and coating, which provide clues to imbalances in qi flow. Then, depending on where the needles need to go, you'll lie face down, face up or on your side during treatment.

DOES IT HURT?

Many people hesitate to try acupuncture for fear that it will hurt. In fact, the needles are so fine that they cause little pain. You may feel a brief uncomfortable sensation—like a pinprick or small electric shock—from the electromagnetic force or "energy grabbing" of the needle. This subsides within seconds, and then you may feel a wave of calmness. If you do feel a strong reaction when a needle goes in, it may mean that you have a lot of qi blockage. The needle disperses that blockage, so with each treatment, discomfort lessens.

Note: The needle should not cause prolonged discomfort. If it does, tell the practitioner so he/she can make adjustments.

The number of needles varies with the condition being treated, your individual needs and the practitioner's training. Needles may be inserted just a tiny fraction of an inch or as deep as an inch or more. They may be left in place for a few minutes, a few hours or even a few days.

A session usually lasts 20 to 60 minutes and costs from $60 to $100 or more, depending on the practitioner and location. Patients generally have a total of six to 10 sessions, going once or twice weekly at first and then gradually increasing the time between appointments as their symptoms improve. Patients may notice improvement during a session, hours after a session or sometimes only after a number of sessions.

Safety: When done by a qualified practitioner, acupuncture is safe for most people.

The practitioner should swab treatment sites with disinfectant, then use sterile, single-use, disposable needles. Occasionally, patients experience very slight bleeding or bruising at a needle site.

Warning: Extra caution must be used when acupuncture is done on patients who have a bleeding disorder or who take a blood thinner. Acupuncture should not be used during pregnancy because there is a slight risk of miscarriage.

Best: Verify that your acupuncturist is certified by the National Certification Commission for Acupuncture and Oriental Medicine (904-598-1005, *www.nccaom.org*)…or by your state's licensing authority. For state-by-state information, visit *www.acupuncture.com/statelaws/state law.htm.*

PROBLEMS OFTEN TREATED WITH ACUPUNCTURE

Acupuncture may ease many conditions, including…

- **Anxiety**
- **Arthritis**
- **Asthma**
- **Back pain**
- **Bladder infections**
- **Blood sugar imbalances**
- **Bursitis**
- **Carpal tunnel syndrome**
- **Dental pain**
- **Depression**
- **Fibromyalgia (widespread muscle and joint pain)**
- **Headache and migraine**
- **Insomnia**
- **Menopausal hot flashes**
- **Menstrual cramps**
- **Postoperative nausea**
- **Sciatica**
- **Seizures**
- **Sinus problems**
- **Stress**
- **Tendinitis**

4

Super Secret Alternative Cures

The Toothpaste Made by Mother Nature

You probably know aloe vera as the cactuslike plant on your kitchen's windowsill. A squeeze of one of its succulent leaves yields a dab of gel, good for soothing minor burns and other boo-boos—so good, in fact, that two common names for aloe vera are "burn plant" and "first aid plant."

Well, maybe aloe should also be dubbed "periodontal plant"—because new research shows aloe vera gel can kill the microbes that cause gum disease.

ALOA VERA KILLS GERMS

A team of Indian researchers tested an aloe vera gel toothpaste to see if it had the same microbe-fighting power as two commercial toothpastes, Colgate and Pepsodent.

And no matter which mouth-inhabiting, disease-causing germ they tested it against—a range of seven bacteria and fungi—aloe vera

held its own, killing as many germs as the commercial toothpastes.

The findings were in *General Dentistry*.

A GREAT ALTERNATIVE

"Aloe vera contains anthraquinones, antimicrobial and anti-inflammatory compounds that kill bacteria and fungi, stop pain and heal tissue," says Dilip George, MDS (Master of Dental Surgery), the study leader. "And because aloe vera doesn't contain the abrasive elements typically found in commercial toothpaste, it's a great alternative for people with sensitive teeth and gums."

However: Not all aloe vera tooth gel contains the effective form of aloe vera.

"To be effective, the product must contain the stabilized gel located in the center of the plant," says Dr. George. "And during manufacturing the gel can't be filtered or treated with

Dilip George, MDS, senior lecturer, Department of Pedodontics and Preventive Dentistry, Pushpagiri College of Dental Sciences, India.

52

excessive heat, which reduces or destroys the active compounds in the gel."

Recommended: Forever Bright Aloe Vera Toothgel, from Forever Living (888-440-2563, *www.foreverliving.com*), the product tested in the study.

Forever Bright Aloe Vera Toothgel is also available at *www.bestaloeveraproduct.com, www.bonanza.com* and other Web sites.

Also helpful: "An aloe vera gel placed directly on gum tissues after periodontal surgery will promote faster healing and prevent infection," says Laura Torrado, DDS, a cosmetic dentist in New York City.

She also recommends applying aloe vera gel any time gum tissue has been "scratched or traumatized."

Plant Remedy for Colds

Some of my patients use Umcka regularly for colds and like it very much. I find that each of my patients tends to find, through trial and error, the remedy that works most effectively for him/her. So, yes, Umcka is worth trying, especially at the first sign of a cold. It's a relatively new remedy that comes from Pelargonium sidoides, a medicinal plant that grows in South Africa. There have been more than 20 clinical studies on this plant, and it has been found to be effective in relieving cold symptoms, sinusitis, sore throats and bronchitis. It's available in liquid, lozenges and chewable tablets.

Brand to try: Nature's Way Umcka (800-962-8873, *www.naturesway.com*). Follow the instructions on the label. There are no side effects, and Umcka is safe for everyone, including children.

Mark A. Stengler, NMD, licensed naturopathic medical doctor in private practice, Stengler Center for Integrative Medicine, Encinitas, California...adjunct associate clinical professor at the National College of Natural Medicine, Portland, Oregon...author of many books and the *Bottom Line/Natural Healing* newsletter. *www.drstengler.com*

Sharks To the Rescue?

A compound derived from sharks (squalamine) appears to be a broad-spectrum antiviral agent that's effective against hepatitis B and C. It is already being tested for cancer and a number of eye diseases.

Proceedings of the National Academy of Sciences Early Edition.

New Scientific Discovery: A Rabbit's Foot Really Works

Srinivasan S. Pillay, MD, assistant clinical professor of psychiatry at Harvard Medical School and author of *Life Unlocked: 7 Revolutionary Lessons to Overcome Fear* (Rodale).

Nancy Mramor, PhD, psychologist in private practice in Pittsburgh, Pennsylvania, and author of *Spiritual Fitness* (Llewellyn). *www.drnancyonline.com*

You stroke a rabbit's foot for good luck. Or jingle a lucky penny in your pocket. Or wear your lucky shirt or blouse on a day when you want to be at your best.

These are superstitious behaviors. Even though you may do them, deep down you know they're nonsense, right?

No, superstitions are practical, say a team of scientists—because they can improve your self-confidence and skill.

THE SUPERSTITION EXPERIMENT

Psychologists at the University of Cologne in Germany conducted an experiment to test the power of superstition to improve performance.

First, they asked 72 volunteers to show up at the laboratory with a "personal lucky charm"—and the volunteers obliged, bringing old stuffed animals, lucky stones and other objects.

When each volunteer arrived, the researchers took away the charm, supposedly to take a photograph of it. But they gave the charm back to only half the volunteers, telling the other half that there was a problem with the camera equipment and they'd return the charm later.

Next, all the volunteers played either a memory game or a word game—and those who still had their lucky charms with them performed much better!

Querying the participants after the two games, the researchers found that the superior performance was probably caused by greater self-confidence—produced by belief in the power of the lucky charm.

In two similar experiments, the researchers found that the ability to sink golf putts improved when people thought they were using a "lucky ball"…and the ability to perform an intricate physical task (quickly putting little balls into little holes) improved when people thought that those watching them had their "fingers crossed" for good luck.

"Activating a good-luck superstition leads to improved performance by boosting people's belief in their ability to master a task," concluded the researchers in the journal *Psychological Science*.

SUPERSTITION, SUPER RESULTS

Superstition can enhance performance in several ways, says Srinivasan S. Pillay, MD, assistant clinical professor of psychiatry at Harvard Medical School and author of *Life Unlocked: 7 Revolutionary Lessons to Overcome Fear* (Rodale). *Superstition can…*

•**Improve your confidence**—the belief that you'll succeed

•**Increase what psychologists call self-efficacy**—the belief you have the abilities to succeed

•**Make you more persistent**—more willing to stick with a task until it's completed

•**Decrease your anxiety,** allowing you to focus more fully on the task at hand

•**Help you feel supported**—you don't think you're taking on the task alone

•**Relieve you of some responsibility for the outcome**—responsibility that can be a mental burden, interfering with ease of performance and success.

In short, superstition improves what Dr. Pillay calls "possibility thinking"—if the lucky charm worked before, it can work again, even if the task seems impossible to achieve. (*Example:* Soon after the long-distance runner Roger Bannister broke the 4-minute mile—a speed thought to be impossible—several other athletes ran 4-minute miles.)

And you can improve the power of superstition to help you achieve your goals, says Nancy Mramor, PhD, a psychologist in private practice in Pittsburgh and author of *Spiritual Fitness* (Llewellyn). "A lucky charm works because of the associations it has with past successes," says Dr. Mramor. *To strengthen those associations…*

1. Hold or rub the object in the same way, every time.

"This convinces the body that the object will work in the way you want it to," she says.

2. Repeat a special word or phrase when holding the object.

"This adds positive associations," she says. Example: Say the word "Success" or the phrase "I will succeed."

3. Remember past successes. "When you use the object, think deeply and clearly about past successes associated with that object—how you felt, what you heard and what you saw. Recalling at least three specifics is very important, she says. "The first convinces your mind, the second convinces your emotions and the third convinces your body."

The Awesome Healing Power of Silver

Mark A. Stengler, NMD, licensed naturopathic medical doctor in private practice, Stengler Center for Integrative Medicine, Encinitas, California…adjunct associate clinical professor at the National College of Natural Medicine, Portland, Oregon…author of many books and the *Bottom Line/Natural Healing* newsletter. *www.drstengler.com*

You know that silver is a precious metal and an industrial commodity—but did you know that it also is a powerful healing agent? Silver has antimicrobial and antibacterial properties, and it has been used throughout the ages to cure infections and help heal wounds. Now interest in silver is growing in the medical community because new studies have found that it can kill a wide range of bacteria and viruses, including the very dangerous E. coli and Staphylococcus.

The form of silver generally used as medicine is colloidal silver, which is the suspension of microscopic particles of silver in liquid.

Before the advent of antibiotics, colloidal silver was used to treat infections. Silver utensils and vessels (with silver linings) were known to kill germs better than utensils and vessels made of other materials. But after antibiotics came into vogue, silver went out of favor with conventional doctors except for a few uses—as a salve for burns and wounds...in nitrate eye solutions to prevent blindness in newborn babies...and as an antibacterial coating in the lining of catheters.

Holistic physicians, however, never stopped prescribing colloidal silver to prevent many types of viral, bacterial and fungal infections, with generally excellent results. Now, with various bacteria strains becoming increasingly resistant to the effects of antibiotics, the rest of the medical community is once again becoming interested in colloidal silver. Because silver attacks microbes in several different ways at once, it's more difficult for these microbes to develop protective mechanisms. In a Taiwanese study published in the journal *Colloids and Surfaces B: Biointerfaces*, colloidal silver was found to kill the potentially deadly superbug *methicillin-resistant Staphylococcus aureus* (MRSA) and *Pseudomonas aeruginosa*, another dangerous superbug, on surfaces (such as doorknobs and light switches, where it is known to colonize and spread among people). A study in *Current Science* found that colloidal silver can boost the effectiveness of standard antibiotics when used in combination with them. Colloidal silver's effectiveness against a range of viruses, including hepatitis C, herpes and HIV, also has been shown in both laboratory tests and in people.

MY APPROACH

I recommend colloidal silver in liquid form, drops or spray to many of my patients with infections of all kinds, including those of the eyes, ears, throat, respiratory tract, digestive tract or urinary tract. To determine how to use

each form of colloidal silver, follow the instructions on the label. *For example, it can be...*

• **Ingested** (one teaspoon of the preparation four times daily, up to seven days).

• **Put into a saline solution to treat pinkeye** (two drops in one-half ounce of saline solution, and rinse the eye with the solution three times daily for seven days).

• **Placed directly in the ear** (two drops in the affected ear three times daily for seven days).

• **Sprayed on cuts.**

Other uses: Colloidal silver often is used by holistic physicians to fight infection intravenously. I frequently prescribe colloidal silver to be taken for several months by patients with Lyme disease...or I recommend it instead of antibiotics for infections. For these types of uses, it is best taken under a doctor's supervision (see below for the risks).

Brand to try: Sovereign Silver (888-328-8840, *www.natural-immunogenics.com*). This high-quality solution contains the smallest particles of any colloidal silver product on the market, with an average diameter of 0.8 nanometers (8 angstroms) per particle. Small particle size is important for several reasons. It enables the particles to penetrate and kill microbe cells more easily...and makes it easier for your body to flush them out of your system once they've done their job.

SAFETY ISSUES

Colloidal silver is safe for children, but it is not recommended for women who are pregnant or breast-feeding, because it has not been studied in these populations.

Ingesting silver products has, in rare cases, been linked to an irreversible condition called argyria, in which the skin turns bluish gray. While this is clearly a side effect that no one wants to encounter, case studies show that this condition occurs only when silver products are consumed for a year or more and/or as a result of ingesting very large amounts—at least one gram, which would require drinking an absurd amount of properly prepared colloidal silver solution (more than 100 quarts daily).

I have never had a case of argyria with the hundreds of patients I have treated with colloidal silver, nor have any of my colleagues witnessed this in their patients. With most commercially made silver products, I consider the risk for argyria to be negligible even with a regimen that lasts for several months (as long as the correct dose is used).

Do not attempt to make a colloidal silver product yourself, and do not ingest someone else's homemade product. A variety of do-it-yourself kits are available. However, these kits create silver particles that are quite large, making them less effec-tive at killing microbes and more difficult for the body's cells to eliminate than smaller particles. Large silver particles are more likely to produce argyria with long-term use.

The Best Beer for Your Bones (Yes, Beer)

Ravin Jugdaohsingh, PhD, senior research scientist in the department of nutrition at King's College, London.

Charles Bamforth, PhD, professor of Food Science in the department of food science & technology at the University of California, Davis, author of *Beer: Health and Nutrition* (Wiley-Blackwell) and many other books about beer and brewing.

You know calcium-rich, vitamin D-fortified milk is good for bones. But beer? It's famous for building bellies, but certainly not bones.

Key fact not widely reported: Beer is the richest dietary source of the mineral silicon—and silicon is a must for healthy bones.

THE SILICON STORY

Nutritional scientists have dubbed iron and zinc essential minerals—but the typical dietary intake of silicon (which is not yet recognized as essential) is twice that of iron and zinc, points out Ravin Jugdaohsingh, PhD, a senior research scientist in the Department of Nutrition at King's College, London.

Kids get most of their daily silicon (68%) from grains.

Men get most of their silicon from beer, which (along with drinking water) supplies the most absorbable or "bioavailable" form of silicon—orthosilicic acid, or OSA. (Beer is rich

in bioavailable silicon because it's made from silicon-rich grains such as barley or wheat that are processed in a way that liberates their OSA.)

Women get most of their silicon from bananas and string beans. But although there's a lot of silicon in those two foods, it's not always bioavailable. (For example, only 4% of the silicon in bananas is absorbed.)

But whatever the dietary source of silicon, a recent study shows that people who have more of it in their diet have stronger bones...

•**Denser hip bones.** Dr. Jugdaohsingh and his colleagues studied nearly 3,000 people and found that those with the most silicon in their diet had hip bones with the highest bone mineral density (BMD), a biomarker for stronger bones.

"Higher dietary silicon intake...may have salutary effects on skeletal health...that has not been previously recognized," he concluded in the *Journal of Bone Mineral Research*.

•**Supplementing with silicon.** New research also shows that adding silicon to the diets of women with osteoporosis (eroded, fracture-prone bones) and osteopenia (pre-osteoporosis) can strengthen bone.

Noting that "mounting evidence supports a role for silicon in bone formation," Dr. Jugdaohsingh and his colleagues studied 134 women with weak bones, giving them supplements of calcium and vitamin D or those two supplements and a silicon supplement. After 12 months, those taking silicon had the biggest boost in bone collagen, a protein in bones. (Calcium makes bones denser. Collagen makes bones more flexible and therefore more fracture-resistant—the bone bends but doesn't break.)

The results suggest that combining silicon with calcium and vitamin D "is of potential use in osteoporosis," concluded the researchers in *BMC Musculoskeletal Disorders*.

PALE ALE, STRONG BONES

But as pointed out earlier, the most bioavailable form of silicon—OSA—is found in beer and water. In fact, a recent study in the *British Journal of Nutrition* showed that 64% of the silicon in beer was absorbed, much more than any other silicon-rich food, and as much as a silicon supplement. *And that well-absorbed silicon is building bone...*

•**More beer, more bone.** In a study of more than 2,400 people, men who drank 1 or 2 bottles of beer a day had hip BMD that was 4% higher than men who didn't drink beer, reported researchers from Tufts University in the *American Journal of Clinical Nutrition.* (However, men who drank more than 2 drinks per day had lower BMD—showing, as have many other studies on alcohol and health, that moderate alcohol intake can be good for you, but heavy intake is almost always bad for you.)

Because beer is such an important source of silicon in the diet, Charles Bamforth, PhD—professor of Food Science in the Department of Food Science & Technology at the University of California, Davis, and author of *Beer: Health and Nutrition* (Wiley-Blackwell) and many other books about beer and brewing—decided to conduct a study to find out exactly which beers supply the most silicon.

His findings were recently reported in the *Journal of the Science of Food and Agriculture...*

•**Malted barley beer is tops.** Beers with high levels of malted barley and hops are the richest in silicon.

•**Pale ales are best.** Among malted beers, pale-colored malts—so-called "pale ales"—have the most silicon (probably because they're heated less than darker malts).

•**Lagers are good.** "Lagers were quite high in silicon as well," says Dr. Bamforth.

•**Wheat beers are worst.** Wheat beers, along with stouts, porters and low-alcohol beers, contain the least silicon.

Bottom line: "First and foremost, drink the beer you enjoy," says Dr. Bamforth. "Trying to force down a beer you don't like for the sake of your bones isn't going to work. After all, even wheat-based beers still have significant levels of silicon in them, compared to other dietary sources. So choose the beer you like the best.

"Beer often gets a bad rap, but it is not empty calories," he continues. "It has nutritive value—and even one, 12-ounce bottle of beer a day can help you make sure you're getting enough silicon for stronger bones."

A BOTTLE OF WATER WORKS TOO

Bottled water from natural sources can also contain high levels of OSA that might help prevent osteoporosis, says Dr. Jugdaohsingh.

Examples: Fiji Water (from Fiji) and Spritzer Water (from Malaysia).

New finding: In a recent study by researchers at the Center for Human Nutrition at the University of California, Los Angeles (UCLA), drinking Fiji Water for three months increased urinary silicon levels.

"Artesian aquifer bottled water is a safe and effective way of providing easily absorbed dietary silicon to the body," concluded the researchers in *Nutrition Journal.* And they recommended future studies to investigate "the mineral's potential as an alternative prevention or treatment to drug therapy for osteoporosis."

Also try: You could also take a silicon supplement—but most of them have low bioavailability, says Dr. Jugdaohsingh.

Best: BioSil, from BioMineral, according to team of Belgian researchers at the University of Antwerp.

It is widely available online and in retail stores where supplements are sold. Follow the dosage recommendation on the label.

Marijuana: The Best Herb for Pain Relief?

Mark Ware, MD, assistant professor of anesthesia and family medicine at McGill University in Montreal, Canada.

Jean Talleyrand, MD, founder and president of Medi-Cann, the country's largest network of medical cannabis doctors, with 21 clinics in California that have treated more than 230,000 patients. *www.medicann.com*

Alaska, Arizona, California, Colorado, Hawaii, Maine, Michigan, Montana, Nevada, New Jersey, New Mexico, Oregon, Rhode Island, Vermont and Washington.

No, those aren't the states necessary to win the electoral college. They're the states where it's legal for a citizen to use medical marijuana—which means 90 million Americans have the herb cannabis sativa as a legitimate medical option.

And a new scientific study shows that it's an option that can relieve pain when all other medical treatments have failed...

NOTHING WORKED BUT CANNABIS

The study was led by Mark Ware, MD, an assistant professor of anesthesia and family medicine at McGill University in Montreal, and reported in *CMAJ* (the *Canadian Medical Association Journal*).

The researchers asked 21 people with long-term nerve pain (chronic neuropathy) caused by surgery or injury to smoke one puff of cannabis, three times a day, for five days. They didn't always smoke the same potency of cannabis, however.

In one five-day period, the cannabis was a placebo: It contained no THC (tetrahydro-cannabinol), the active ingredient. In three other five-day periods, the marijuana contained either 2.5%, 6% or 9.6% THC.

Results: When participants smoked the cannabis with 9.6% THC, they had a small but significant decrease in pain compared with smoking cannabis without THC.

But that small decrease was a huge relief to the people in the study—no other medication had worked to decrease their neuropathy, a pain problem that afflicts 15 million Americans. "We were surprised to see this degree of pain relief in this group of patients, for whom all other standard treatments had failed," says Dr. Ware.

Also important: this relatively low dose of THC did not make the participants "high"—their daytime functioning was normal while using medicinal cannabis. (And their nighttime functioning was better—they fell asleep faster and woke up less often during the night.) In fact, researchers measured the participants' blood levels of THC and found it was less than half that of blood levels typically seen in recreational users of cannabis.

"Our study showed that low doses of cannabis can relieve pain and has medical value," says Dr. Ware. "Cannabis may offer physicians and their patients another tool in treating neuropathic pain."

How it works: The body has a built in cannabinoid system—cannabinoid molecules and cannabinoid receptors on cells that regulate a variety of functions, including movement, appetite, mood, memory, and pain, explains Dr. Ware. Many of those cannabinoid receptors sit on the end of nerve cells, where they regulate messages sent from nerve to nerve. In neuropathy, there's an abnormal level of nerve activity, producing electric pain, burning, and hypersensitivity. Medical cannabis can calm down that activity, decreasing pain.

CANNABIS COMMONSENSE

The American Medical Association—noting that studies show smoked cannabis reduces pain, improves appetite in cancer patients and helps relive spasticity and pain in people with multiple sclerosis—issued a statement urging more clinical research on marijuana and the "development of cannabinoid-based medicines." The American College of Physicians issued a similar statement, supporting research into the medical use of marijuana.

But maybe you live in one of the 15 states that has legalized medical marijuana, and you don't want to wait for more research—like the 15% of people with chronic pain who already use cannabis for relief (according to a survey by Dr. Ware), you may want to use medical cannabis now. What should you do?

Here are recommendations from Jean Talleyrand, MD, founder and president of MediCann in California (*www.medicann.com*), the country's largest network of medical cannabis doctors...

• **First, talk to your doctor.** "If conventional medicines aren't solving your problem—as was the case in the study with patients with chronic neuropathy—consider medical cannabis as an option," says Dr. Talleyrand. "Discuss your illness with your doctor, and see if it makes sense for the treatment plan to include a recommendation for cannabis."

Who can benefit: The National Institutes of Health lists the following conditions in which medical cannabis appears to have benefits...

• **Pain management for a wide variety of painful conditions**

• **Stimulating appetite and relieving cachexia,** the extensive muscle loss and wasting away of cancer sufferers and AIDS patients

• **Control of nausea and vomiting in cancer chemotherapy**

• **Decreased intraocular pressure inside the eyeball,** for the relief of glaucoma

• **Reducing symptoms in neurological and movement disorders,** such as the spasticity of multiple sclerosis and cerebral palsy

• **Temporary relief of anxiety**

The conditions most treated by medical cannabis in the MediCann clinics are…

• **Low back pain**
• **Anxiety**
• **Depression**
• **Migraine headaches**
• **Insomnia**
• **Neck pain**
• **Muscle spasms.**

• **Understand the modes of delivery.** There are many different ways to use medicinal cannabis, explains Dr. Talleyrand. You can smoke it, consume edibles (such as cookies and brownies) and use an herbal tincture, a vaporizer or even a topical preparation for local pain relief.

• **Start with a small dose.** To find out what level of intake is effective, you need to dose yourself and see if the medical cannabis helps or not. If the low dose doesn't work, slowly increase the dose, via your chosen method of intake, until you find a level that's effective for your problem.

• **Be aware of the potential side effects.** Although smoking cannabis is safer than tobacco, smoking any plant material creates tars and combustion byproducts that may harm the lungs, says Dr. Talleyrand. There is also slowed reaction and loss of coordination, which is why you should never use medical cannabis at work, or while driving or operating machinery. There are also possible withdrawal symptoms, such as irritability, insomnia, mood swings and mild depression.

• **Have a follow-up with your doctor.** After using medical cannabis for several months, see your doctor for a follow-up visit, to discuss the effect of the medication and its possible continued use.

A Surprising, Easy Way to Detox

Mark A. Stengler, NMD, licensed naturopathic medical doctor in private practice, Stengler Center for Integrative Medicine, Encinitas, California…adjunct associate clinical professor at the National College of Natural Medicine, Portland, Oregon…author of many books, including *The Natural Physician's Healing Therapies* and coauthor of *Prescription for Natural Cures* (both from Bottom Line Books)…and author of the *Bottom Line/Natural Healing* newsletter. *www.drstengler.com*

I often tell my patients about an easy, at-home way to clear toxins from the body—one that actually feels good and is inexpensive. It's a technique known as dry brushing. There are many ways to detoxify the body through different organs, but using a dry brush to detoxify via the skin, the body's biggest organ, has many benefits. *What you should know…*

• **How it helps.** When you dry brush, you exfoliate dead cells and give the body a gentle massage. This improves circulation…gives you glowing skin…and energizes you. But the most therapeutic benefit involves activating the lymphatic system, which is part of the immune system. The light pressure of brushing encourages movement of lymph fluid under the skin. This fluid carries away impurities that then are eliminated by the body. The movement of the lymph fluid, which results in lymphatic drainage, is a major component of your detoxification system. Dry brushing is safe for everyone, including pregnant women. And it leaves you feeling invigorated!

• **How to do it.** The best time to dry brush is before or during a shower. The water washes away dead cells exfoliated during the treatment. It's important that you always brush toward your heart because this is the natural direction of your circulation and the natural flow of lymph fluid. I recommend that you brush your skin from your head to your heart on the upper body and from the hands and arms in toward your torso. Then brush from your feet up your legs toward your torso. Long sweeping strokes are best. Dry brushing should take about five to 10 minutes daily. You can either go up and down your body several times or brush each body part several times before moving to the next one.

• **Choosing a brush.** Look for a brush that has a long handle and relatively soft bristles. (The amount of pressure you apply is more important than the bristles' softness.) Most wooden-handled brushes, available at health-food stores, cost about $6. Or you can use a loofah, which is a coarse sponge, although it may be too rough for your skin. You also can get a detox effect if you move a loofah toward your heart in the shower.

Magic Muscle-Cramp Cures from Your Kitchen

Barry Wiese, DC, board-certified chiropractic neurologist in private practice in Rochester, New York.

Sometimes muscle cramps aren't so easy to get rid of and, in fact, sometimes they are a sign of a serious illness. And, of course, not everyone knows about my magic cure...so I thought this was a topic you might like to know some more about.

WHO GETS MUSCLE CRAMPS?

Muscle cramps are a common problem—medically speaking, a muscle cramp is a sudden, involuntary contraction of one or more muscles that can be very painful, sometimes leaving tenderness for up to 24 hours after the cramp subsides. Aging and overuse of the muscles are two common causes, but other triggers can include dehydration...low blood sugar...calcium, sodium and/or magnesium deficiency...underactive thyroid...kidney or liver dysfunction...peripheral vascular disease (which restricts blood flow to the legs)...nerve compression...Lou Gehrig's disease (ALS)...brain tumors/cancer...multiple sclerosis...well, you get the picture.

WHAT YOU NEED TO KNOW

To get some useful advice, we contacted Barry Wiese, DC, board-certified chiropractic neurologist in private practice in Rochester, New York, whose specialty work with geriatric patients and background as a marathon

runner have given him especially unique expertise on this topic. Cautioning that there is no surefire, works-every-time solution, he told me how to differentiate a run-of-the-mill (if excruciating) cramp from one that you must tell your doctor about.

Here's a list of questions to ask yourself...

• **Are my cramps random?** According to Dr. Wiese, a cramp that comes on suddenly and inexplicably is usually not a problem. Noting that the majority of random cramps are no big deal, he suggested that it's fine to try the "old standby" cures, including eating a banana (for potassium)...drinking more water to counter dehydration...light stretching of the affected area...self-massage...and heat packs to relieve pain and tenderness.

• **Are my cramps becoming more frequent and/or following a pattern?** Cramps that begin to establish themselves in a predictable pattern—such as at a particular time of day or when you walk—may be a worrisome sign that you should discuss with your doctor.

Did I do something that might explain this cramp? If you realize that you are getting cramps often, even predictably in certain situations, start a log of when they strike including time of day...what you've eaten...how long they last...how painful they are (consider a score between one and 10)...and what you were doing before and during the episode. Share this information with your doctor.

• **Should I see my doctor?** With persistent or worsening muscle cramps, you need to see your doctor to discuss potential causes and treatments. Though muscle cramping represents abnormal function, it's only rarely serious, Dr. Weise said. However, he pointed out that "many disease processes include cramping in their list of symptoms...and for many of those, the earlier you get treated, the better the outcome—so it pays to follow a conservative, cautious route until proven otherwise."

You'll be asked about your medical history, and your doctor may suggest some tests, including blood work, to find the root cause. Treatment options could range from vitamin B supplementation...to prescription medications, such as diltiazem (a calcium-channel blocker) and baclofen (a potent muscle relaxant sometimes used to treat muscle spasms in patients with MS and ALS)...and possibly even quinine, the malaria treatment, though it's used only in extreme cases because of the potential adverse side effects.

KITCHEN CURES

We learned that pickle juice contains acetic acid, salts and other ingredients that help neutralize the compounds or electrolyte deficiencies that may cause cramps. Other helpful remedies you may be able to pull out of your kitchen cabinets include apple cider vinegar (mix two teaspoons with one teaspoon of honey into a glass of warm water), which works much like the pickle juice...and chamomile tea, which contains glycine, an amino acid that helps relieve muscle spasms.

Get Out On the Dance Floor

Volunteers who participated in dance therapy improved their balance and gait, say University of Missouri researchers, who maintain that these improvements could reduce the risk for falls. Move to the music—and it will improve every move you make throughout the day and for years to come.

Mark A. Stengler, NMD, licensed naturopathic medical doctor in private practice, Stengler Center for Integrative Medicine, Encinitas, California...adjunct associate clinical professor at the National College of Natural Medicine, Portland, Oregon...author of many books and the *Bottom Line/Natural Healing* newsletter. *www.drstengler.com*

Swear at Your Pain— You'll Feel Better

Richard Stephens, PhD, lecturer in the School of Psychology at Keele University in England.

He accidentally hit his hand with a hammer while building a garden shed— and swore.

His wife was in the most difficult part of his daughter's birth—and she swore. A lot. (The midwives told him it was a normal part of the process.)

After those two events, Richard Stephens, PhD, a lecturer in the School of Psychology at Keele University in England, started wondering why the readiest words out of our mouths when we're suddenly in pain usually contain four letters. Does swearing soothe the hurt?

To find out, he conducted a first-of-its-kind study, involving buckets of freezing water and a lot of expletives...

THE CURSING CURE

Dr. Stephens recruited 64 students for his study, asking them to keep one hand in a bucket of ice-cold water for as long as possible, and swear away, using their favorite expletive.

Then they were asked to repeat the process—this time, saying a word they'd typically use to describe a table. (Flat, brown, hard, etc.)

Cursing was curative...

Results: When the students swore, they could keep their hands in the icy water for an average of two minutes. When they didn't swear, the average was one minute and 15 seconds. Later, the students rated the intensity of their pain during the two immersions—and there was less self-perceived pain when they swore. The findings were published in *Neuro Report*.

Why it works: Dr. Stephens admits that he doesn't know. But he has a theory. Those who swore had a higher heart rate. That means swearing might help trigger the fight-or-flight response, the body's automatic response to immediate threat, which includes increased heart rate, decreased respiration, tighter muscles, slower digestion—and lower sensitivity to pain.

DON'T WEAR OUT SWEARING

Dr. Stephens has two recommendations if you want to use swear words to help decrease pain.

•**Relief is a four-letter word.** "If you hurt yourself, swear." That's obvious.

But this isn't...

•**Don't swear all the time.** "If you want to use the pain-lessening effect of swearing to

61

your advantage, you need to do less casual swearing," he says. "Swearing is an emotional language. But if you overuse it, it loses its emotional significance. Without emotion, all that's left is saying the swearword itself—and that's unlikely to reduce anyone's pain."

Heal Wounds with Honey

Mark A. Stengler, NMD, naturopathic medical doctor and founder and medical director of the Stengler Center for Integrative Medicine, Encinitas, California... adjunct associate clinical professor at the National College of Natural Medicine, Portland, Oregon...the author of many books, including *The Natural Physician's Healing Therapies* and coauthor of *Prescription for Natural Cures* and *Prescription for Drug Alternatives* as well as author of the *Bottom Line/Natural Healing* newsletter. *www.drstengler.com*

Manuka honey from bees feeding on the manuka bush in New Zealand is more than deliciously sweet to eat. It also has antibacterial properties that have been found to help heal many types of wounds and skin problems.

Using honey to heal wounds is an ancient practice. Recently, researchers have observed that when used as a wound dressing, manuka honey helps clear infection...reduce inflammation...aid in shedding dead tissue...and induce healing by stimulating the growth of new tissue and capillaries. Manuka honey does not damage surrounding tissue, which can occur with topical antibiotics after several days of use. It is useful in treating skin ulcers, cuts, scrapes, burns and infections and can help with acne, eczema and cracked skin.

Manuka honey is one of the few honeys that has been tested for its antibacterial properties. Unique Manuka Factor (UMF) is the term used by manufacturers to determine whether a manuka honey product has enough of the antibacterial component. A rating of 10 or more indicates that the honey can be used medicinally.

Brand to try: UMF 16+ Active Manuka Honey, $35.95 (866-289-9233, *www.honeybee*

therapy.com*). To use, clean the area. Then apply a dab of honey and cover with a bandage.

Got Goat, Sheep or Buffalo Milk?

Andrew L. Rubman, ND, founder and director, Southbury Clinic for Traditional Medicines, Southbury, Connecticut. *www.southburyclinic.com*

He made his first diagnosis at age seven. *Daily Health News* contributing editor Andrew L. Rubman, ND, told his parents, "No more milk." Sure enough, that spelled the end of his trouble with fatigue, runny nose and other allergy symptoms, not to mention the beginning of a lifelong habit of challenging accepted health-care wisdom.

Dr. Rubman is still not a milk drinker, but he agreed to share his thoughts about the slew of "new" milks on the shelves of health-food stores and even mainstream supermarkets. For a variety of reasons, milk from other animals—including goats and sheep—might be more beneficial to your health than cow's milk. And, believe it or not, the FDA recently removed the legal barriers that have thus far prevented milk from camels, llamas, reindeer, moose and donkeys from being sold in the US—though I'd be very surprised if those show up in many retail stores anytime soon, since distributors must prove that those milks are processed according to the same standards that are required for cow's milk.

WHY DRINK MILK?

Most of us grew up hearing that we should drink lots and lots of milk—three glasses a day—to help us grow big and strong. The health claims are not without merit. Cow's milk, and indeed all mammalian milks, naturally contain a mixture of healthful compounds, including protein, fat, calcium and other minerals and vitamins. However, each species produces the specific blend of nutrients best-suited for its own offspring, Dr. Rubman explains—calves grow best with cow's milk, lambs with sheep milk and so on. It's therefore no surprise that for humans, milk from an animal—any animal—is more allergenic and difficult to digest than what nature intended, which is, of course, milk from our own mothers.

Practically everyone knows that some people have trouble digesting milk, but not so many people realize that there are actually two different reasons why that's so. Some people have sensitive or allergic reactions to one or more proteins found in one or more types of milk, while others cannot tolerate the sugar (called lactose) that is found in all mammalian milk. Why? With age, some people lose the natural ability to produce lactase, the digestive enzyme that breaks down lactose. Symptoms of both problems are the same—intestinal gas, diarrhea, runny nose, nasal congestion, asthma, wheezing, vomiting and skin rash.

COW'S MILK—THE WORST!

Economics are a key reason why cow's milk became so popular—cows produce more milk than goats and other mammals, and at a lower cost.

However, with high levels of alpha-S1 casein protein (a major allergen), lactose and large fat globules, cow's milk happens to pose the greatest challenge of all milks to humans. Dr. Rubman said that some who can't tolerate cow's milk do fine with milk from another animal, however.

NEXT BEST: GOAT'S MILK

You may be surprised to hear that worldwide, more people drink goat's milk than cow's milk, and lately I've noticed cartons of it in the dairy section of my local supermarket. Easier for many people to digest, goat's milk contains a bit less lactose and higher amounts of protein and fat and in forms that are more digestible than cow's milk.

Milk from goats contains more of other nutrients than cow's milk as well. For example, it has 13% more calcium and greater amounts of healthful short- and medium-chain fatty acids. Proponents prefer its tangy flavor and like that it is usually produced on small farms, free of antibiotics and growth hormone. (To verify, look at the label for certification that the production method is antibiotic and/or growth-hormone free.) Expect to pay more for

milk from goats—one popular brand, Meyenberg (*www.meyenberg.com*), is double the price of cow's milk... but enthusiasts say they don't mind, since they like the taste and the increased nutrition. People who like and easily tolerate goat milk will likely also find that goat cheeses, yogurts and ice creams go down easily.

SHEEP AND BUFFALO MILK: UP NEXT?

If you can find them in your health-food store, sheep and buffalo milks are a tasty—but considerably more expensive—alternative. Both resemble cow's milk in taste but have a thicker, creamier texture. Like goat's milk, milk from ewes has more short- and medium-chain fatty acids than cow's milk and smaller fat globules, which makes it healthier and easier to digest for humans. It also packs more calcium, phosphorus, potassium, magnesium and vitamins A, B (especially B-6 and B-12) and E. Buffalo milk has more calcium than milk from cows, goats or sheep... contains more butterfat and protein than cow's milk...and is a rich source of phosphorus, vitamin A and iron.

On the other hand, both sheep and buffalo milk have more lactose than cow's milk, so avoid these (and other products made from them) if you are lactose-intolerant. Common sheep milk products include yogurt, ice cream and cheeses (Feta from Greece, Roquefort from France, Pecorino Romano from Italy, Manchego from Spain, etc.). As for the buffalo, in addition to the milk you can find yogurt, ice cream and cheeses including, of course, the gourmet buffalo mozzarella.

CAMEL MILK

While camel milk is popular in the Middle East and Africa, the FDA still hasn't approved its sale in the US—but camel milk enthusiasts, especially one in particular, are working on that. Holistic health practitioner Millie Hinkle, who "fell in love with camel milk" on a trip to the United Arab Emirates, has made it her mission to market it here in the US.

If camel milk marketers can get over the FDA approval hump, they face a few other challenges—one is its somewhat salty taste, and the other is that camels are pretty uncooperative about being milked. The milk can boast some major nutritional advantages over cow's milk, however—it has less lactose (as much as half)...three times as much vitamin C...and slightly higher levels of iron, unsaturated fatty acids and B vitamins. Camel milk afficionados also insist that their beverage of choice is an aphrodisiac—and you can bet that claim will make it into their marketing materials! You can find out more about camel milk at *www.camelmilkusa.com.*

Super-Green "Shot"

Mark A. Stengler, NMD, licensed naturopathic medical doctor in private practice, Stengler Center for Integrative Medicine, Encinitas, California...adjunct associate clinical professor at the National College of Natural Medicine, Portland, Oregon...author of many books and of the *Bottom Line/Natural Healing* newsletter. *www.drstengler.com*

I have many patients who say that they benefit from regularly consuming wheatgrass, a food prepared from young wheat plants. Wheatgrass is gluten-free because gluten does not form in the young plant, and it is one of several "super greens" that is a great detoxifier. Consuming wheatgrass makes people feel more energetic...have better immunity...and have healthier-looking skin. It is available at health-food stores in capsule and powder form. You also can buy it as a juice—or juice it yourself. A nutritional powerhouse, wheatgrass is rich in the plant pigment chlorophyll, which provides a healthful dose of antioxidants, as well as the vitamins A, C, E, K and B complex, iron, calcium, magnesium, selenium and amino acids. It really does smell and taste like grass, so I like to combine it with carrot juice rather than as a straight "shot," which many people do. One study found that it was helpful for reducing the symptoms of ulcerative colitis. Since wheatgrass contains vitamin K, patients taking prescription blood thinners, such as Coumadin, should use it with caution and while supervised by a doctor.

Tune Up Your Heart—With the Right Music

Alice H. Cash, PhD, LCSW, clinical musicologist and social worker in Louisville, Kentucky. *www.healingmusicenterprises.com*

"Music hath charms to soothe a savage breast, to soften rocks, or bend a knotted oak," wrote William Congreve, seventeenth-century English poet and playwright.

"Music induces a continuous, dynamic change in the cardiovascular system," concluded Luciano Bernardi, MD, twenty-first-century Italian scientist.

It's taken a couple of centuries, but the scientists have finally caught up to the poets—they've proved that music can soothe a breast, chest and the heart inside it, providing a buffer against high blood pressure, heart disease and stroke.

LOUDER MUSIC, FASTER HEARTBEAT

Researchers in Italy conducted a study in which they found that music with a fast tempo sped up heart rate, boosted blood pressure and triggered more rapid breathing—and that music with a slow tempo had the opposite effect.

In their most recent study, the same researchers played several tracks of classical music (from Puccini, Bach, Verdi and Beethoven) to 24 people, while monitoring the electrical activity of their hearts. This time, they wanted to see how the heart responds to crescendos and decrescendos—gradual increases and decreases in the volume of music.

Result: Like fast music, the crescendos increased heart rate...narrowed blood vessels...increased blood pressure...and increased the respiration rate. And the louder the crescendo, the greater the changes. In the decrescendo, all of those parameters returned to normal.

But Dr. Bernardi isn't the only scientist studying music's effect on the heart.

Standout scientific evidence: Researchers at the Art and Quality of Life Research Center at Temple University, Philadelphia, recently analyzed 23 studies that looked at how music affects stress and anxiety level in people with heart disease. "Music listening can have a beneficial effect on blood pressure, heart rate, respiratory rate, anxiety and pain in persons with coronary heart disease," the researchers concluded.

ENTRAINING YOUR HEART TO HEALTH

"Music can calm the heart because of the principle of entrainment—just as nearby metronomes equalize to the same beat, so the rhythms of the body, such as heartbeat and breathing, quickly synchronize or 'entrain' with the tempo and mood of a piece of music," says Alice H. Cash, PhD, LCSW, a clinical musicologist and social worker in Louisville, Kentucky.

"Music alone isn't going to prevent or reverse heart disease," she adds. "But it can be one of many tools for protecting and improving the health of the heart." Her recommendations…

• **Change your "musical diet" from stressful to restful.** "If you're trying to prevent or control heart disease, you're probably focusing on changing your diet," says Dr. Cash. "Well, you can also focus on changing your 'musical diet,' as a way of calming down, and reducing the stress that can cause or complicate heart problems.

"Become aware of the music that calms you, relaxes you and makes you smile—whether it's classical, country or another style—and listen to more of that."

• **Use music to help you exercise.** Regular exercise is crucial to the health of your heart—and music can make regular exercise a lot more enjoyable, says Dr. Cash. "I always listen to music when I exercise. I particularly like athletics-inspired music, such as 'Chariots of Fire' from Vangelis, or the theme from *Rocky*."

Newest research: German researchers divided 20 people into two groups—one group exercised on a treadmill while listening to music through headphones, and one did the same exercise without music. Those listening to the music had less of a sense of unpleasantness during exercise and exercised harder.

• **Listen to calming music before, during, and after angioplasty or heart surgery.** People who are undergoing a stressful heart procedure such as angiography or heart surgery should listen through headphones to relaxing music with a slow, steady, heart-calming tempo of sixty beats per minute, such as music by the baroque composers Bach, Handel and Pachelbel, says Dr. Cash.

"Studies show that you will probably need less anxiety medication before the surgery, less anesthesia during surgery, less pain medication after the surgery and that you'll recover faster."

Important: Research shows that at some level of awareness you do hear sound during surgery, even though you're supposedly "unconscious," says Dr. Cash.

That's why it's necessary to listen to music before, during and after surgery.

Resource: The "Surgical Serenity System"—a pair of self-contained, wireless headphones that are preloaded with calming "surgical music." You can also program the headphones with music of your own choosing.

It's available at *www.surgicalheadphones. com*, or 502-419-1698.

Newest research: Swedish researchers studied forty people the day after open-heart surgery—half listened to soft, relaxing music through an MP3 player, and half didn't.

The music group had higher levels of oxytocin (a hormone linked to feelings of relaxation and peace), and said they felt more relaxed.

"Music intervention should be offered…to patients who have undergone cardiovascular surgery," they conclude.

In another Swedish study, patients who listened to music before surgery had a greater decrease in anxiety than those who took anti-anxiety medication.

The Rise of Vitamin "T"— The Amazing Healing Properties of Tocotrienols

Mark A. Stengler, NMD, licensed naturopathic medical doctor in private practice, Stengler Center for Integrative Medicine, Encinitas, California…adjunct associate clinical professor at the National College of Natural Medicine, Portland, Oregon…author of many books, including *The Natural Physician's Healing Therapies* and coauthor of *Prescription for Natural Cures* (both from Bottom Line Books)…and author of the *Bottom Line/Natural Healing* newsletter. *www.drstengler.com*

Ten years ago, food scientist Barrie Tan, PhD, was on a trip to South America investigating plant pigments when he stumbled across a colorful, lipstick-red plant—and couldn't take his eyes off it. Dr. Tan knew that the annatto plant (*Bixa orellana*) was phototropic, meaning that it moved and turned its blossoms toward the sun. Usually plants with blossoms this color don't follow the sun—if they did, they would be harmed by overexposure to UV rays. What was in this plant that protected it?

Dr. Tan discovered, to his surprise, that the plant's protector was tocotrienols, one of two main groups of compounds that constitute vitamin E. It was the first time a plant had been found to be a source of pure tocotrienols—and the discovery called into question everything that was previously known about vitamin E, the vitamin we have been taking for years. Dr. Tan found that the tocotrienols in the annatto plant (the purest form ever found) consisted of 90% delta-tocotrienol and 10% gamma-tocotrienol. And they helped to prevent cardiovascular disease, cancer and certain eye diseases.

Tocopherols, the other main compound that constitutes vitamin E, do not provide these same benefits.

Even today, most vitamin E supplements are made mainly of tocopherols. Alpha-tocopherol is most often used, and most vitamin E research has focused on this subtype. (Tocotrienol and tocopherol include subtypes called alpha, beta, delta and gamma.) Alpha-tocopherol is the most common form of vitamin E in the body and the only form found in blood plasma.

THE TAIL TELLS THE STORY

Both types of vitamin E neutralize disease-causing free radicals, but the key functional difference between tocopherols and tocotrienols lies in their "tails." Tocopherol molecules have longer, stiffer tails that anchor them in place in the body's cell membranes, while tocotrienol molecules have shorter, more flexible tails that enable them to move around the cell to more effectively neutralize free radicals. It is estimated that tocotrienols are 50 times more potent than tocopherols.

HOW TO BENEFIT

How tocotrienols can help you…

• **Cardiovascular disease protection.** *Tocotrienols seem to protect cardiovascular health by…*

• Lowering LDL cholesterol and triglycerides. Tocotrienols inhibit the same LDL (bad) cholesterol–producing enzyme that is targeted by statin drugs but without statins' side effects, such as fatigue and muscle pain. In one study, people with high cholesterol took 25 milligrams (mg), 50 mg, 100 mg or 200 mg daily of tocotrienols in combination with a heart-healthy diet. The researchers found that 100 mg daily provided optimal benefit, since it lowered LDL cholesterol levels by 25% and triglycerides (blood fats) by 12%. It also raised HDL (good) cholesterol slightly in some studies. More than 100 mg provided no additional benefit.

• Preventing atherosclerosis. This effect stems from the inhibitory effect of tocotrienols on molecules that help plaque adhere to artery walls. In a landmark study at Elmhurst Medical Center in Queens, New York, 50 people with atherosclerosis of the carotid arteries, a major risk factor for stroke, were given 240 mg daily of tocotrienols (along with 60 mg of alpha-tocopherols).

Result: Eighty-eight percent showed either stabilization or regression of arterial plaque, while only 8% in the placebo group had stabilized or improved amounts of plaque. About 60% in the placebo group had plaque buildup during the study. (Alpha-tocopherals on their own do not reduce atherosclerosis.) Tocotrienols also have been found to reduce the formation of blood clots that can lead to heart attack and stroke.

• **Anticancer activity.** Tocotrienols appear to fight cancer in several ways. They neutralize vascular endothelial growth factor (VEGF), the chemical that stimulates development of new blood vessels needed for tumor growth—an effect known as anti-angiogenesis. Tocotrienols also interfere with the processes that tumor cells use to multiply. Clinical trials are currently under way to study the safety of delta-tocotrienol for treating breast and pancreatic cancers. Because preliminary studies are promising and there is no toxicity related to tocotrienols, it seems that cancer patients may benefit when taking 300 mg daily of tocotrienols.

• **Eye health.** Tocotrienols' anti-VEGF effects appear to inhibit the sight-damaging growth of blood vessels associated with macular degeneration and diabetes-related retinopathy (damage to the retina).

Dose: 50 mg to 100 mg daily.

For these conditions, a concentrated form of vitamin E is best—namely, a supplement made of "pure" annatto-derived tocotrienols consisting of 90% delta- and 10% gamma-tocotrienols.

Brands to try: A.C. Grace Unique E Tocotrienols, 125 mg (800-833-4368, *www.acgrace. com*)...Doctor's Best Tocotrienols, 50 mg (800-333-6977, *www.drbvitamins.com*, for a store locator)...and Nutricology Delta-Fraction Tocotrienols, 50 mg and 125 mg (800-545-9960, *www.nutricology.com*).

IF YOU ARE HEALTHY

Tocotrienols are found in small amounts in foods such as coconut and wheat germ—but not enough to provide the benefit of supplements. People who are healthy (and don't have one of the conditions described above) are helped by taking a multivitamin or a full-spectrum vitamin E product that contains a blend of tocopherols and tocotrienols (5 mg is a good amount), which is still the best choice for disease prevention.

If you are healthy but have elevated cholesterol, try taking 50 mg to 100 mg of tocotrienols daily in addition to your multivitamin.

Caution: Tocotrienols inhibit blood clotting, so people on blood-thinners should consult their doctors before taking them.

5

Remedies for a Healthy Family

How to Tell a Child He Has a Psychiatric or Learning Disorder

Approximately 15 million American children and teens suffer from a psychiatric disorder, such as autism, Asperger's syndrome, Tourette's syndrome, attention-deficit/ hyperactivity disorder (ADHD), anxiety disorder or depression. An even greater number suffer from a learning disorder, such as dyslexia. Parents of these children often struggle to decide when and how to tell their kids about their conditions. *Here's how to do it right...*

DISCUSS IT

It is important to share this information with the child. While parents sometimes imagine that keeping such problems from children spares them from feeling different, it usually does no such thing. Once children with psychiatric or learning disorders start school, they

generally figure out very quickly that they are different from their classmates. Often they are picked on by or socially isolated from their peers, too.

Not discussing the disorder with the child will not spare him/her from experiencing fear about it, either. Children are very good at sensing when their parents are worried, and they know that trips to see doctors usually mean that something is wrong. When parents won't explain what's happening, these children often assume the worst—and with their parents not discussing it, they must face these fears alone, adding to their confusion and sense of isolation.

Besides, when parents fail to discuss these disorders, children sometimes learn that they

---

Harold S. Koplewicz, MD, a child and adolescent psychiatrist who is founding president of the Child Mind Institute in New York City and editor in chief of *Journal of Child and Adolescent Psychopharmacology*. He previously served as director of the Nathan S. Kline Institute for Psychiatric Research and as founder and director of the NYU Child Study Center. His books include *It's Nobody's Fault: New Hope and Help for Difficult Children and Their Parents* (Three Rivers). *www.childmind.org*

have them anyway, by overhearing conversations. Without a proper explanation, these children cannot understand what it means to have the condition—except that if everyone is hiding it from them, it must be very bad.

It often comes as a tremendous relief to the child to learn that there is a reason why he is the way he is and that there are others like him—but only if the parent gets this crucial conversation right.

THE RIGHT TIME

Children younger than eight generally cannot grasp abstract concepts such as psychiatric or learning disorders, but those as young as age four or five often can understand the behaviors that their disorders cause.

Example: A child of five with ADHD will be confused by the words "attention-deficit/hyperactivity disorder," but he likely can understand that he has more trouble sitting still in school than his classmates.

If the child has started school and is having trouble making friends…is getting picked on by other kids…or seems to sense that he is different, that's a good time to have a conversation about the behaviors caused by the disorder. If these issues do not arise, plan to have this conversation around age eight, when the child is better able to understand abstract concepts.

THE RIGHT WORDS AND TONE

To increase the odds that this conversation makes the child feel reassured, not frightened…

•**Maintain a calm, positive tone and expression.** Young children pick up on their parents' moods even more than they hear their words. If your mood is sad or negative, the child will assume his condition is very bad no matter what you say. If you cannot discuss the child's disorder without breaking down or choking up, postpone the conversation until you can or let your partner handle it.

•**Describe the most obvious or problematic behavior(s) caused by the disorder,** then tell the child that the reason he does this or feels this way is because he has a particular condition. If there are any positive elements to the condition, immediately mention these as well. If not, just say that the child has strengths and weaknesses like everyone else, and this is just an area that's a challenge for him.

Example: "You know how you have trouble having conversations with other kids? That's because you have what's called Asperger's syndrome. But you know how you have an incredible memory and you are really, really interested in trains? That's part of Asperger's, too."

•**Clarify that differences are not flaws and that challenges aren't disasters.** Explain that everyone is different from everyone else, and this is just one of those differences. True, this difference might cause some challenges, but everyone faces challenges.

Add that the child still is the same person that he always has been…this isn't anything horrible…and you and your partner are always there to help.

Example: "You're still John, the same boy you always have been. Everyone has obstacles that he has to overcome. This just happens to be yours. We'll all work together to make sure it's no big deal."

Explain that there are millions of people who have the same condition. Encouraging the child to feel like part of a large group can reduce the sense of isolation and loneliness that he may feel.

Before this conversation, investigate whether there are any celebrities that the child knows of who share the condition. If so, cite them. A Google search using the name of the disorder and a term such as "famous" or "celebrities" should help you locate examples.

•**Provide hope.** Say that you understand that this condition sometimes makes certain things difficult or embarrassing for the child, but that you're going to take him to see a doctor who can help the child with his problems. If there is any medicine that helps control the condition, say this, too.

•**Return to this topic later.** This should be an ongoing dialog, not a onetime talk. Your child will have questions and misunderstandings about the condition as he mulls over what you've said now and as he grows older. Check in with the child regularly on this topic, and make sure that you have uninterrupted quality time together so that the child can ask questions or raise concerns.

Among the questions kids often ask during or after this initial conversation...

• **Will it last forever?** Be honest if the condition will never go away—but add that we can help to make it better and that the symptoms can be treated so that it no longer is such a problem for the child.

• **Does anyone else I know have this?** If the answer is "No" or "Not that I know of," say so, but add that millions of other people do have the condition and are coping well with it.

• **Why did I get this?** Am I being punished? Reassure the child that it is not his fault. Tell him that nothing he did was the cause—it's just the way he was born.

Dial "MOM"!

Young girls in a high-stress situation had the same reduction in stress hormones when they talked to their mothers on the phone as when they received an in-person hug.

University of Wisconsin-Madison.

Anxiety Through Generations

Golda Ginsburg, PhD, child psychologist, Johns Hopkins Children's Center, Baltimore, and leader of a study of 40 children, published in *Journal of Consulting and Clinical Psychology.*

Children of adults with anxiety disorders are more likely to develop anxiety themselves. Anxiety affects up to one-fifth of children in the US but often is not recognized—and delays in diagnosis and treatment can lead to depression and substance abuse. A recent study suggests weekly family sessions of cognitive behavioral therapy may prevent children from developing the same problems with anxiety that their

parents struggle with. Parents should seek help if they notice early signs of anxiety in children, such as physicial complaints with no medical cause, avoidance of daily activities and too much worry.

Resources to find cognitive behavioral therapists: Anxiety Disorders Association of America (*www.adaa.org*)...Association for Behavioral and Cognitive Therapies (*www.abct. org*)...Academy of Cognitive Therapy (*www. academyofct.org*).

Kids Are Getting Their Drugs from YOU

Robert Stutman, 25-year veteran of the Drug Enforcement Administration (DEA). He served as special agent in charge of several DEA field divisions, including the New York field division, the nation's largest. In 1990, Stutman founded The Stutman Group, a consulting company that designs and implements substance-abuse prevention programs, Boca Raton, Florida. He is special consultant on substance abuse for CBS News and speaks to more than 100 groups a year. *www.thestutmangroup.com*

America's drug problem is staggering. Illegal drug use has climbed to 20 million Americans.

Even more shocking: Many addicts began abusing drugs or alcohol as kids under the watchful eye of well-intentioned parents.

Parents fail to take steps that might steer their kids away from addiction because they don't understand how much drug use has changed since they were young. Today there are different drugs, different dangers and a different demographic of young people at risk. *Here's what parents need to know now...*

• **Drug abuse begins early.** A generation ago, the average age of first drug use among eventual users was 15. Today that average starting age is alarmingly low—12 or 13. This is a huge problem because the younger people are when they first try drugs, the greater the odds that they will become addicted.

Important: Start talking with your kids about the dangers of drugs before they set foot in junior high school. By high school, it may be too late.

The drugs teens abuse today are not the ones your generation used. Today young people are much more likely to abuse prescription medications than marijuana or LSD. In fact, one in five high school students have taken a prescription drug that they didn't get from a doctor. Teens almost always get their pharmaceutical drugs from their parents' medicine cabinets or the cabinets of friends' parents.

Dozens of different pharmaceuticals can be abused. As a rule of thumb, if there's a sticker on a pill bottle warning against driving after use, it's likely that teens take the drug to get high. Even over-the-counter medications such as cough suppressants are abused.

If anyone in your house is prescribed a medication that has a warning sticker about driving after use, buy a lockbox or a safe and lock up these pills. Do this even if you trust your kids completely—you don't want your kids' friends or your babysitter to be tempted.

●**Abusing prescription drugs often is riskier than abusing illegal drugs.** Many teens—and even parents—incorrectly assume that anything prescribed by a doctor can't be all that dangerous. In truth, many prescription medications are extremely dangerous when not used as intended.

Example: OxyContin is a time-release pill designed to suppress pain over six to eight hours. Drug abusers crush these pills into powder so that the full dose is absorbed all at once.

Fact: Either this year or next, fatalities from misuse of prescription medications are likely to surpass auto accidents as the single leading cause of accidental death in the US.

Drug abuse is not just a problem for cities, minorities, the poor and kids who underachieve in school. Rural and suburban kids are just as likely as city kids to abuse drugs or alcohol—perhaps even slightly more likely.

White kids are as likely as African-American kids to do so. Private school kids are as likely as public school kids. Teens on sports teams are just as likely to use drugs as any other teen. Kids who do well in school are somewhat less likely to abuse drugs and alcohol than those

who do poorly, but good grades are not the ironclad evidence of nonuse that many parents imagine them to be. Even smart kids can be drug users, and some of them are smart enough to maintain their grades after they start using.

●**Those who start drinking as teens are almost twice as likely to become alcoholics.** Alcohol is the most socially acceptable drug in our culture, but that doesn't mean it's not dangerous. Consuming one or two alcoholic drinks is not a problem for most adults, but when teens drink, they almost never stop at just one or two—they drink until they are intoxicated.

The teenage brain is especially prone to addiction, including alcohol addiction, because it is still developing. Those who start drinking as teens or preteens are approximately twice as likely to become alcoholics as those who wait until their 20s.

Do not drink to get drunk in front of your child—even if your child is still too young to fully understand what drinking means. As early as age two, children begin forming lifelong beliefs and behaviors based on what they see their parents doing.

Certainly never allow your teens to get drunk in your presence. Some parents permit their teens to drink at home because they think this is safer than the teens drinking elsewhere and then driving home. I am somewhat sympathetic to this thinking, though studies suggest that teens who drink with their parents are slightly more likely to become alcoholics than those who do not. I am not sympathetic when parents allow kids to drink to the point of drunkenness at home. That only increases the odds of future drinking problems.

WHAT EVERY PARENT MUST DO

Many parents believe that nothing they do or say about drugs gets through to their teens. While it's true that parents cannot control their teens completely, all kids learn important life lessons from their parents—even when neither parent nor child realizes that learning is taking place.

●**Have dinner as a family as often as possible.** Families that eat together are much less likely to have kids who become addicts. Children who have dinner with their parents

71

at least three times a week are less likely to develop drug or alcohol problems.

•**Tell your children regularly and emphatically that you want them to stay away from drugs,** including alcohol and prescription medications. Your teens might roll their eyes, but at some level, your words are likely to have an effect—studies show that kids who know their parents care whether they use drugs are less likely to use them.

Helpful: For information about talking with children about drugs, read *How to Raise a Drug-Free Kid* by Joseph Califano, Jr. (Fireside)...and explore the links section on my Web site (*www.thestutmangroup.com*, then click "Links").

•**Confront your teen if you smell cigarette smoke on his/her clothes or discover other evidence of tobacco use.** Teens who use tobacco are at greater risk than nontobacco users of becoming drug addicts. If you smoke, quit.

•**Inform your teens that if one of their peers ever passes out from drinking or drug abuse in their presence,** they should immediately roll this person onto his/her side (to prevent suffocation if the person vomits), then call 911. Thousands of lives would be saved if every teen knew this.

Honesty Is the Best Policy On Drug Use

How do you warn kids about drugs if you used them yourself? Be honest, and tailor your message to your child, who may want lots of information or only a little. Say immediately that you do not want him/her using drugs, and explain why. Explain your own drug use directly—for instance, you might say that you tried them because other kids did...or that you made a mistake and ended up doing things you are not proud of. Listen as much as you talk—ask what your child thinks and what his friends think.

Recommendations from the Partnership at Drugfree. org. *www.drugfree.org*

What to Say If Your Child Is Gay

Robert A. Bernstein, JD, former attorney for the US Justice Department and former national vice president of Parents, Families and Friends of Lesbians and Gays (PFLAG), a national nonprofit organization. He lives in Bethesda, Maryland, and is the father of a gay daughter and author of *Straight Parents, Gay Children* (Thunder's Mouth), which won the Gustavus Myers Center for the Study of Human Rights in America's Best Scholarship on the Subject of Intolerance Award.

Coming out to a parent is a pivotal moment in the lives of many homosexuals, so the parent's first response will not be soon forgotten. Trouble is, a less-than-ideal initial reaction could cause lasting damage to the parent-child relationship.

A poor reaction from a parent even could make a young person who already feels socially isolated because of sexual orientation believe that he/she is completely alone, increasing the odds of depression or suicide.

My younger daughter came out to me the summer between her sophomore and junior years of college. Since then, I have talked with hundreds of parents and young people about what to do if your child tells you he is gay or if you suspect that's the case...

THE COMING-OUT CONVERSATION

Whatever your initial feelings when your child says that he is gay, your best response is one of love and acceptance.

Example: "You're our child. We love you no matter what."

Acceptance is what your child needs from you right now, and as a parent, your primary responsibility is to give your child what he needs.

It can help to add, "Thanks for telling me/us." Your child has taken an obviously difficult step that allows you to know him better. Your acknowledgment of this increases the odds that the child will keep you in the loop on future developments in his life.

One way to further emphasize your desire to be supportive is to suggest that you attend a meeting together of Parents, Families and Friends of Lesbians and Gays (PFLAG). PFLAG is a nonprofit organization with more than 350 chapters located in all 50 states (202-467-8180, *www.pflag.org*). Attending meetings could help you and your child answer any questions that you might have about homosexuality. And suggesting this sends a message of acceptance and family unity to your child.

Also, ask your child whether you should share the news with friends, and if so, how he wants the news shared. Just because your child came out to you does not necessarily mean that he is ready for everyone to know.

"ARE YOU SURE?"

Parents sometimes are taken completely by surprise when their children decide to come out. *Some reasons for this include...*

• **This child's general behavior or prior relationships might have led the parents to think that the child was heterosexual.** While some homosexuals exhibit interests or mannerisms that lead their families to suspect that they might be gay, others do not. It's relatively common for those who later come out to first date and sometimes even wed members of the opposite sex, either because they are not yet fully aware of or willing to confront their true sexuality or because they wish to hide it from others.

• **Some relatively young children come out before their parents even realize they're thinking about sex.** Young people know more about sex and relationships and mature faster these days than they did in past generations, and some might come out at age 11 or 12 or even earlier. (Others come out as teens or college students, and still others not until well into adulthood.)

• **Surprised parents might be tempted to respond to their child's coming out with words of doubt,** such as, "Are you sure?"..."How do you know?"..."But you've always dated girls" (or boys, as the case may be). Some parents even will say, "It must be just a phase." However, if your child has reached the point of coming out to his/her parents, there probably is no doubt.

If you do blurt out words of doubt, as soon as possible explain that this was just shock talking—and immediately express your love and acceptance of your child.

IF YOU SUSPECT
BUT HAVEN'T BEEN TOLD

While some parents are taken by surprise by the news that a child is gay, others have suspected as much for years. These parents might be tempted to broach the subject if only to assure the child that he will be loved regardless of his sexual orientation. But it's better to wait for the child to come to you with this information. Even if you are correct, the child might not yet be ready to face his sexual orientation, much less share it with others.

But there is something constructive you can do. Voice words of acceptance when homosexuality comes up, such as on TV or in the community. This will not necessarily cause your child to come out any sooner, but it could make coming to terms with homosexuality less stressful for the child and will strengthen your bond with him.

QUESTIONS PARENTS ASK

Among the questions and issues that often cross parents' minds when their kids come out...

• **What will we tell Grandpa?** (Or some other family member known for negative feelings about homosexuals.) Let your child decide when and whether to break the news to relatives who might not be accepting. If such a person is informed and responds poorly, make it clear that the rest of the family accepts this child and will not appreciate disparaging comments.

One father decided to send a family photo Christmas card, which included his daughter and her partner and their children. In an accompanying letter, the father explained that his daughter and her partner had been together for six years, and he wrote, "I love my daughter, and I admire her and have been enriched by her life experiences. I accept her without any reservation, and I want you to accept her and her family with the warmth that you have always extended to me. That's my Christmas wish."

• **What about AIDS?** Yes, AIDS still is an especially serious concern for male homosexuals—but it's also a serious concern for straight people. Whatever your child's sexual orientation, you should help him understand the threat of AIDS and how to stay safe.

•**Where did I go wrong?** Some parents feel guilt when they learn that their child is gay. They worry that being gay will make that child less happy in life, and they wonder whether their parenting style led to this sexual orientation. It did not. Research strongly suggests that homosexuality might have a significant genetic component and, in any event, is strongly influenced by biochemical events prior to birth. So parenting has nothing to do with it.

•**I accept that you're gay, but do you have to flaunt it?** This is a statement of nonacceptance. Truly accepting a child's homosexuality does not just mean accepting it in the abstract—it also means endeavoring to make this child feel like a fully accepted member of the family. If your gay child does not feel permitted to bring a same-sex partner to family gatherings—and to kiss or hug this partner just as openly as heterosexual family members do with their partners—then the family has not truly accepted his homosexuality.

•**Can he change?** In a word, no. Being gay is not a choice your child is making that can be reversed, nor is it a medical problem that can be "cured." Some religious groups do claim that it is possible to "cure" homosexuality, but there is no evidence to support this. If you suggest to your gay child that his sexual orientation can be changed, all you do is send a powerful message of disapproval.

Family Dinners Are Key

Family dinners encourage responsible behavior among teens. Recent finding: Teens who have dinner with their families at least five times a week are less likely to abuse alcohol and/or drugs than teens who have dinner with their families three or fewer times a week. Teens who are less involved with their families are twice as likely to use tobacco or marijuana...more than one-and-a-half times

more likely to use alcohol...and twice as likely to try drugs.

"The Importance of Family Dinners V," a report by The National Center on Addiction and Substance Abuse at Columbia University, New York City. www. casacolumbia.org

Kids Can Get Kidney Stones, Too

The painful stones typically occur in middle-aged adults, but they are being seen more often now in children.

Possible reasons: Drinking too little water ...consuming too much sodium...eating a lot of chocolate or nuts or drinking a lot of herbal or regular tea, all of which are high in oxalate, a substance that is commonly found in kidney stones.

Self-defense: Be sure your child has about eight eight-ounce glasses of liquids a day—as much as possible from water. Limit sodium in children's diets by cutting back on processed meats, frozen meals, fast food, packaged snack foods and convenience foods.

Alicia M. Neu, MD, clinical director of pediatric nephrology, Johns Hopkins Children's Center, Baltimore.

Caution With Hand Sanitizers

Keep hand sanitizer out of reach of small children. If swallowed, the alcohol content in hand sanitizers—usually about 65%, or 130 proof—is high enough to cause alcohol poisoning in children under age five.

Better: Encourage hand-washing with regular soap and water whenever possible. If you have a poisoning emergency, call the American Association of Poison Control Centers, 800-222-1222.

Alfred Aleguas, Jr., PharmD, clinical manager, Regional Center for Poison Control and Prevention, Children's Hospital Boston.

Lack of Sun Hurts Kids' Eyes

Studies in the US, Singapore and China have found a consistent link between the time spent outdoors and myopia (nearsightedness). Children who spent the most time outdoors—10 to 14 hours a week—were half as likely to have myopia as children who were outdoors only three to six hours a week. Avoiding the outdoors causes a lack of retinal dopamine, which can lead to myopia.

Kathryn Rose, PhD, associate professor, Faculty of Health Sciences, University of Sydney, Australia, and coauthor of a study of 4,132 children, published in *Ophthalmology*.

Dog Bite Prevention

Half of all children in the US are bitten by a dog before they reach age 12—and the most seriously injured kids are those under age seven.

Teach children to avoid dog bites by showing them proper behavior and explaining basic rules: Never approach a dog you do not know or one that is alone, without an owner nearby. Ask the owner's permission before petting a dog. Do not go near a dog that is sleeping, eating, nursing puppies or playing with a bone or toy. Do not tease a dog in any way—the dog may not realize that you are being playful.

American Humane Society recommendations, published in *Dog Fancy*.

A Better Test for Food Allergies

Kids diagnosed with food allergies may not have them at all. Blood and skin tests do not necessarily indicate a true allergic response. These tests measure the level of the antibody immunoglobulin E (IgE), which the body may make in response to a food. But having IgE antibodies does not necessarily mean that a person will develop allergic symptoms from eating the food.

More accurate: An oral food challenge test, in which doctors give a child tiny amounts of various foods to ingest and closely watch for signs of a reaction. But food challenge tests are time-consuming and expensive, so parents usually prefer the quicker and easier blood and skin tests.

Hugh Sampson, MD, professor of pediatrics, division of allergy and immunology, Mount Sinai School of Medicine, New York City.

Family Meals Help Kids with Asthma

Family mealtimes help asthmatic children by reducing their anxiety—so their lung function improves. Children with asthma often have separation anxiety—they worry about being away from their parents in case of a breathing emergency. Positive interaction at family meals reduces asthmatic children's worries and can help them breathe more easily.

Barbara H. Fiese, PhD, professor of human development and family studies, University of Illinois, Chicago, director of the university's Family Resiliency Center and leader of a study published in *Journal of Child Psychology and Psychiatry*.

Beach Sand Alert

Digging in beach sand can make kids sick. Children under age 11 who dig in beach sand have a 44% greater risk for diarrhea than those who do not dig in the sand.

Reason: Beach sand can contain dangerous bacteria, including E.coli and enterococcus from sewage outfalls, storm-water runoff and domestic and wild animals.

Chris Heaney, PhD, epidemiologist, researcher, University of North Carolina at Chapel Hill, and leader of a study of 27,365 people who had visited seven US beaches, published in *American Journal of Epidemiology*.

Keep Calm

Remain calm when dealing with an irritable child. Often, the child is upset when he/she feels as if the world is demanding more than he is capable of. His behavior is not directed at you personally. Don't attempt a quick fix. Authoritative directives, such as "Sit down and be quiet," don't teach the child any new coping skills. Empathize with the child—saying that you understand will help to soothe him. Encourage the child to communicate with you. Ask questions to understand what is bothering him. Teaching a child how to identify and express his feelings helps him learn to cope when he is upset.

Psychology Today, 115 E. 23 St., New York City 10010, *www.psychologytoday.com*.

Warning on Teen Drivers And Cell Phones

Half of teenagers talk on cell phones while driving...and one-third of teens of driving age send text messages while driving. This is despite mounting evidence showing the dangers of inattention and distraction when driving. Talk to your teen about the dangers.

Amanda Lenhart, senior research specialist, Pew Research Center's Internet & American Life Project, University of Michigan, Ann Arbor, and author of a study of 800 teens, published at *www.pewinternet.org*.

Parenting Your Parents

John Bertschler, PhD, a mediator, licensed psychologist and co-owner of Northcoast Conflict Solutions, a mediation practice based in Seven Hills, Ohio. He also trains mediators and is coauthor of *Elder Mediation: A New Solution to Age-Old Problems* (NCS). *www.ncsmediation.com*

Teenagers aren't the only ones who argue with their parents. Full-grown adults sometimes disagree with their aging parents. When these conflicts involve a parent's safety or financial security, the adult children often refuse to yield despite the parent's wishes.

These disagreements can grow so heated that it almost seems as if a referee needs to be called in to avoid ruining the relationship.

Here are ways to increase the odds of a peaceful resolution when grown children and their parents disagree...

Include close family members in the conversation with the parent, and meet with those family members beforehand. Family members who are close to this parent are more likely to oppose your position if they feel excluded from the decision-making process. Also, parents are more likely to respect an opinion shared by many family members than that of just one adult child.

Schedule the conversation for morning or early afternoon if the parent experiences "sundowning"—reduced mental clarity as evening approaches. People in the early stages of dementia often are mentally sharpest and best able to contribute to important conversations early in the day.

Have ready specific examples of why you believe something needs to be done. Examples can increase the odds that the parent and other relatives will agree that action is required.

Example: "It's not just my opinion that your driving skills have slipped. You've had three fender benders in the past year."

Raise an issue by saying it might be time to discuss the available options, not by saying it's time to take the specific action that you, personally, consider best. Pushing your opinion at the outset only increases the odds that the parent will dig in his/her heels.

Example: Say, "I think it's time we discussed what sort of help you might need in the future," rather than, "I think it's time we thought about moving you into a nursing home"—even if you think a nursing home is the best choice.

Once a parent agrees to take part in the discussion, it is more likely that he will listen when you provide evidence that the option you favor is worth a look.

If family discussions about elder issues become rancorous, find a mediator. The National Eldercare Mediator Network (*www.eldercare*

mediators.com) or the Association for Conflict Resolution (*www.acrnet.org*) can help you locate a professional mediator in your region who has experience dealing with elder issues. Mediators typically charge from $150 to $500 an hour, depending on the region and their experience. If this is cost prohibitive, perhaps the family can agree on a respected family member, family friend or religious counselor to serve as a mediator.

Among the issues involving elderly parents that often become sources of family strife...

HOW MUCH CARE

Conflict: Some family members believe an elderly parent needs more assistance from professional caregivers, possibly even a nursing home—but the parent disagrees.

Strategy: Cite the specific dangerous incidents that are causing your concern—falls or ovens being left on, for example. Keep the term "nursing home" out of the conversation—it carries too much negative baggage in many people's minds. Instead, explain that there are many other possible care options, ranging from having someone look in on the parent regularly...to an assisted-living facility. Say that your goal is to find the option that gets the parent the amount of assistance needed to live the life he wants.

If that fails—or if you are the elderly parent and you truly believe that your current living arrangements are appropriate—suggest that the family arrange a geriatric assessment. This provides an unbiased, informed evaluation of what level of assistance is appropriate for a senior. It is typically offered through hospitals and geriatric care centers. The parent's doctor might be able to recommend someone. If not, your state's Adult Protective Services department might be able to help you find one. (Put "Adult Protective Services" and your state's name into any search engine to find contact information for this government agency.)

SHOULD THE PARENT DRIVE?

Conflict: An aging parent's driving seems unsafe to one or more family members, but the parent won't surrender the car keys.

Strategy: Do not just ask a parent to give up the car keys—present a plan for how the parent will get around without a car. If you are the parent, explain that you might be willing to discuss giving up driving if such a plan could be arranged. Research the region's public transit, senior shuttles and taxi services. Or explore whether family members and friends who live in the region could provide rides when needed.

Example: A man agreed to sell his car when his son suggested that some of the money from this sale be put into an account with a local cab company.

If the parent still considers himself a safe driver, suggest that he retake the driving test through the state department of motor vehicles to settle the matter objectively...and/or suggest that he take driving lessons designed for aging adults given by organizations such as Keeping Us Safe (877-907-8841, *www.keeping ussafe.org*)...and AAA (202-638-5944, *www. seniordrivers.org*).

LIVING TOGETHER

Conflict: Family members may get under one another's skin when an elderly parent moves in with an adult child.

Strategy: Neither parent nor child should attempt to impose "house rules." Instead, say that everyone will have to work together to develop a system that keeps family members from annoying one another. Propose that the first month be treated as an adjustment period, and choose a date and time of month in the future for family members to discuss what policies need to be implemented.

Example: An older man often got up in the middle of the night for a snack, then left his son's kitchen a mess. During the follow-up meeting, he agreed to clean his dishes before returning to bed. He hadn't realized this was annoying because his late wife had never complained about it.

If the parent has diminished mental capacity and cannot help but do things that annoy the rest of the family, search for ways you could alter the living arrangements to minimize these annoyances. Perhaps the parent could move into a room in the basement so that his late-night noise is less disruptive. If no solution presents itself, the adult child must decide whether the behavior can be endured or whether it is so disruptive that the only solution is to find alternate living arrangements for the parent.

How to Stay Close to Your Kids

Scott Haltzman, MD, clinical assistant professor of psychiatry and human behavior at Alpert Medical School of Brown University, Providence. He is the medical director of Northern Rhode Island (NRI) Community Services in Woonsocket, Rhode Island, and author of *The Secrets of Happy Families: Eight Keys to Building a Lifetime of Connection and Contentment* (Jossey-Bass). *www.drscott.com*

In our mobile modern society, many adult children live hundreds or thousands of miles from their parents. Unfortunately, that geographical distance tends to be highly correlated with emotional distance from our kids and grandkids.

Even extended families whose members still live near one another face challenges, with ever-increasing demands on their time.

The good news: Parents can overcome these challenges and build strong relationships with their adult children no matter where they live. *Five ways to make that happen...*

SHOW RESPECT

Make your respect for your grown kids a recurring theme of the relationship. Adult children want one thing from their parents above all else—respect. The more you provide, the greater the odds that your children will want to remain close with you.

One way to show respect is to shower your grown kids with praise just as you did when they were young. Search for any excuse to offer a compliment. Make "I'm proud of you" and "You handled that very well" your mantras.

It also is important not to criticize your grown children when it seems as if they have failed. Criticism will only drive them away from you.

Helpful: If you catch yourself being critical, make at least five positive comments or actions before the end of your call or visit. Research has shown that a positive-to-negative interaction ratio of five-to-one or better can help maintain closeness in our relationships with our children (and our own spouses, too).

BUILD TRADITIONS

A family's traditions help to define it as well as preserve it. These traditions might include a distinctive way of celebrating a holiday or something as simple as gathering each year to watch an annual event on TV. Sure, your kids are busy with their own families and maybe there's been some bickering—but everyone still gathers at your house to watch the Super Bowl because it's a tradition.

It's never too late to create new family traditions. Whenever the extended family gets together and has a good time, single out something distinctive about the occasion—perhaps the place that the family gathered...the board game the family played...or the day of the year on which the gathering occurred. Suggest that the family try this again, perhaps the following year. If everyone has as much fun the second time, it could become a tradition.

Warning: Never make family traditions seem like requirements. If you hold it against your son that he spent Thanksgiving with his in-laws, the holiday could become a source of anxiety, driving your family apart, rather than a tradition that holds you together.

DON'T GIVE ADVICE

Resist the urge to give advice, even when it is requested. Receiving guidance from a parent can make adults feel like helpless children again. They tend to rebel against this unpleasant feeling by pulling away from the parent—even if they asked for advice.

If your adult child requests your advice, say, "I'm happy to help you sort through the pros and cons, but it's your decision to make, and I know you'll make the right choice."

One way to provide guidance to grown children is to ask them to teach you how they do something. Rather than criticize your adult children's decisions or methods, express an interest in these and ask if they could explain them to you. Listen attentively and without criticism, then casually mention that a different method was taught back when you were learning this task. Briefly describe your method and its advantages, then ask whether this strategy is still used. If your child doesn't wish to pursue the discussion any further, let it drop. This should dodge the psychological pitfalls of providing parental advice because the child gets to act as teacher first…and your guidance is presented as something that someone else taught you.

Example: When your son comes to you enthusiastically intending to buy junk bonds, you can ask about the company and its financial health, even look it up online with him. Then you can share how exciting it is to take a risk, as well as how you have learned not to invest any more than you can afford to lose.

Provide direct advice only if the adult child is about to make a massive and potentially irreversible misstep, such as driving an unsafe vehicle or buying an older home without a home inspection.

BEFRIEND YOUR CHILD'S SPOUSE

Search for ways to support and praise your sons- and daughters-in-law—even if you don't really care for them. It's your relationship with your children and grandchildren that will suffer the most if you don't get along with your kids' spouses. Your grown kids might decide it's easier to cut you out of their lives than to deal with the problems created when you and the spouse are together. And your child's spouse is likely to come up with excuses for the child's family not to visit you or invite you over.

Warning: The fact that your child criticizes his/her spouse to you does not mean that you are free to criticize that spouse, too. What you take as serious criticisms might just be your child venting normal marital frustrations. He actually might love and respect this partner very deeply. If so, your criticisms might damage your relationship with your child.

DON'T INTRUDE

Select noninvasive communication methods. Frequent phone calls or drop-in visits from parents can seem overbearing to adult children. *Better options…*

• **E-mail and social-networking Web sites.** Modern technology lets families keep in touch without interfering with one another's schedules. You can write as much as you like in an e-mail message or on a Facebook page—and your kids can read it whenever they like.

• **Care packages.** Young kids away at summer camp aren't the only ones who appreciate care packages. A batch of cookies that arrives unexpectedly in the mail can be a great way to remind your adult child of your love. My mother sent me clothes that she found on sale for a full decade after I married. My wife and I both appreciated it.

Warning: Do not follow up your packages with calls. These calls could make it seem like you are fishing for a thank-you or an invitation to visit. Gifts are most effective as relationship builders when there are no strings attached.

Also, be sure that gifts won't be misconstrued as subtle hints that your children or their spouses don't measure up. Books about dieting or a free session with a marriage counselor will be seen by your kids as signs of your disapproval, even though in your eyes, you're just trying to help.

Family Link to Alzheimer's Disease

According to a recent study, people whose mothers had Alzheimer's may be at greater risk for developing the disease than people whose fathers had it. For people with a maternal link to Alzheimer's, it may help to keep weight and blood pressure down, and stay mentally active.

Lisa Mosconi, PhD, research assistant professor of psychiatry, New York University School of Medicine, New York City, and leader of a study of 49 cognitively normal people, ages 50 to 80, published on-line in *Proceedings of the National Academy of Sciences of the United States of America.*

Happy Marriage May Lower Stroke Risk for Men

Researchers who tracked marriage and health data of 10,059 men for 34 years found that single or unhappily married men were 64% more likely to die from a stroke than happily married men.

Theory: Having a supportive life partner increases the likelihood that a man will seek regular medical attention, eat healthfully and take medications as required.

Uri Goldbourt, PhD, professor of epidemiology, Neufeld Cardiac Research Institute, Tel Aviv University, Israel.

Help for the Grieving

When 18 people received weekly, 25-minute foot and/or hand massages for eight weeks following the death of a loved one, researchers found that the massages helped diminish feelings of loneliness and provided physical comfort.

Journal of Clinical Nursing

One Big Happy Family— Secrets to Staying Close To Married Kids

Susan Forward, PhD, therapist in private practice in Westlake Village, California. She has served as therapist, instructor and consultant for many Southern California psychiatric and medical facilities. She is author of several best-selling books, including *Toxic In-Laws* (Harper). Her Web site is *www.susanforward.com.*

A wise person once said, "Parenting is the only love where the goal is separation."

When a child grows up and gets married, the transition can be difficult for parents. Well-meaning parents may not realize that some of their actions may be undermining the new marriage as well as their relationships with their children. *What to do…*

• **Focus on the positive.** It is normal to feel a sense of loss that you are no longer number one in your child's life. While acknowledging this feeling of loss, be willing to shift your attention to the benefits. To do so, ask yourself love-based questions rather than fear-based questions.

Fear-based questions focus on what you are giving up. They grow out of the assumption that there is not enough love to go around.

Examples: Will we still have family holidays together? Is my child's partner a threat to me? Will I never see my son?

Love-based questions focus on what you have to give and gain. They grow out of the assumption that love is unlimited.

Examples: What do my children and their new partners bring to my life? How does what I say or do affect them? How can I make the new person in the family feel welcome and at ease?

• **Don't give unsolicited advice.** Even your best-intentioned suggestions are likely to be perceived as criticism. Instead, ask the couple, "Would you like some help with this?" or "I have some ideas about this situation—would you like to hear them?" Respect the answer. If they do ask for advice, do not expect or pressure them to follow it.

Helpful: Whenever you catch yourself saying or thinking the word *should*, stop. You are likely to be imposing your values on the couple. Even if you are certain that you are right, your input will not be welcome and may create a chasm between you.

Better: Pause before you speak. Take a deep breath…count silently to three…and ask yourself, What are the potential effects of what I am about to say?

Keeping quiet can be especially difficult where grandchildren are concerned. You may worry or disapprove when your children make child-rearing choices that you disagree with. Unless a child's safety is at risk, it is better to keep your opinions to yourself.

• **Be willing to apologize.** An apology is one of the greatest gifts parents can give their children. When you apologize, you change the balance of power. The parent becomes less formidable, more accessible. Whether you said or did something thoughtless or innocently pushed someone's hot button, take responsibility for doing so. If you're not sure what you did wrong, use a calm, friendly tone and the phrase "Can you help me understand...?"

Example: "I am so sorry that I upset you. Can you help me understand what about it bothered you?"

•**Keep a healthy distance.** The line between inclusiveness and smothering can be hard to discern. Some families enjoy a great deal of contact, such as a tradition of having Sunday dinner together every week. Others are more hands-off.

No matter what your custom has been, do not assume that these traditions will continue unchanged. The young couple may want to create their own traditions.

Better: Invite, but don't pressure. Have an honest discussion about what the couple would prefer.

Example: "We would love to have you at our family dinners, but we want to respect your needs, too. How much extended-family time feels comfortable to you?" Do not be surprised if their needs continue to change over time.

And never drop by for a visit unannounced, even if you used to do so before your child got married.

•**Work on yourself, Develop interests apart from your child.** Take classes, join clubs and expand your circle of friends. Having a support system outside your immediate family keeps you from relying on your children to make you happy.

Despite all your best efforts, misunderstandings can arise because you or your child or your child's partner still has unresolved family conflicts that are triggered by others' behavior. Self-development is a lifelong process. Rather than assuming that you have everything under control, be willing to talk to a counselor or clergy person about issues that you could learn to handle better.

•**Don't get caught in the middle.** Never talk about your child's spouse behind his/her back. And if your child comes to you to complain about his/her spouse, avoid taking sides. The situation may only escalate, and you could be blamed.

Better: Say, "Honey, I support you and I'm here for you, but I'm not a professional and I'm not going to give you advice about what to do. If the two of you can't sort this out, I encourage you to talk it over with a counselor."

•**Keep expectations realistic.** While some sons- and daughters-in-law become beloved friends and confidants, many do not. You lack a shared history, and your preferences and tastes may be very different.

If you feel that there's a distance between yourself and your child's partner, make a point to share some of your own experiences. Encourage the partner to tell you more about himself. You may never be best buddies, but the more he finds out about your life and you about his, the closer you two are likely to be.

If you feel that your child's spouse is not nice to you, put it out on the table. Say, "I will always try to treat you with courtesy, and I really would appreciate the same."

Make Older Relatives Comfortable at Family Gatherings

There are several things you can do to make the oldest members of your extended family more comfortable at family get-togethers. First, offer to drive them to your home if they need assistance. Grandchildren who recently obtained their driver's licenses may be willing to help—which can lead to intergenerational bonding. Also, seat older people with physical challenges appropriately—for instance, place someone with hearing loss close to a person who can repeat parts of conversations to him/her. And, ask older adults about their life experiences so that they feel included in conversations. Consider bringing out old photograph albums for everyone to review and discuss together—another bonding experience.

Rheta Rosen, PhD, coordinator, Interpersonal Skills Teaching Centre, Ryerson University, Toronto.

Is Your Spouse Making You Sick?

Marjory Abrams, president, Boardroom Inc., *www.bot tomlinepublications.com*

I once saw an episode of the TV sitcom *Everybody Loves Raymond* in which Raymond's father was in the hospital. Every time Ray's mother walked into the hospital room, his father's blood pressure would skyrocket. When she walked out, his pressure quickly came down. It was hilarious to watch, but in real life, such marital tension is nothing to laugh at, says Yale Medical School professor emeritus Howard M. Spiro, MD. Dr. Spiro is author of *The Power of Hope: A Doctor's Perspective*, among other books, and has been happily married for 60 years.

Tension between spouses affects more than the heart. Dr. Spiro notes that marital stress might aggravate the situation of people predisposed to chronic fatigue syndrome, lupus, rheumatoid arthritis and other autoimmune disorders. Stress also decreases immunity to upper respiratory infections. It worsens irritable bowel syndrome, depression and many other ailments.

Women in strained marriages are at increased risk for metabolic syndrome, a cluster of symptoms—such as high blood pressure and low HDL (the "good" cholesterol)—that can lead to heart disease, stroke and diabetes.

Marital hostility even can affect the teeth. A Brazilian study linked low-quality marriages with a significant increase in dental cavities and periodontal disease.

All this makes marriage sound bad for your health—but research suggests that those in happy marriages live longest. If you are struggling in a strained marriage, I encourage you to seek counseling to get things back on a happy track or help you figure out if it's time to amicably part ways.

When Couples Don't Agree on Where to Retire

Dorian Mintzer, MSW, PhD, licensed social worker and psychologist and career/life transition and executive coach in Boston, and Roberta K. Taylor, RNCS, MEd, a licensed psychotherapist and career, life and relationship coach in Waltham, Massachusetts. They are coauthors of *The Couple's Retirement Puzzle: 10 Must-Have Conversations for Transitioning to the Second Half of Life* (Lincoln Street). *www.couplesretirementpuzzle.com*

For most of our adult lives, we live where our careers take us. When we retire, we finally have the freedom to live wherever we like—perhaps near a beach or near our grandkids—or so we imagine. Trouble is, our spouses might have other ideas.

Many couples don't discuss where they will live in retirement until it is almost upon them. Some assume that their partners share their visions...while others suspect their partners have different destinations in mind and put off these conversations to avoid arguments. Even couples who have discussed and decided where to retire might need to revisit this issue if changing financial circumstances, priorities and/or health status forces a reevaluation.

Example: A couple who enjoyed hiking bought land in the mountains and agreed to build their retirement home there. As retirement neared, however, the husband realized that his worsening arthritis made hiking less fun and his other health problems made proximity to a good hospital a priority.

In generations past, the relatively small number of retirement-destination options made these discussions fairly simple. Most retirees either stayed put or moved someplace warm, such as Florida or Arizona. Today's retirees see many more options. In addition to the Sun Belt and their current communities, retirees are heading to college towns, urban centers and even foreign countries. It's wonderful to have options, but more options mean that it's more likely that partners' retirement visions will differ.

Where to live during retirement should be an ongoing conversation throughout marriage. However, if retirement is near and this issue has not been settled, it's time to sit down for a serious discussion on the subject. Try to schedule the meeting in advance so that both partners have time to think it through.

SEEKING A COMPROMISE

When preferred retirement destinations differ, it can seem as though the only option is for one or the other partner to yield. That can result in heated arguments.

There is more room for compromise in retirement-destination decisions than couples tend to realize. The important thing is to put the "where should we retire" debate on hold for the moment and focus instead on "what factors are most important to each of us in a retirement destination." What is it about the place where you want to retire that makes you want to retire there? Both partners should list and rank their top priorities in a retirement location.

Common priorities include proximity to…

• **Kids and grandkids.**

• **Elderly parents.**

• **Friends.**

Warning: This is more important than many preretirees realize. If you move away from your friends in retirement, you might find that it's not so easy to make new friends and you end up relying totally on your spouse, which can stress even a strong relationship.

• **Specific cultural amenities,** such as theaters, concert halls and interesting restaurants.

• **Natural attractions and recreational facilities,** such as beaches, national parks, golf courses or fishing lakes.

• **Quality health-care facilities.**

• **A major airport.**

Other priorities could include…

• **Certain population density**—which might mean urban excitement, rural tranquillity or something in between.

• **A sense of community or proximity to a specific religious community.**

• **A specific climate.**

• **A sense of safety.**

• **Affordability.**

Some people can and want to "live high" in retirement. Others may want to spend very sparingly.

Couples should compare lists, then brainstorm about locations that combine each partner's top priorities.

Example: Perhaps one partner's top priority is tranquillity, while the other primarily wants culture. This couple might consider Oregon or the Carolinas. Greater Portland and Ashland, Oregon…Charleston, South Carolina, and the Raleigh-Durham area of North Carolina all combine a relaxed feel with lots of culture. Or move to a tranquil town that's near a train station, providing quick access to a vibrant city…or consider a relatively rural town near a large university (large universities offer a multitude of cultural options).

CREATIVE COMPROMISES

If a mutually satisfactory retirement destination does not suggest itself, consider these five potential solutions…

• **Sample possible retirement destinations rather than make a decision now.** Rent a home or condo for three months or longer in each candidate region before choosing. Extended visits will take some of the fear and mystery out of moving somewhere new, and they increase the odds of finding someplace that both of you love.

Warning: "We went there on vacation and I liked it/didn't like it" is not enough on which to base a decision. The experience of living in a place for months is very different from the experience of visiting as a tourist for a week or two.

• **Divide your retirement between two locations.** It's fairly common for retired couples to spend winter months in a warm-weather location and summer months up north, but that's not the only possible way to divide your retirement time. You could have a house in the country and a pied-à-terre in the city, for example.

Not everyone can afford to buy and maintain two homes, of course, but the costs come down considerably if you trade one big home for two smaller ones. Many retirees discover that they are just as happy in a smaller home now that the kids are grown and gone.

Warning: If you maintain two residences, consider making at least one a condo or rental.

Otherwise, you'll have to handle every home-maintenance chore twice over. That can be a burden, particularly as you get older.

•**If proximity to kids or grandkids is a major sticking point,** perhaps renting a home near the kids for a month or a season each year would provide sufficient family togetherness. Perhaps you could plan multigenerational trips with your kids and grandkids to keep the relationship close rather than live nearby. Or perhaps if you retired someplace that's interesting and near an airport, your kids would come visit you regularly even if you weren't nearby.

Warning: If your kids are a key factor in your retirement plans, include them in the retirement-destination discussion. You don't want to choose a retirement region close to your children only to discover that they might soon move. Also, note that grandkids often have less time for their grandparents as they grow up.

•**Form an "intentional community."** If proximity to a close circle of friends is important to you, staying in your current home might not be a perfect solution—those friends might retire somewhere else even if you don't. Discuss retirement destinations with these friends. Perhaps some or all of the group can agree to retire to the same region, bringing your own community with you.

•**Live apart part-time.** This might seem extreme, but some time apart actually can strengthen relationships strained by spending 24 hours a day together in retirement.

Example: A New England woman in her 70s rents a condo in Florida each winter. Her husband, who doesn't care for Florida, stays in New England but takes short trips down to visit.

How Being Too Supportive Can Harm Your Marriage

Being too supportive may harm a marriage. Giving too much support—usually as un-

wanted advice—is a bigger risk factor for marital unhappiness than not giving enough support.

Reason: Someone who does not get enough support from a spouse can get more from family and friends—but someone who is given too much support cannot escape it.

Erika Lawrence, PhD, associate professor, department of psychology, University of Iowa, Iowa City, and leader of a study of 103 husbands and wives, published in *Journal of Family Psychology.*

Touch Reduces Stress

Married couples who give each other back rubs or touch each other affectionately in other ways for at least 30 minutes three times a week have 34% lower levels of stress. Researchers found that being affectionate releases the hormone oxytocin, which may protect against stress-related illnesses.

Julianne Holt-Lunstad, PhD, assistant professor, department of psychology, Brigham Young University, Provo, Utah, and leader of a study published in *Psychosomatic Medicine.*

When Spouses Disagree About their Kids

Marjory Abrams, president, Boardroom Inc., *www.bottomlinepublications.com*

I have found—on both ends of the parent/child relationship—that disagreements between spouses about their children don't stop as children evolve into adults. Instead of conflict about limits on TV or junk food, parents may argue about the "child's" career choice or love relationships.

Such conflict is unavoidable, says Nancy Samalin, director of the New York City–based Parent Guidance Workshops (*www.samalin.com*). One spouse's style may be authoritarian, the other laissez-faire...one may be more controlling than the other.

Nancy advises parents to agree to disagree. Important strategies…

• **Discuss differences, but do it out of earshot of your kids.** You don't always have to present a united front, but by discussing issues prior to talking to your child, you'll be more apt to respect your spouse's point of view.

• **Find a compromise position.** Let's say your adult child loses his/her job and needs to move back home. One parent may want to indulge "his/her baby"…the other may expect the child to be more like a boarder while living in the home. Parents need to discuss their views, then meet with the child to discuss everyone's expectations for the situation and come to an agreement. For example, instead of paying rent, the child could handle some household repairs, cleaning or lawn care.

• **Stay out of the middle.** If your child complains to you about the other parent, tell him that the issue is between the two of them, and encourage him to speak directly to the parent he's complaining about.

Nancy, for her part, sees a parent's role as that of a harbor, not a rescue vessel. You are always there for the boat to sail back in, but you shouldn't steer or chase after it.

New Fathers Suffer from Postpartum Depression

James F. Paulson, PhD, assistant professor of pediatrics, Eastern Virginia Medical School, Norfolk, and leader of a study of 28,004 men, published in *The Journal of the American Medical Association*.

About 10.4% of American men become depressed either during their mate's pregnancy or within the year following the baby's birth.

Reason: Pregnancy and new parenthood are times of immense change and stress for both parents—including an overall rethinking of life roles, from being independent adults to parents who are responsible for an infant. Symptoms include persistent sadness and/or irritability…low energy…changes in sleep and appetite…persistent negative thinking…feelings of hopelessness…and loss of interest in hobbies.

Self-defense: Learn about the symptoms at the Web site of the National Institute of Mental Health (*www.nimh.nih.gov*) and/or by speaking with your primary care physician or a specialty mental health professional.

6

Natural Beauty Cures

Skin Care from the Inside Out

To take care of their skin, most people reach for sunscreen, lotions and creams to protect, smooth and moisturize. These products can help, but beautiful, healthy skin starts with what goes into your body, not what you rub on it. Research shows that good nutrition may reduce the effects of sun damage...minimize redness and wrinkling...and even protect against some skin cancers.

FIRST STEP: HYDRATE

The single most important nutritional factor for keeping skin healthy is water. Staying hydrated keeps cells plump, making skin look firmer and clearer. When cells are dehydrated, they shrivel and can make your skin look wrinkled. Think of it this way—when you dehydrate a juicy grape, you get a raisin. In addition, water transports nutrients into skin cells and helps flush toxins out of the body.

To stay hydrated, drink whenever you feel thirsty.

Helpful sign: If your urine is pale yellow, you are adequately hydrated—but if it is bright or dark yellow, you may need to boost your fluid intake.

Good news: Drinking unsweetened tea helps keep you hydrated, plus you get the benefit of antioxidant nutrients called polyphenols, which may help prevent sun-related skin cancers. Green, white, black and oolong teas provide more polyphenols than herbal teas. It is your choice whether to drink caffeinated or decaffeinated tea. Although caffeine is a mild diuretic (increasing the amount of urine that is passed from the body), the relatively small amount in tea doesn't affect its ability to keep skin hydrated and healthy.

Joy Bauer, MS, RD, CDN, nutritionist/dietitian in private practice in New York City. She is the nutrition expert for the *Today* show and nutritionist for the New York City Ballet. She is author of several bestselling books, including *Joy Bauer's Food Cures: Treat Common Health Concerns, Look Younger & Live Longer* (Rodale). *www.joybauer.com*

Avoid: Teas sweetened with a lot of sugar — excess sugar can make skin dull and wrinkled.

SKIN-HEALTHY FOODS

Everything we eat is reflected in the health of our skin—for better or for worse. *Among the best nutrients for the skin…*

•**Beta-carotene,** a powerful antioxidant which, once ingested, is converted to vitamin A, a nutrient necessary for skin tissue growth and repair.

Skin-smart: Have at least one serving per day of beta-carotene–rich foods—for instance, orange carrots, sweet potatoes and tomatoes …green arugula, asparagus and spinach…and fruits such as cherries, grapefruit, mangoes and watermelon.

•**Omega-3 fatty acids,** healthful fats that are important building blocks of the membranes that make up cell walls, allowing water and nutrients to enter and keeping out waste and toxins.

Skin-smart: Eat at least three servings of omega-3–rich foods each week—such as wild salmon (farm-raised salmon may have higher levels of potentially dangerous contaminants) …mackerel (not king mackerel, which has too much mercury)…anchovies, herring and sardines. Good fats also are found in smaller amounts in flaxseed, soybeans and walnuts. If you don't eat enough of these omega-3 foods, consider taking daily supplements of fish oil providing 1,000 mg of combined *eicosapentaenoic acid* (EPA) and *docosahexaenoic acid* (DHA), the most biologically active and beneficial components. Look for brands that have been tested for purity, such as VitalOils 1000 (877-342-3721, *www.myvitalremedymd.com*) and Ultimate Omega by Nordic Naturals (800-662-2544, *www.nordicnaturals.com*).

•**Selenium,** a mineral with antioxidant activity thought to help skin elasticity (which means you'll look younger longer) and prevent sun-related skin damage and cancers.

Skin-smart: Eat at least one serving a day of a selenium-rich food—canned light tuna (which has less mercury than canned albacore or white tuna), crab, tilapia…whole-wheat breads and pasta…lean beef…chicken and turkey (breast meat is lowest in fat).

Caution: Taking selenium in supplement form may increase the risk for squamous cell skin cancer in people with a personal or family history of the disease. Selenium in food is safe and healthful.

•**Vitamin C,** an antioxidant that helps build collagen and elastin (proteins that comprise the skin's underlying structure)…and also protects against free radicals (molecules in the body that damage cells) when the skin is exposed to sunlight.

Skin-smart: Eat at least one serving a day of any of these vitamin C-rich foods—cantaloupe, citrus fruits, kiwifruit, papaya, pineapple, strawberries, watermelon…and bell peppers, broccoli, brussels sprouts, cabbage, cauliflower, kale and kidney beans.

•**Zinc,** a mineral that helps maintain collagen. People with zinc deficiencies often develop skin redness and lesions.

Skin-smart: Eat at least one serving of a zinc-rich food daily—chicken or turkey breast, crab, lean beef, pork tenderloin (lower in fat than other cuts)…peanuts and peanut butter …fat-free dairy products (cheese, milk and yogurt).

Wise for everyone: A daily multivitamin that contains 100% of the daily value for vitamins A, C, E and zinc and no more than 70 mcg of selenium.

WHAT TO AVOID

•**Sugar.** Research suggests that sugary foods (such as soda and cookies) may contribute to skin blemishes. These "bad carbs" may promote harmful inflammation throughout the body, which can trigger breakouts. Limit your indulgence in sweet treats to no more than one small serving per day.

•**White flour.** Minimize white-flour foods (such as white bread and pasta) in your diet by choosing whole-grain breads and rolls, cereals, crackers and pasta.

•**Dairy foods.** Milk may contain hormones (especially if cows are pregnant) and iodine from iodine-fortified feed. Although uncommon, both of these components can cause pimples. If you are prone to acne, try going off dairy for a while to see if your skin improves.

•**Cigarette smoke, including secondhand smoke.** It fills your body with toxins, inflammation causing irritants and free radicals that damage every cell they touch...and also limits blood flow, so skin cells don't receive the oxygen and nutrients they need.

More from Joy Bauer...

Hair Care from the Inside Out

Foods that are healthy for skin also are healthy for hair. *In addition, hair requires...*

• **Iron-rich protein.** Hair is made primarily of protein. Without enough of it, hair can weaken, grow more slowly or fall out. Iron helps red blood cells carry oxygen throughout the body, including to hair-growth cells. Eat at least one serving per day of protein foods high in iron, such as clams, oysters, shrimp...duck, lamb, lean beef, pork, turkey...eggs...fortified whole-grain breads and cereals...tofu and legumes (beans, peas, etc.).

• **B vitamins.** Folate, biotin, vitamin B-6 and vitamin B-12 are needed to make red blood cells. Without enough of these vitamins, hair follicles can become starved for nutrients and oxygen, and your hair can fall out. Eat two servings a day of foods that contain one or more of these nutrients.

Good choices: Fortified whole-grain breads and cereals...broccoli, leafy dark green vegetables and legumes...eggs and fat-free dairy products...peanut butter...and wild salmon.

Curry Cream Erases Wrinkles

Bharat Aggarwal, PhD, professor of cancer research, biochemistry, immunology and experimental therapeutics, director of the Cytokine Research Laboratory, MD Anderson Cancer Center, Houston, Texas, and author of *Healing Spices: How to Use 50 Everyday and Exotic Spices to Boost Health and Beat Disease* (Sterling).

"The spice turmeric is a kitchen staple in India, found in just about every dish that crosses the table, including curries—and it's one of nature's most powerful healers," says Bharat Aggarwal, PhD, profes-

sor of experimental therapeutics at MD Anderson Cancer Center in Houston and author of *Healing Spices* (Sterling).

"Turmeric owes it preventive and curative skills to curcumin, its active ingredient," he continues. "Curcumin is a compound so diverse and powerfully rich in antioxidant and anti-inflammatory actions that it has been shown to protect and improve the health of virtually every organ in the body."

And that includes the body's biggest organ—your skin.

New finding: In studies presented at the annual meeting of the American Academy of Dermatology (AAD), a turmeric-based moisturizing cream reduced fine lines, wrinkles and age spots.

ANTI-WRINKLES, ANTI-SPOTS

"For the first time, we've shown clinically relevant anti-aging benefits from a turmeric extract," says Cheri Swanson, PhD, the leader of the two studies.

• **Smoothing fine lines.** In the first study, 89 women, aged 40 to 60, applied a turmeric-containing skin cream to one side of their face twice daily, and a placebo cream to the other side.

Results: Dermatologists evaluated photographs of the women's faces at the beginning of the study and after eight weeks of using turmeric—and found the turmeric-cream was "significantly better at reducing the appearance of fine lines and wrinkles" than the placebo cream.

• **Erasing age spots.** In a similar study, 105 women aged 25 to 55 used the skin cream or the placebo cream for eight weeks. But this time they were evaluated for age spots, or what dermatologists call hyperpigmentation.

Results: The turmeric-based cream reduced the appearance of age spots by 15%. "Even a 10% change is very noticeable," says Dr. Swanson.

• **Confirming the mechanism of action.** In another study, Dr. Swanson and her colleagues found that a turmeric extract activated 11 different "antioxidant genes" and deactivated genes involved in the production of oxidizing free radicals. They also found the extract was anti-inflammatory. "Antioxidant and anti-inflammatory properties of turmeric" were confirmed, the scientists told dermatologists at the AAD meeting.

Product: The colorless, odorless "Turmeric Complex" used in the studies is contained in several Doctors Dermatological Formula (DDF) products from Procter & Gamble. *They include…*

- **DDF Advanced Firming Cream**
- **DDF Advanced Eye Firming Concentrate**
- **DDF Advanced Micro-Exfoliation Cleanser**

You can find DDF products on the Web at *www.ddfskincare.com* and other online stores, and at beauty and skin care retailers such as Sephora.

WRINKLE-REDUCING TURMERIC MASK

If you don't want to spend money on over-the-counter skin care products, you can make your own turmeric-containing, wrinkle-reducing facial mask, says Dr. Aggarwal.

"My wife and many other Indian women use such a facial mask to keep the face smooth, radiant and free of wrinkles and blemishes," he says.

To make the mask, Indian women use sesame oil made in India, but any odorless oil, such as vegetable or canola, will do. "To use sesame, you must get the sesame oil found in Indian markets, as the sesame oil generally found in supermarkets has a strong smell and is expensive," says Dr. Aggarwal.

"This formula should last for several uses, and feels fresh and clean as a spa facial—at a fraction of the cost!" he says.

TURMERIC FACIAL MASK

Ingredients…

½ cup garbanzo (chickpea) flour

1½ tablespoons turmeric

Odorless cooking oil

Water Instructions…

1. Mix the flour and turmeric in a container with a tight fitting lid. Store container in a dry place.

2. To make the mask, mix about 1 tablespoon of the flour mixture in a small dish with about 5 drops of oil. Add enough water

to make a paste. It should be the consistency of cake batter.

3. Pull your hair back or cover it with a towel. Using your fingertips, spread the mixture on your face and neck, making sure to stay clear of the eyes. Let the mixture stay on your face until it dries, about 15 minutes. Wash it off in the shower.

Anti-Wrinkle Foods

When dietary data for 4,025 women was analyzed in a recent study, those with high intakes of vitamin C and the essential fatty acid linoleic acid had fewer wrinkles than women with lower intakes.

Theory: Vitamin C is an important component in collagen synthesis (which keeps skin supple), and linoleic acid promotes normal skin structure.

For younger-looking skin: Eat vitamin C–rich fruits and vegetables, such as oranges and broccoli, and foods high in linoleic acid, such as soybeans and sunflower oil.

Maeve C. Cosgrove, PhD, research scientist, Corporate Research, Unilever Colworth Science Park, Bedford, UK.

What Your Skin Is Trying to Tell You

Andrew Bronin, MD, associate clinical professor of dermatology at Yale School of Medicine in New Haven, Connecticut. A dermatologist in private practice in Rye Brook, New York, he also is editor-in-chief of *DermClips*, an American Academy of Dermatology (AAD) continuing medical education publication, and a recipient of AAD's Presidential Citation award, given to major contributors in the field of dermatology.

A rash here and an itch there may seem minor—and usually they are. Yet sometimes symptoms that appear to be "only skin deep" actually are warning signs of serious health problems. This is one reason why it is important to get regular skin checkup

This is one reason why it is important to get regular skin checkups, typically yearly. Of course your dermatologist looks for skin cancer, including the potentially deadly malignant melanoma…but during a full-body exam, the doctor may spot subtle signs indicating a problem inside the body.

Below are symptoms that your dermatologist should look for during a checkup—and that you should report promptly if you notice them first. Your dermatologist may treat the problem if he/she feels that it is primarily a skin disorder…or, if an underlying condition is suspected, you may be sent to a specialist or back to your primary care doctor for a full diagnosis and treatment.

To locate a dermatologist in your area who is a member of The American Academy of Dermatology, go to *www.aad.org*.

RED NOSE AND CHEEKS

Skin problem: Often the cause is rosacea, a chronic inflammatory skin disorder sometimes characterized just by facial redness…and sometimes by small red bumps on the face. Though it cannot be cured, rosacea is not dangerous. Usually it can be controlled with topical and/or oral antibiotics.

Below-the-skin problem: Systemic lupus erythematosus sometimes causes a butterfly-shaped red rash that goes across the bridge of the nose and onto the cheeks. Lupus is a chronic autoimmune disorder that affects nine times as many women as men. The rash does not respond to acne drugs and may be exacerbated by certain antibiotics, such as sulfa drugs or tetracycline. Untreated, lupus can damage the joints, kidneys, heart, lungs, digestive tract and nervous system.

Action: If lupus is suspected, a rheumatologist orders diagnostic blood and urine tests. There is no cure, but prompt treatment with medication (such as steroids) and lifestyle changes (including avoiding alcohol and excessive sunlight) minimizes symptoms and reduces risk for complications.

BREAST RASH

Skin problem: A patch of itchy, bumpy redness on the breast could be atopic dermatitis (also called eczema), an inflammatory skin condition common in allergic individuals. Atopic dermatitis frequently affects other areas, too—especially the crooks of the elbows and the backs of the knees. Symptoms often can be controlled with topical medication, such as steroid cream.

Below-the-skin problems: If a scaly rash appears on or around the nipple, it may be Paget's disease of the breast, a rash that can signify underlying breast cancer or intraductal carcinoma (abnormal cells in the breast duct that may become invasive cancer). If the breast is swollen and warm and its skin is discolored or pitted (like an orange peel), this may signal inflammatory breast cancer, most often diagnosed in women in their 50s. A breast rash caused by cancer may not respond to topical creams, though sometimes symptoms spontaneously abate briefly.

Action: A biopsy is needed to confirm the diagnosis. An oncologist provides guidance on treatment options, including surgery, radiation and/or chemotherapy.

UNDER-EYE CIRCLES

Skin problems: Dark circles worsen with age as skin thins and loses elasticity, making veins more visible. Excess sun darkens the area further by increasing production of the skin pigment melanin.

Recommended: Daily use of sunscreen helps prevent sun-related changes.

Below-the-skin problem: Darkening of the skin around the eyes could be "atopic shiners," which sometimes occur in people who have allergies. One theory suggests that atopic shiners result from chronic rubbing of itchy skin in the eye area. Additional allergy-related skin symptoms include rough, dry skin…cracked skin on the hands and feet…and tiny, hard red or white bumps called keratosis pilaris on the upper arms, thighs, buttocks and face.

Action: An allergist can perform skin tests to determine what you are allergic to and then recommend avoidance strategies, medication and/or immunotherapy injections to minimize allergic symptoms, such as asthma or hay fever.

But: Often the skin signs of allergy, such as atopic shiners, persist even when other symptoms respond to treatment.

ITCHING

Skin problem: Common causes include dry skin, sunburn, allergic reactions, insect bites, scabies infestation, poison ivy, bacterial or fungal infections, psoriasis or stress. Treatment depends on the specific condition. For quick temporary relief, it helps to run cool water or place a cold compress on the area…soak in an oatmeal bath…use an over-the-counter cream with camphor, menthol, calamine, benzocaine, hydrocortisone or triamcinolone…and/or take an oral antihistamine.

Below-the-skin problems: *Persistent itchiness could signal any of the following…*

•**Hodgkin's lymphoma.** Intractable itchiness that does not respond to treatment can be an early sign of this cancer, which starts in the cells of the immune system. Other symptoms include swollen lymph nodes, cough, fever, night sweats, fatigue and/or unintended weight loss.

Action: An oncologist confirms the diagnosis with blood tests, imaging tests and lymph node biopsy. Treatment generally includes chemotherapy and radiation.

•**Liver disease.** A number of liver problems—including a viral disease, such as hepatitis, or the metastasis (spread) of cancer to the liver—can produce intense itching.

Action: A gastroenterologist does tests, such as blood work, imaging studies and/or biopsy, to determine the exact nature of the problem. Treatment depends on the specific diagnosis.

•**Thyroid disorder.** Thyroid hormones regulate metabolism. Both hyperthyroidism (overactive thyroid gland) and hypothyroidism (underactive thyroid) can produce generalized itching. Other symptoms of hyperthyroidism include a rash and swelling on the shins, sudden weight loss despite an increased appetite, rapid or irregular heartbeat, hand tremors, fatigue and/or increased sensitivity to heat. Untreated hyperthyroidism can cause severe heart problems and osteoporosis. Hypothyroidism often is accompanied by dry skin, weight gain, muscle aches and fatigue. Untreated hypothyroidism may lead to infertility and heart disease.

Action: An endocrinologist orders blood tests to measure hormone levels. With medication to regulate thyroid hormones and sometimes with surgery, symptoms generally subside and complications are prevented.

Makeup Without Risky Chemicals

Find out which cosmetics have chemicals linked to cancer, allergies or other harmful substances. You can browse lists of lipsticks, nail polishes, etc., and sort the lists by product name or level of hazard, or search for a specific manufacturer, ingredient or product. The site also maintains databases on baby-care and oral-care products. Visit Environmental Working Group's Skin Deep database at *www.cos meticdatabase.com.*

Money, Time-Life Building, Rockefeller Center, New York City 10020.

Skin Cancer Warning

A persistent itch may be a sign of skin cancer. Any skin irritation that persists for weeks may be early-stage skin cancer, especially if it increases in size, changes color or bleeds. See a dermatologist—he/she usually can tell quickly whether an irritation is benign or cancerous.

Perry Robins, MD, dermatologist and professor emeritus of dermatology at New York University Medical Center, New York City, and president of The Skin Cancer Foundation.

Better Acne Control

Patients who had moderate to severe acne showed significant improvement after applying a specially formulated 3% green tea solution to their skin twice daily for 12 weeks. The solution cleared skin as effectively as the conventional acne medication benzoyl peroxide but with less itching, peeling and other side effects. Green tea cream is available at health-food stores.

Jennifer Gan-Wong, MD, dermatologist, Chinese General Hospital and Medical Center, Manila, the Philippines.

Clothes That Can Save Your Skin

Ascension Riva, PhD, professor, Universitat Politècnica de Catalunya, Terrassa, Spain.

Cynthia Bailey, MD, dermatologist in private practice in Sebastopol, California. *www.otbskincare.com*

Here comes the sun, and it's all right, sang the Beatles.

But if the band members had been four dermatologists, they would have been singing, Here comes the sun, and it's not all right for you to be outside without adequate protection.

Warning: A lifetime of exposure to the ultraviolet-B (UVB) rays of the sun can scramble the DNA in skin cells, triggering a squamous cell or basal cell carcinoma, the two skin cancers that account for 95% of all cases. (The link between sun exposure and melanoma—the deadliest skin cancer—is still a matter of debate among scientists, though most believe that excessive sun exposure raises the risk for some types of this cancer.)

And even if you don't get cancer, you get older faster. Those DNA-damaging rays gradually shred protein fibers in the skin called elastin. Eventually, once-firm skin stretches and sags, creasing your body with wrinkles. (Sun damage can also cause age spots, dilated blood vessels and sallow coloring.)

Maybe you're sun-savvy and slather on sunscreen every day, particularly during the summer, when UVB rays are at their most direct and damaging.

But can the color of the clothes you wear provide maximum protection from UVB?

A new study from scientists in sunny Spain provides the answer.

STUDY DETAILS

The team researchers tested different colored cotton clothing to find out which were the best at blocking UVB rays.

The winners: blue and red.

The loser: yellow.

"The color of cotton woven fabrics is a factor that has a remarkable influence on their protection against ultraviolet rays," say the scientists, in Industrial & Engineering Chemistry Research.

What happens: Darker colors absorb more UVB rays, explains Ascension Riva, PhD, the study leader. (Even though it wasn't tested in this study, black is the most protective color, she says.)

"People think that any piece of clothing will sufficiently protect them from the UV radiation of the sun, and that's not true," she adds. "The lighter and more porous the fabric, the less it will protect."

WHAT TO DO

"Yes, the sun's UV rays can go right through your clothes," says Cynthia Bailey, MD, a dermatologist in private practice in Sebastopol, California.

Problem: One-third of what you wear during the summer does not protect you, she adds.

That includes clothes with these types of fabrics…

- **Light colors**
- **Lightweight and thin**
- **Cotton**
- **Linen**
- **Rayon**
- **Wet and stretched** (*example*: wet cotton T-shirt)

However: "Fuzzy, new, unbleached cotton sometimes provides good sun protection when it's dry," she says.

Wear protective fabrics as much as possible. To provide maximum protection, consider wearing fabrics that are more protective, she says. *They include...*

- **Dark colors**
- **Thick and tightly woven threads**
- **Polyester**
- **Nylon**
- **Wool**

Unfortunately, points out Dr. Bailey, these are just the type of clothes you're least likely to wear during the summer.

But don't give up. You can wash some extra sun protection into your light-colored, lightweight summer clothes.

- **Wash your laundry in Sun Guard.** "This product contains Tinosorb, which binds to fabric and absorbs UV rays," says Dr. Bailey. "I've used it many times—in the washing machine, and in a hotel sink to wash a new cotton knit shirt while on vacation—and it's never damaged or changed the look of a fabric."

The protection lasts for 19 launderings, she says.

- **Use a laundry detergent with an "optical brightener."** The optical brightener absorbs UV rays, releasing the energy as "fluorescence"—which is why your clothes look brighter, she explains.

- **Don't bleach.** It decreases sun protection, so try to avoid it, especially for cotton and rayon, she says.

- **Buy sun-protective clothing.** For sun-intensive activities—like hiking, gardening and cycling—consider buying special sun protective clothing from companies such as REI, Sun Precautions or Coolibar, says Dr. Bailey. "Sun protective garments often contain hidden vents and zippers that open for ventilation, plus other clever tricks to keep you cool in sunny, hot places."

Resources: The Web site of REI is *www.rei.com*, and includes a store locator. The Web site of online retailer Sun Precautions is *www.sunprecautions.com*. The Web site of online retailer Coolibar is *www.coolibar.com*.

Follow these other sun-guarding precautions. Dr. Bailey counsels her patients—many of whom have precancerous lesions, or who have already had skin cancer—to make use of the following strategies to minimize sun exposure...

- **Use multiple forms of sun protection, rather than just one.** "Wear sunscreen, a hat, sun-protecting clothes and stand in the shade," says Dr. Bailey. "It's these multiple forms of sun protection that allow you to avoid having to reapply sunscreen every two hours, which is the standard recommendation, but which few people ever do." (However, she adds, multiple applications are important if you're out in the sun for extended periods of time, or after you've gotten wet.)

- **Be prepared in advance.** Put your sunscreen on first thing in the morning, and keep an extra hat and sun umbrella in the car, she says.

- **Use the best sunscreen ingredient.** It's 5% micronized zinc oxide. It provides excellent protection, she says, has almost no risk of side effects (unlike chemical sunscreens) and blends into the skin completely, without leaving a white residue. And it provides protection from ultraviolet-A (UVA), which also damages skin, and is a year-round threat.

Bottom line: "Learn the practical strategies that work for you in everyday life to minimize sun exposure, and put them into place," says Dr. Bailey.

Apply Twice as Much Sunscreen as You Think You Need

FDA testing calls for about twice as much as most people apply. To be able to count on the protection listed on the label, apply sunscreen, wait 20 minutes, then apply it again. It takes two to three tablespoons per application to cover exposed adult skin adequately. Look for sunscreens labeled broad spectrum or ones that protect against both UVA and UVB rays.

Vincent A. DeLeo, MD, chairman of the department of dermatology, St. Luke's–Roosevelt Hospital Center and Beth Israel Medical Center, New York City.

The Salad Cure for Sun-Damaged Skin

Alan C. Logan, ND, naturopathic doctor and author of *Your Skin, Younger* and *The Clear Skin Diet* (Cumberland House). His scientific articles have appeared in *Archives of Dermatology*, the *International Journal of Dermatology*, the *Journal of the American Academy of Dermatology* and the *British Journal of Dermatology*. *www.drlogan.com*

Julia T. Hunter, MD, holistic dermatologist and medical director of Skin Fitness Plus in Beverly Hills, California. *www.skinfitnessplus.com*

What are the hottest ingredients in skin care that can help protect you from the ravages of the sun, such as wrinkles and sags…and even skin cancer? Tomatoes, carrots and broccoli.

What you may not know: According to recent scientific studies, what you put in your body—the foods you eat—may be just as important for youthful, healthy skin as any skin care ingredients that you put on your body.

"High-quality nutrition provides all the raw materials necessary for both structure and functioning of skin—and a steady stream of optimal nutrients goes a long way in supporting healthy skin over the course of a lifetime," says Alan C. Logan, ND, a naturopathic doctor and author of *Your Skin, Younger* (Cumberland House).

NEWEST RESEARCH

"A diet rich in a variety of colorful vegetables and fruits can put the brakes on the skin's aging process," says Dr. Logan. *The latest studies show he's right…*

• **Tomatoes.** Researchers from the University of Manchester in England studied 17 women aged 21 to 47, dividing them into two groups—one group ate a "scientific snack" of about two ounces of tomato paste with olive oil every day, while the other group just consumed olive oil. At the beginning of the study and after three months, a small section of skin on the women's buttocks was exposed to a dose of skin-aging ultraviolet (UV) radiation (the same type of radiation from the sun), to see how much UV light it took to produce damaging redness.

Results: After eating tomato paste every day for three months, it took 28% longer for the UV radiation to produce redness. There was no difference in the women who just ate the olive oil.

And those who ate the tomato paste also had lower levels of skin damage and healthier skin when they were exposed to UV light. *Specifically, they had…*

• **Less damage to fibrillin-1,** a protein that helps form elastin, the fiber that maintains the elasticity of skin (so that it doesn't sag).

• **Less buildup of matrix metalloproteinase,** enzymes that damage collagen, protein fibers that help maintain the firmness and youth of skin (so that it doesn't wrinkle).

• **More procollagen,** the molecule that forms collagen.

• **Less DNA damage in skin cells.**

In short, they had less of what dermatologists call photoaging—damage from the sun's UV radiation.

"Tomato paste provides protection against acute and potentially longer-term aspects of photoaging," concluded the researchers in the *British Journal of Dermatology*.

Why it works: Tomatoes contain the carotenoid lycopene, an antioxidant and pigment that has UV-protecting properties, says Dr. Logan. "Lycopene is abundant in tomato products, and also in apricots, pink grapefruit, guava and watermelon. If you decide to incorporate lycopene in your diet, consider eating tomatoes or taking a tomato-extract supplement."

Example of a tomato extract supplement: Lyc-O-Mato, from LycoRed (*www.lycored.com*).

• **Carrots, sweet potatoes, romaine lettuce, spinach and kale.** Beta-carotene is another carotenoid, found abundantly in carrots, sweet potatoes, winter squash, romaine lettuce, spinach, kale, dandelion greens, collard greens and turnip greens.

And like lycopene, it can protect skin.

The study: Korean researchers in the Department of Dermatology at Seoul National University studied the skin of 30 women aged 50 and over, who took beta-carotene for three months.

"Beta-carotene improved facial wrinkles and elasticity significantly," reported the researchers in the medical journal *Dermatology*. The women also had four times more procollagen.

"30 mg/day of beta-carotene supplementation is demonstrated to prevent and repair photoaging," they concluded.

You can get 30 mg of beta-carotene in about five servings of red, orange or dark green vegetables.

• **Broccoli sprouts.** Researchers in the School of Medicine at Johns Hopkins University conducted an experiment with two groups of hairless mice, feeding one group an extract from broccoli sprouts, and then exposing both groups to 17 weeks of UV radiation.

Results: The broccoli-eating mice developed 25% less skin cancer, and the tumors they developed were 70% smaller. The results were reported in *Photochemical & Photobiological Sciences*.

Why it works: Broccoli sprouts are the richest dietary source of *sulforaphane glucosinolate* (SGS), containing 50 times more than mature broccoli—and SGS is the precursor to sulphoraphane, a powerful anti-cancer compound.

• **Berries and nuts.** Ellagic acid is an antioxidant found in blackberries, raspberries, strawberries and cranberries, and also in walnuts, pecans and in pomegranates.

The study: Korean researchers conducted studies with human skin cells and experimental animals, and found that ellagic acid could reduce the breakdown of collagen...reduce inflammation from UV exposure...and help prevent the formation of wrinkles and age-related skin thickening.

"Dietary interventions with berries rich in ellagic acid may be a promising treatment strategy for interrupting skin wrinkling and inflammation associated with chronic UV ex-

posure," concluded the researchers in the journal *Experimental Dermatology*.

And in another animal study, researchers from the Department of Dermatology at the University of Wisconsin found that a pomegranate fruit extract rich in ellagic acid reduced seven different biomarkers of skin cancer.

The extract "affords substantial protection from the adverse effects of UVB radiation" wrote the researchers in the journal *Photochemistry and Photobiology*.

• **The Mediterranean diet.** All the foods just discussed are found in abundance in the Mediterranean diet, which is rich in vegetables, fruits and nuts. And an Israeli researcher thinks the Mediterranean diet is very good for your skin.

"Foods such as colorful fruits and vegetables—as well as olive oil, fish and yogurt—fight the oxidizing effect of the sun," says Niva Shapira, PhD, RD, of the Stanley Steyer School of Health Professions at Tel Aviv University, in the journal *Nutrition Reviews*. "The presence of these foods in the traditional Greek-style Mediterranean diet may have contributed to the low rates of melanoma in the Mediterranean region, despite high levels of solar radiation."

To help prove her point, Dr. Shapira conducted a study, dividing participants into two groups—for two weeks, one group drank an antioxidant-rich fruit beverage supplemented with the antioxidants vitamin C, vitamin E and selenium, and one group didn't drink the beverage. During the two weeks, both groups had four to six hours of sun exposure a day.

At the end of two weeks, those drinking the antioxidant-rich beverage had no increase in blood levels of *malondialdehyde* (MDA), a biomarker of skin-damaging oxidation—while those not drinking the beverage had a 50% increase.

She also cites a study which links the following features of the Mediterranean diet to less risk for skin cancer...

• **Weekly consumption of fish** (omega-3 fatty acids in fish protect the skin)

• **Daily drinking of tea** (both black and green tea are rich in antioxidants)

- **High intakes of vegetables** (particularly carrots, broccoli and other cruciferous vegetables, and leafy green vegetables)
- **High intakes of fruit**
- **High intakes of carotenoids** (such as found in tomatoes).

"If you provide the body with sufficient and relevant antioxidants, you can reduce damage from sun exposure," she concludes.

Bottom line: "The health of your skin starts with what you eat," says Julia Hunter, MD, a holistic dermatologist and medical director of Skin Fitness Plus in Beverly Hills, California. "Food is your medicine—along with external sun protection, it's a crucial way to prevent the aging of skin, and to rejuvenate skin that has aged. And the more anti-inflammatory antioxidants in your diet, the better."

Beta-Carotene for Better Sun Protection

Andrew L. Rubman, ND, medical director, Southbury Clinic for Traditional Medicines, Southbury, Connecticut. *www.southburyclinic.com*

In a recent meta-analysis of seven studies, researchers at Münster University Hospital in Germany found that oral beta-carotene supplements help protect against sunburn. How long you take these is key, however—protective benefits kicked in at 10 weeks, and the longer a person had been taking supplements, the more protective benefit they received. Scientists also stressed that beta-carotene alone is not the answer to sunburn prevention. With an equivalent SPF (sun protection factor) of four, at most, it should be used in addition to—not instead of—regular sunscreen.

Andrew L. Rubman, ND, explains that as an antioxidant, beta-carotene helps your body better withstand a variety of free radical challenges, including those posed by exposure to the sun's ultraviolet (UV) rays. UV radiation consists of particles of energy called photons—when these strike and penetrate your skin, they set off oxidative changes that can damage tissue. Beta-carotene makes your skin more resistant to these harmful effects.

PRACTICE SUN SMARTS

Sun exposure is a must for good health. Your body needs a daily dose of at least 15 minutes to produce the vitamin D you need for bone growth, immune resistance and other physiological and mental processes. It's nonetheless important to avoid painful and potentially dangerous sunburn—apply water-resistant sunscreen with an SPF of at least 15 every two hours...wear protective clothing such as wide-brimmed hats and long-sleeved cover-ups...and seek shade as appropriate, especially when the sun's rays are at their most intense between 10 a.m. and 4 p.m.

If you want to add beta-carotene to your sun protection plan, a daily dose shouldn't exceed six to 15 milligrams. Better than supplements, however, is to get your beta-carotene from dietary sources—consume five servings of fruits and vegetables daily, which naturally provide six to eight milligrams of beta-carotene. Carrots, green leafy vegetables, sweet potatoes, winter squash, cantaloupe and broccoli are all rich dietary sources.

Exercise and Coffee May Fight Skin Cancer?

Skin cancer develops in cells whose DNA has been damaged by UV radiation—but damaged cells often die before becoming malignant. The death rate of precancerous skin cells in mice that received exercise and oral caffeine was nearly 400% greater than in mice that had neither exercise nor caffeine.

Allan H. Conney, PhD, professor of pharmacology and director of the Susan Lehman Cullman Laboratory for Cancer Research, Rutgers State University of New Jersey, Piscataway, and coauthor of a study published in *Proceedings of the National Academy of Sciences*.

Green Tea Combats Skin Cancer

Polyphenols, a type of antioxidant found in green tea, protect skin from the sun's damaging ultraviolet radiation and help prevent the formation of skin tumors.

Best: Drink five to six cups of green tea a day—the fresher, the better. Fresh green tea leaves have a light yellow or green color. A brownish hue indicates that the tea has undergone oxidation, which destroys antioxidants. Tea bags and loose leaves are better than instant and bottled teas.

Santosh Katiyar, PhD, associate professor of dermatology, University of Alabama, Birmingham, and leader of a study of green tea and skin tumor development in mice, published in *The Journal of Nutritional Biochemistry.*

Beware of Melanomas on Your Feet or Ankles

Melanomas on the feet or ankles have a higher mortality rate than other melanomas. That's because the cancer tends to be diagnosed at a later stage.

Self-defense: Check the entire foot monthly—ankles, tops of feet, soles (use a mirror), between the toes and around the toenails. Look for small areas of pigmented skin, moles that have changed in size or appearance and any unexplained discoloration under a toenail. If you see any of these signs, consult a doctor.

Neil A. Campbell, DPM, podiatrist in Yoakum, Texas, is a spokesperson for the American College of Foot and Ankle Surgeons.

Freckle Faders

Jessie S. Cheung, MD, associate director of cosmetic dermatology and assistant professor of dermatology, Langone Medical Center, New York University, New York City.

If you like your freckles, there's no need to worry. Freckles are harmless pockets of the skin pigment melanin that become promi-

nent on sun-exposed areas of the body. Abundant freckling does not mean that you will develop skin cancer, but it does suggest that your skin is sun-sensitive and your risk for skin cancer may be elevated. Use sunscreen, wear a wide-brimmed hat and limit exposure to midday sun to help prevent existing freckles from darkening, keep new freckles from developing and reduce your skin cancer risk. If any freckle or other spot looks strange—lumpy, scaly, reddish, unusually large—see your dermatologist.

Don't even think of rubbing lemon juice on freckles in an attempt to lighten them. This old folk "remedy" can make skin blister or break out in a rash when you're in the sun. Instead, try an over-the-counter fade cream, such as Ambi or Porcelana, with 2% hydroquinone… or a prescription 4% hydroquinone cream. These work by blocking the synthesis of new melanin (not by bleaching existing spots)—so it may take several months of daily use for old melanin to migrate out through the natural process of exfoliation.

For faster and more thorough results, see your dermatologist for laser therapy. It works by using specific wavelengths of light to break down the melanin, which is then expelled from the surface and also carried away by your body's lymphatic system. Most people experience mild discomfort from the laser procedure, so your doctor may use a numbing cream on your skin before starting. Usually one session eliminates or substantially reduces existing freckles (though future sun exposure may create new ones). A session typically costs $500 to $1,500, depending on the size of the area treated, and generally is not covered by medical insurance.

The Whole-Body Cure For Chronic Hives

Kamila Kingston, certified practitioner of Traditional Chinese Medicine (TCM) and cofounder of the White Lotus Cosmetic Acupuncture and Longevity Center in Brisbane, Australia. *www.whitelotus.com.au*

If you're one of the millions of Americans with repeated outbreaks of hives—histamine-sparked eruptions of raised, red and very itchy bumps—you've probably been to doctor after doctor, trying to find relief.

You've received prescriptions for antihistamines to short-circuit the outbreaks, and for topical medications such as steroid creams to ease the itching.

You've had allergy tests to detect the allergen—the food, food additive, medication or other factor that is supposedly triggering the outbreaks. But if you're like 95% of people with hives, the allergen was never found.

Maybe you even have to carry an EpiPen with injectable epinephrine (adrenaline), just in case an outbreak of hives cascades out of control into anaphylactic shock, with your tongue and throat swelling up so much you can't breathe.

And in spite of all that, your hives still aren't under control. In fact, you feel really bad. And not just when you're having another one of those maddeningly itchy outbreaks.

"I've never seen a case of chronic hives where the person isn't also generally ill—with allergies, digestive problems and constant fatigue," says Kamila Kingston, a certified practitioner of Traditional Chinese Medicine (TCM) at the White Lotus Cosmetic Acupuncture and Longevity Center in Brisbane, Australia. "Most of these people have been in the medical mill for 10 to 15 years, seeing doctor after doctor, trying everything that's medically recommended, while their problem gets worse and worse."

But a recent scientific study shows that an alternative treatment for chronic hives may be more effective than the conventional treatments of modern medicine.

That treatment is acupuncture—small, pain-free needles are placed strategically along invisible channels of energy called meridians, unblocking and balancing the flow of energy, which restores ease and harmony to the body, alleviating symptoms.

70% REDUCTION

Doctors in the Department of Acupuncture and Moxibustion at the Chinese Academy of Chinese Medical Sciences in Beijing treated 31 people with chronic hives. Their patients were 4 to 82 years old, and hives had bothered them anywhere from one month to 30 years.

The doctors explain that acupuncture treats both the hives—"the incidental"—and the imbalances underlying the hives—"the fundamental." And the treatment works.

Of the 31 people treated, eight were cured—they had no more outbreaks.

Another 17 were improved—they had at least a 70% reduction in number of hives, longer time between outbreaks and their symptoms (such as itching) were alleviated.

Overall, 25 of the 31 people treated—81%—experienced significant relief.

How it works: In their study, the doctors point out that the main cause of hives is a body weakened by deficiencies of *qi* (pronounced CHEE) and blood.

"Qi is the fundamental energy in the body and in the universe," explains Kingston. "When there isn't enough qi, the body isn't able to make sufficient blood. A deficiency of qi and blood causes fundamental weakness in the internal organs, which produces symptoms such as hives."

BETTER THAN WESTERN MEDICINE

"In my experience, Chinese medicine is better than Western medicine at treating long-standing problems such as chronic hives," says Kingston.

• **Find a practitioner.** She recommends finding a practitioner of Traditional Chinese Medicine (TCM) who specializes in skin disorders, and who uses both acupuncture and Chinese herbal medicine, which she says go hand-in-hand in treating qi and blood deficiency.

Resource: To find a practitioner of TCM near you, go to the Web site of the National Certification Commission for Acupuncture and Oriental Medicine (*www.nccaom.org*) and click the link "Find a Practioner." You can then search by country, state and zip code.

Understand the treatment isn't short-term. In the study, the doctors followed up on the patients six months later, and found that those experiencing a recurrence of hives had stopped their acupuncture treatments after about one month, as soon as the outbreaks cleared up. "This suggests that continuous treatment after alleviation of the symptoms is effective for decreasing recurrences of hives," they say.

"Treatment for a chronic problem is not short-term," agrees Kingston. "Within the first month, you should start to notice an improvement in the frequency and intensity of your outbreaks. But for long-term relief—to address the underlying qi and blood deficiency, so that the problem doesn't come back—you probably need a minimum of three to six months of acupuncture, with a treatment every three to four weeks.

"Your health and energy levels are going to improve so much, that you'll probably be happy to continue the treatments!"

•**Don't stop conventional treatment on your own.** "As symptoms decrease, it will be natural to use less medication, with your dermatologist's approval and supervision," says Kingston.

"Since most conventional doctors have tried everything for their patients without avail, they're usually very happy to cooperate with the TCM practitioner in this way. And once the medications are lessened, the practitioner can begin to introduce Chinese herbal medicines.

"Acupuncture and Chinese herbal medicine—by addressing the symptoms and the imbalances causing the symptoms—can give hope to hopeless, suffering people with chronic hives, who've probably concluded nothing will ever solve their problem."

For Your Next Facial, Try Acupuncture. Yes, Really!

Martha Lucas, PhD, LAc, Mei Zen acupuncture practitioner in private practice in Denver and author of *Vanity Calamity: Your Guide to Cosmetic Acupuncture for Anti-Aging* (InstantPublisher.com). *www.acupuncture woman.com*

Maybe you wouldn't feel squeamish if a friend said that she was getting an acupuncture facial... but I did. Could the results really be worth the "ick" factor of having needles in your face?

Absolutely yes, I was told by Martha Lucas, PhD, LAc, a practitioner of Mei Zen ("beautiful person") cosmetic acupuncture. "Typically,

the practitioner first places very thin needles at specific points in the body to correct imbalances in qi (energy), then puts in the facial needles. The treatment causes no discomfort other than an occasional slight prick, and in fact, it can be quite relaxing," she assured me.

An acupuncture facial addresses several types of cosmetic problems. *It can help...*

•**Soften deep lines and eliminate fine lines.**

•**Reduce sagging on the cheeks, chin and neck.**

•**Lighten age spots...reduce redness...and make skin tone more even.**

•**Slightly lift the eyelids and brows.**

•**Improve acne and rosacea.**

How it works: "From the traditional Chinese medicine perspective, facial acupuncture brings more qi to the face and improves facial blood flow, providing extra oxygen and nutrients to the skin and underlying muscles. From the modern medicine perspective, the needles create micro-traumas—and in response, the body sends in fibroblast cells to repair the collagen and elastin, the supporting connective tissues that give skin its structure," said Dr. Lucas.

Typically, Dr. Lucas uses about 60 needles in the face. Additionally, a few other needles are placed in the body to help regulate the endocrine system and counter the effects of age-related declines in estrogen levels...stimulate production of mood-boosting endorphins... and alleviate stress and enhance sleep, so there is less anxiety and fatigue reflected in the face.

Results vary, depending on a person's overall health and skin condition. Some people notice improvement after just one session, while for others it may take four to six sessions to see results. A typical course of treatment is 10 twice-weekly sessions followed by maintenance sessions every month or two. Cost: About $100 to $120 per session.

When performed by a qualified professional, facial acupuncture is completely safe. The only potential side effects are slight discomfort and bruising. However, if you have a chronic health condition or have recently undergone chemotherapy, check with your doctor first. Referrals: To find a certified cosmetic acupuncture practitioner near you, contact the American Association of Acupuncture & Oriental Medicine, 866-455-7999, *www.aaaom online.org*, or go to Acupuncture Referral Service, *www.acufinder.com*. To find a certified Mei Zen practitioner near you, go to *www.cos meticacupunctureseminars.com*.

Cold-Weather Skin Care

Brandith Irwin, MD, board-certified dermatologist and internist, and director of the Madison Skin & Laser Center in Seattle. She has been a guest medical expert on *The Oprah Winfrey Show* and is author of *The Surgery-Free Makeover: All You Need to Know for Great Skin and a Younger Face* (Perseus). *www.skintour.com*

Winter is lizard-skin season—when skin turns dry, scaly, itchy and flaky. But don't blame the cold weather.

Real culprits: Low humidity outdoors... and dry, heated air indoors, which draws moisture out of the inner layers of skin. In addition, normal shedding of skin cells slows with age because cells become less active—so you end up with visible layers of dead, scaly skin. *What helps...*

•**Shorten your shower.** Though it seems counterintuitive, excess water dries out skin by breaking down its natural oils. The hotter the water, the worse it is.

Best: Use lukewarm water, and limit showers to no more than five minutes.

•**Take an Epsom salt bath.** Epsom salts contain magnesium, which helps slough off dead skin cells. Once or twice a week, add one to two cups of Epsom salts to a tubful of lukewarm water and soak for 10 to 15 minutes.

•**Use cleansing lotion, not soap.** Soap is alkaline and can strip skin of moisture.

For face and body: Try Cetaphil Gentle Skin Cleanser or Purpose Gentle Cleansing Wash.

•**Exfoliate—gently.** Use a loofah in the shower or bath to manually remove dead skin cells from your body. Allow the loofah to dry completely after each use to minimize bacteria. On your face, use a mildly abrasive facial exfoliating cream, such as Dermalogica Daily Microfoliant (310-900-4000, *www.dermalog*

ica.com). I recommend exfoliating no more than twice weekly to avoid irritating the skin.

•**Slather on a body moisturizer with a high oil-to-water ratio.** Choose a brand that feels rich and slick, such as Éminence Honeydew Body Lotion (888-747-6342, *www.emin enceorganics.com*). Apply liberally while skin is still damp from your shower or bath. Reapply at least once more per day, first dampening skin with a wet washcloth.

•**Spritz your face with water.** Do this before applying makeup and again before bed. Follow with moisturizer, such as Cetaphil Daily Facial Moisturizer.

•**Avoid irritating laundry products.** Use detergent that has no bleach or fragrances, such as All Free or Cheer Free. Never use dryer sheets—even the unscented ones leave tiny irritating fibers on clothes.

How to Get Rid of Spider Veins

Ronald Moy, MD, professor of dermatology at the David Geffen School of Medicine at the University of California, Los Angeles, and founder and medical director of Moy Cosmetic Laser Surgery, with four locations in Southern California. *www.moycosmeticlaser.com*

Spider veins are small blood vessels near the skin's surface that are visible as thin red, blue or purple lines. They most often appear on the legs but can occur on the face and elsewhere. In addition to being unsightly, spider veins may ache, swell or burn.

Age is one culprit—over time, veins get larger and skin gets thinner and more transparent. A propensity for spider veins runs in families, though they also can be caused by injury. Home remedies cannot get rid of spider veins, but two types of medical treatment can.

•**Sclerotherapy involves injecting spider veins with a salt-based solution.** This collapses the veins and cuts off blood flow, causing them to fade and easing discomfort. Pain is minor because the needle is very small. A single injection can destroy many interconnected veins, though you may need several injections and/or sessions. After sclerotherapy, healthy veins take over for destroyed ones.

Cost: About $200 per treatment.

• **Laser treatment uses pulses of energy to heat and shrink the veins.** Each laser pulse feels like a rubber band snapping on your skin, and many pulses are needed along the length of the vein. Facial spider veins generally respond best to laser treatment.

Cost: $300 or more per treatment.

Side effects are rare but may include sores, red marks and scarring.

Contact the American Academy of Dermatology, 866-503-7546, *www.aad.org.*

Beware of Infections From Pedicures

Skin infections from spa pedicures are becoming common.

Self-defense: Broken skin should not come in contact with foot-bath water. Don't shave, wax or use hair-removal cream on legs in the 24 hours before going to a foot spa. Don't go to the spa if you have skin damage, such as cuts or bug bites, on your feet or lower-leg area. Ask salon workers if foot spas are disinfected after each customer and again at night with a hospital disinfectant.

Recommendations from the US Environmental Protection Agency.

Eat Your Way to Skin Health

Mark A. Stengler, NMD, licensed naturopathic medical doctor in private practice, Stengler Center for Integrative Medicine, Encinitas, California...adjunct associate clinical professor at the National College of Natural Medicine, Portland, Oregon...author of many books and the *Bottom Line/Natural Healing* newsletter.

Summer is in full swing, and that means a lot more sun exposure and increased vitamin D levels! But one of the primary health concerns during the summer is preventing sun damage. I'm sure you already wear sunscreen regularly—preferably one that does not contain potentially harmful chemicals such as oxybenzone or retinyl palmitate. But did you know that you can consume foods that help protect your skin from sun damage?

Brightly colored fruits and vegetables are rich in carotenoids, which are potent antioxidants that help to prevent the breakdown of collagen, the body's main protein. In fact, the brighter the food, the greater the concentration of carotenoids.

Examples: Cantaloupe, watermelon, apricots, papaya, peaches, cherries, tomatoes, peppers (all colors), kale, sweet potatoes and carrots. While these foods are good for your skin year-round, they are especially helpful when you are exposed to the sun. I recommend consuming at least two servings daily of carotenoid-rich foods for the rest of the summer—and on into the early, sunny days of fall. Your skin will be better for it.

Quick Cure for Those Dry, Winter Hands

To quickly ease the cracked, dry skin that can irritate hands during the winter, try the homeopathic remedy Petroleum (not to be confused with petroleum jelly). Take two 30C pellets twice daily for seven days, then use as needed. It may seem counterintuitive to take an oral remedy, but it really helps. Petroleum is available in health-food stores and is safe for everyone. This remedy is for the hands only.

Mark A. Stengler, NMD, licensed naturopathic medical doctor in private practice, Stengler Center for Integrative Medicine, Encinitas, California...adjunct associate clinical professor at the National College of Natural Medicine, Portland, Oregon...author of many books and the *Bottom Line/Natural Healing* newsletter.

Rosacea

Mark A. Stengler, NMD, licensed naturopathic medical doctor and leading authority on the practice of alternative and integrated medicine. He is founder and medical director of the Stengler Center for Integrative Medicine, Encinitas, California, and associate clinical professor at the National College of Naturopathic Medicine, Portland, Oregon. He is author of the newsletter *Bottom Line Natural Healing, www.drstengler.com*

About 14 million adult Americans have acne rosacea, a skin condition characterized by redness, visible blood vessels and small pustules on the cheeks, forehead, nose or chin. Flare-ups can be caused by too much sunlight exposure, exercise, hot baths or saunas, spicy foods, hot beverages, alcohol and steroidal medications. For women in mid-life, hormone imbalance also can be a trigger. I recommend avoiding spicy foods and alcohol—and having a food sensitivity test given by a holistic physician to see what might be contributing to the problem. Natural treatments that can help include fish oil and gamma linoleic acid (GLA) supplements, which can help reduce skin inflammation. A topical cream consisting of alpha lipoic acid (3%) and vitamin C (5%) applied to the face at bedtime can improve this condition quickly.

Example: Reviva Labs' Alpha Lipoic Acid, Vitamin C Ester and DMAE Cream (800-257-7774, *www.revivalabs.com*). It also is available with a prescription at a compounding pharmacy. Menopausal women may be helped by supplementing with bioidentical progesterone.

My Rules for Natural Skin Care

Jamison Starbuck, ND, naturopathic physician in family practice in Missoula, Montana. She is a past president of the American Association of Naturopathic Physicians and a contributing editor to *The Alternative Advisor: The Complete Guide to Natural Therapies and Alternative Treatments* (Time-Life).

Americans spend up to $5 billion a year on skin-care products, but, in my opinion, many of these lotions, balms and gels are not necessary. *Here's a natural approach that not only helps keep your skin supple and vibrant, but also improves your overall health...*

1. Hydrate. For skin to function properly as a protective layer and a vehicle for eliminating toxins, the body must be hydrated. With dehydration, the skin loses its "turgor," or fullness, and begins to sag. For good skin health, consume one-half ounce of water per pound of body weight daily. (Some of this can come from herbal tea.) You will need more water if the temperature is above 90°F or if you are perspiring a lot.

2. Use a dry brush. Using a natural bristle brush or loofah (the dried interior of fruit from the loofah plant)—both are available at most drugstores—brush your skin with small, circular motions for two minutes before getting into the shower or bath several times a week. Dry brushing improves circulation to your skin and removes old, dead skin cells.

3. Take cod-liver oil. My favorite omega-3 fish oil choice for people who have skin conditions is cod-liver oil. It not only contains essential fatty acids necessary for healthy skin, but also vitamins A and D, which are both fundamental to good health.

Daily dose: 1,500 mg in capsule or liquid form, taken with a meal. Be sure the label says the oil has been purified—and consult your doctor before exceeding 10,000 international units (IU) of vitamin A daily from all supplement sources.* If you have skin problems and already take fish oil, check the label to determine the fish source. If it's not cod, consider switching.

4. Reduce your toxic load. The skin is an organ that, like the liver, kidneys and lungs, helps excrete toxins. The health of your skin declines in proportion to the amount of toxic substances you ingest through medication and food and/or are exposed to via pollution, herbicides and household chemicals. Don't smoke, and don't allow others to smoke in your home. Use naturally based cleaning products, such as baking soda and vinegar. Consider buying a high efficiency particulate air (HEPA) filter, available at most home stores, for your home and/or office.

5. Eat turmeric. Curry, the traditional Indian dish, is often made with turmeric, which contains curcumin, a substance that has antioxidant, anti-inflammatory and anticancer properties. Curcumin may help prevent acne and sun damage.

Caution: If you have a stomach ulcer, avoid curry.

6. Choose the right sunscreen. Use a sunscreen that contains zinc oxide as its main sun-blocking agent, as well as vitamins E and C and the mineral selenium, and has a sun protection factor (SPF) of 15 or higher. Researchers have found that sunscreens containing these antioxidants are more likely to prevent skin damage than sunscreens without these protective compounds.

*Pregnant or lactating women should check with their doctors before using cod-liver oil.

7

Cancer Fighters

Wheat Germ Extract: A Promising New Cancer Fighter

Wheat germ was one of the original health foods. The "germ" is the most nutritious part of the wheat seed. Today *fermented wheat germ extract* (FWGE) is showing promise as a potential breakthrough for treating cancer patients.

The evidence: A number of cell, animal and human studies support the use and benefits of FWGE as an adjunct therapy, meaning one that is used as part of a broader treatment program.

• **Colorectal cancer.** A study of 170 patients who had received conventional treatments for colorectal cancer found that those who also took 9 grams (g) of FWGE daily for six months had less risk of developing new cancers. The cancer spread among only 8% of the patients receiving FWGE, compared with 23% of those getting only conventional treatment.

• **Oral cancer.** Researchers compared 22 patients with oral cancer who took FWGE with 21 patients not receiving the supplement. FWGE reduced the risk for cancer progression by 85%.

• **Melanoma.** For one year, FWGE was given to 22 patients with advanced (stage 3) melanoma, and their progress was compared with 24 similar patients not receiving FWGE. Patients taking FWGE were half as likely to die from melanoma during this time.

• **Chemotherapy-induced infections.** Researchers studied 22 children and teenagers with different types of cancer. The 11 children

Mark A. Stengler, NMD, licensed naturopathic medical doctor in private practice, Stengler Center for Integrative Medicine, Encinitas, California...adjunct associate clinical professor at the National College of Natural Medicine, Portland, Oregon...author of many books, including *The Natural Physician's Healing Therapies* and coauthor of *Prescription for Natural Cures* (both from Bottom Line Books)...and author of the *Bottom Line/Natural Healing* newsletter. *www.drstengler.com*

who received FWGE had significantly fewer infections and fevers while receiving chemotherapy.

• **Animal studies.** Numerous studies suggest benefits from FWGE for leukemia as well as breast, ovarian, gastric and thyroid cancers. In one study, laboratory rats received both FWGE and vitamin C in the treatment of lung, skin and colon cancers. The combination prevented the cancer from spreading, but vitamin C alone did not. In another study, FWGE worked better alone than it did with vitamin C to treat kidney cancer.

HOW IT WORKS

FWGE appears to work by starving cancer cells of glucose, prompting their death...and by enhancing immune cell activity. Wheat germ contains chemicals that seem to have anticancer properties, and fermentation increases their concentration.

Note: FWGE is very different from the regular wheat germ you can buy at health-food stores. It comes in a powder and is sold in health-food stores and online.

Good brands: Avemar (*www.avemar-alternativetherapy.com*) and OncoMAR (800-647-6100, *www.xymogen.com*).

MY ADVICE

If you would like to begin taking FWGE, check with your physician about incorporating it into your treatment program. I recommend one packet a day, which equals 9 g. You can mix it into a glass of cold water and then drink it—or substitute a non-citrus juice, such as apple or cranberry (citrus can deactivate FWGE's active ingredient).

FWGE is not cheap—it costs about $160/month—but I think the expense is worth it, given the early indications that it may improve cancer survival rates.

Good news: FWGE is generally safe, and any side effects, such as diarrhea and flatulence, occur only occasionally.

Apple Skins Fight Alzheimer's Disease and Cancer

They contain high levels of *quercetin*, an antioxidant that may fight cell damage linked with these diseases.

Best: Eat at least one red apple a day. Quercetin also can be found in onions, raspberries, cherries, red wine, red grapes, citrus fruits, broccoli, leafy greens and green and black tea.

Chang Y. Lee, PhD, professor, department of food science, Cornell University, Geneva, New York.

Magical Food Combos That Fight Cancer

Karen Collins, MS, RD, registered dietitian and nutrition adviser to the American Institute for Cancer Research (*www.aicr.org*). A syndicated newspaper columnist and public speaker, she maintains a private nutrition counseling practice in Washington, DC.

Researchers know that some foods can help prevent cancer. Now there is growing evidence that certain food combinations may offer more protection against cancer than any one specific food.

The following combinations of foods are especially beneficial. *Eat them regularly—either at the same meal or separately throughout the week...*

TOMATOES AND BROCCOLI

Results of an animal study presented at the American Institute for Cancer Research International Research Conference showed that rats with tumors that were given a diet of tomatoes and broccoli had significantly smaller tumors than animals fed one of these foods.

The *lycopene* in tomatoes is an antioxidant. Antioxidants are crucial for preventing cancer because they help prevent unstable molecules, called free radicals, from damaging cell structures and DNA. Broccoli contains chemical compounds known as *glucosinolates*, which may be effective in flushing carcinogens from the body.

Also helpful: Combine broccoli or other cruciferous vegetables, such as brussels sprouts and cabbage, with foods that are high in selenium, such as shellfish and Brazil nuts. A study published by the UK's Institute of Food Research found that the combination of broccoli's glucosinolates and selenium has more powerful anticancer effects than either food eaten alone.

BRUSSELS SPROUTS AND BROCCOLI

These potent cancer-fighting vegetables also are rich in vitamin C and folate, as well as phytonutrients that deactivate carcinogens. When eaten in combination, brussels sprouts and broccoli may provide more protection than either one eaten alone.

Brussels sprouts have the phytonutrient *crambene*, which stimulates phase-2 enzymes, substances that help prevent carcinogens from damaging DNA. Broccoli is high in *indole-3-carbinol*, a phytonutrient that also stimulates phase-2 enzymes—but in a different way.

ORANGES, APPLES, GRAPES AND BLUEBERRIES

Each of these foods is very high in antioxidants. In a recent laboratory analysis, researchers measured the amount of antioxidants in each of these fruits individually. Then they combined them and still took additional measurements.

Result: The mixture of fruits was more powerful against free radicals than any one fruit alone.

CURCUMIN AND QUERCETIN

Curcumin is a phytonutrient found in the spice turmeric. *Quercetin* is a phytonutrient that is abundant in yellow onions, especially in the outermost rings. According to a small study in *Clinical Gastroenterology and Hepatology*, people who consumed large amounts of these two phytonutrients had a reduction in the number of colon polyps, growths that may turn into cancer.

The study looked at a small number of people with *familial adenomatous polyposis*, a hereditary condition that increases the likelihood of developing polyps. The phytochemical combination reduced the number of polyps by 60%. It also caused some polyps to shrink.

The researchers used concentrated forms of curcumin and quercetin. You would have to eat two-and-a-half tablespoons of turmeric daily to get a comparable amount. To get the necessary amount of quercetin, you would need to have about two-thirds cup of chopped onions daily.

Recommended: Eat a variety of herbs and spices to get the most phytonutrient protection. Even small amounts used frequently will impact your health over time. Among herbs, rosemary and oregano rank among the best phytonutrient sources. Ginger is another powerful spice.

TOMATOES AND FAT

The lycopene in tomatoes is particularly effective against prostate cancer—but only when it's consumed with a small amount of fat. Lycopene, like other members of the carotenoid chemical family, is a fat-soluble substance. The body can't absorb it efficiently in the absence of fat.

It takes only three to five grams of fat (about one teaspoon of oil) to improve the absorption of lycopene from tomatoes. For example, you could have a salad with an oil-based dressing. The type of fat doesn't matter for absorption of lycopene and other carotenoids, but you might as well choose a fat that promotes health. Olive oil and canola oil are good choices.

MORE VARIETY, LESS CANCER

In a recent study published in *The Journal of Nutrition*, researchers divided 106 women into two groups. All of the women were asked to eat eight to 10 servings of fruits and vegetables daily for two weeks. However, one of the groups (the high-diversity group) was told to include foods from 18 different botanical groups, including onions and garlic from the allium family, legumes, cruciferous vegetables, etc. The other group (the low-diversity one) was asked to concentrate all its choices among only five major groups.

Results: Women in both groups showed a decrease in *lipid peroxidation*—important for reducing the risk of cancer and heart disease. However, only the women in the high-diversity group showed a decrease in DNA oxidation, which is one of the steps that initiates cancer development.

The ways that chemicals work in the body, known as metabolic pathways, have a rate-limiting effect. This means that beyond a certain point, eating more of a specific food won't provide additional protection. Eating a wide variety of foods brings more metabolic pathways into play, thus bypassing this limiting effect.

A Medicinal Mushroom For Cancer?

Mark A. Stengler, NMD, licensed naturopathic medical doctor in private practice, Stengler Center for Integrative Medicine, Encinitas, California...adjunct associate clinical professor at the National College of Natural Medicine, Portland, Oregon...author of many books, including *The Natural Physician's Healing Therapies* and coauthor of *Prescription for Natural Cures* (both from Bottom Line Books)...and author of the *Bottom Line/Natural Healing* newsletter. *www.drstengler.com*

Researchers have been studying the health benefits of *Agaricus blazei* (A. blazei), an edible mushroom native to Brazil.

A. blazei appears to act as an antioxidant, to balance glucose within the body, prevent abnormal cell growth, bolster the immune system and attack existing tumor cells. Is it worth taking in supplement form?

HEALTH BENEFITS

Studies show the benefits of A. blazei for the following conditions...

• **Cancer.** In one study, patients with cervical, ovarian or endometrial cancer were treated with chemotherapy, plus either an oral A. blazei extract or a placebo. The activity of tumor-fighting cells was significantly higher in those taking A. blazei compared with those who took the placebo. Most striking: Patients taking A. blazei also suffered fewer side effects of chemotherapy, including hair loss, weakness and decreased appetite.

• **Hepatitis C.** A study in *Japanese Pharmacology & Therapeutics* suggests that A. blazei extract may be effective in treating hepatitis C. In 80% of study participants, A. blazei extract appeared to reduce levels of the liver enzyme *gamma-glutamyl transpeptidase* (GGT), an indicator of liver damage.

MY ADVICE

For those with any type of cancer (particularly those noted above) or hepatitis C, I recommend 1,500 milligrams (mg) to 3,000 mg daily of A. blazei. Have your doctor determine the dose and monitor your response, including blood glucose levels. (A. blazei can improve insulin resistance, a condition in which the body doesn't use insulin properly.)

Caution: A. blazei should not be taken by anyone on immune-suppressing transplant medications—these patients do not want their immune system to reject the new organ. Avoid A. blazei if you have an autoimmune disease (such as rheumatoid arthritis) in which the immune system already is overactive. Good choice: Nutraceutics Rx AgariPure Agaricus Blazei Murrill extract at American Nutrition (800-454-3724, *www.americannutrition.com*, $29.95 for 120 500-mg capsules).

Another Reason to Love Olive Oil

Henrik E. Poulsen, MD, professor of clinical pharmacology and the head of the department of clinical pharmacology at Rigshospitalet, University Hospital, Copenhagen, Denmark.

It's no news that omega-3 fatty acid and phenolic-rich olive oil is good for your heart. However, the virtues of olive oil seem now to extend into the rest of the body as well, according to new research. Noting that the incidence of breast, large bowel, ovary and prostate cancer is lower in Mediterranean countries than in Northern Europe —and that the association between olive oil and cancer reduction has been established— researchers wondered whether olive oil with higher amounts of phenolic compounds may be even more protective.

WHAT'S HEALTHY ABOUT OLIVE OIL?

Researchers believed it was probably the phenolic compounds—healthful plant compounds, abundant in olive oil—that were delivering the cancer-fighting benefits, so they tested three different olive oils with three different phenolic concentrations—high, medium and low. For the study, they divided 182 healthy European men between 20 and 60 years old, from five different countries (Denmark, Finland, Germany, Italy and Spain) into three groups. Each group consumed 25 milliliters (0.84 oz.) of one kind of the olive oils at a time. After three weeks on each of the three olive oils, with a two-week washout period in between, their urine was tested for presence of a substance (8oxodG) considered a reliable measure of oxidative damage.

It turned out to not even matter which kind of olive oil the men had been consuming, since all had noticeably reduced measures of 8oxodG. It seems to have been the olive oil itself that had made the difference, regardless of phenol content. "It is likely the monounsaturated fat in the olive oil is the protective element," one of the study's co-authors, Henrik Poulsen, MD, professor of clinical pharmacology, Rigshospitalet, University Hospital, Copenhagen, Denmark, told me, since it is known to have anti-inflammatory properties. Dr. Poulsen speculates that other oils high in monounsaturated fat, such as macadamia nut oil and almond oil, may be cancer-protective as well, though this study only examined olive oil.

EXTRA VIRGIN WORTH EXTRA INVESTMENT

Phenolic compounds are always touted as one of the virtues of extra-virgin olive oil, since they are better preserved than in the other, less expensive olive oils. I asked Dr. Poulsen if there was any benefit to paying the higher price for these. Yes, he said, the extra virgin olive oil is worth the extra investment. Not only is it subject to the least processing and heat exposure, but it also works harder for your health than regular or light olive oils. "Our other research shows that the high phenolic content of extra virgin olive oil is what's protective against arteriosclerosis," he told me. "Extra virgin olive oil gives you the best of both worlds."

Exercise and Coffee May Fight Skin Cancer

Skin cancer develops in cells whose DNA has been damaged by UV radiation—but damaged cells often die before becoming malignant. The death rate of precancerous skin cells in mice that received exercise and oral caffeine was nearly 400% greater than in mice that had neither exercise nor caffeine.

Allan H. Conney, PhD, professor of pharmacology and director of the Susan Lehman Cullman Laboratory for Cancer Research, Rutgers State University of New Jersey, Piscataway, and coauthor of a study published in *Proceedings of the National Academy of Sciences.*

Lentils May Prevent Breast Cancer

Women who ate one-half cup of lentils at least twice a week were 24% less likely to develop breast cancer, compared with women who ate the same amount of lentils less than once a month or not at all.

Theory: Lentils' protective effects may be due to particular types of phytochemicals. One-half cup of lentils has 9 grams (g) of protein, 8 g of fiber, 3 milligrams of iron and only 115 calories. And they are inexpensive. Add lentils while cooking soups and whole grains, and use cooked lentils in salads.

Clement A. Adebamowo, MD, DSc, associate professor of epidemiology and public health, department of epidemiology and preventive medicine, Institute of Human Virology, member of the Greenebaum Cancer Center, School of Medicine, University of Maryland, Baltimore, and coauthor of a study of 90,630 women, published in *International Journal of Cancer*.

Cancer-Prevention Pill

Mark A. Stengler, NMD, licensed naturopathic medical doctor in private practice, Stengler Center for Integrative Medicine, Encinitas, California...adjunct associate clinical professor at the National College of Natural Medicine, Portland, Oregon...author of many books, including *The Natural Physician's Healing Therapies* and coauthor of *Prescription for Natural Cures* (both from Bottom Line Books)...and author of the *Bottom Line/Natural Healing* newsletter. *www.drstengler.com*.

Some people don't have the time—or taste buds—for a full day's worth of fruits and vegetables. That's when the capsule form of the cancer-fighting compound *sulphoraphane glucosinolate* (SGS) comes in handy. I recommend it for people with a family history of cancer...as a complement to ongoing cancer treatments (with your doctor's approval)...for those who have been exposed to toxins...and for all who want to reduce their risk of cancer.

The supplement company Xymogen (*www.xymogen.com*) markets OncoPlex SGS, which contains 30 mg of SGS per capsule. Though it does not require a prescription, it is not sold in health-food stores and usually is purchased through holistic doctors.

In general, I advise taking one capsule daily. If you have had cancer or are undergoing cancer treatment, increase to two to four capsules daily, under the supervision of your doctor.

Red Wine—It's Like the New Green Vegetable

Jeffrey B. Schwimmer, MD, director, Fatty Liver Clinic Children's Hospital, and assistant professor of pediatrics and director, quality improvement, division of gastroenterology, hepatology, and nutrition, department of pediatrics, University of California, both in San Diego, California.

Red wine seems to be the new "green vegetable"...good for practically everything. New research points to a surprising and counterintuitive connection between moderate wine consumption and the lower risk of a certain kind of liver disease...plus, I recently saw another study that suggests serving red wine with steaks can help diminish the harmful effects associated with eating red meat. Once again it appears that modern science is confirming age-old wisdom, in this case those who revered the "nectar of the Gods."

SHALL WE DRINK TO THAT?

Of course, experts are quick to point out that wine is beneficial to your health in moderation only. *That said, following are a sample of the many benefits that moderate wine consumption may confer upon your health...*

• **Lowers risk of liver disease.** Considered by some to be an emerging epidemic, *nonalcoholic fatty liver disease* (NAFLD) has become the most common chronic liver disease in the United States today, due in large part to our Western lifestyle and obesity, notes study author Jeffrey B. Schwimmer, MD, at the University of California, San Diego. He and his colleagues found that moderate wine drinkers are significantly less likely to develop NAFLD than nondrinkers, even after controlling for other possible contributing factors.

• **Healthier heart.** Wine in particular possesses potent heart-healthy benefits, according to a large-scale study, published in 2000, which included Copenhagen City Heart Study data. Researchers found the risk of death significantly lower than for people who did not drink wine and believe it's due to ethanol and the substances in wine. Other research shows that the high polyphenol content in red wine protects the linings of cardiovascular blood vessels and may inhibit plaque formation.

• **Prostate cancer protection.** Men who drink four to seven glasses of red wine weekly are half as likely to be diagnosed with prostate cancer as men who do not drink red wine, according to research from the Fred Hutchinson Cancer Research Center in Seattle. Doctors speculate that healthful antioxidant compounds such as flavonoids and resveratrol are responsible for this effect. White wine was helpful too, but not as much as red wine, which is a richer source of these health-promoting compounds.

• **Kidney care.** Drinking at least two glasses of red wine a week may lower the risk of kidney cancer, say doctors at the Karolinska Institutet in Sweden. Beneficial effects were also found with white wine and strong beer, but not liquor. Other research, conducted in part at Harvard Medical School, suggests that men who consume seven or more drinks weekly have a 29% lower risk of developing kidney problems.

• **Longer life.** One day resveratrol may prove to be the key to unlocking the secret of lasting youth. Laboratory tests demonstrate that this antioxidant compound in red wine prevents early death in mice that were fed high-fat diets. Yet so far no human research has taken place, so further study is needed.

TO YOUR HEALTH

So it seems there's some merit to such toasts as "salud" (health) and "l'chaim" (to life). Enjoying a glass of red wine with your evening meal may indeed improve your health and extend your life -- but do so with restraint, and drink at mealtime, since food slows alcohol absorption. Most experts suggest that an intake of one to two glasses of wine a day for men and one for women is optimal for health benefits. More, however, may increase the risk of some of the consequences of excessive alcohol consumption. Red wines have more polyphenols than white (which, as noted above, can also be beneficial) but not all red wines offer equal potency of this health-promoting

compound. A study in the scientific journal *Nature* reported that the most powerful heart-healthy polyphenols are procyanidins, which is the main source of the vascular health benefits in red wine. Wines from Southern France and Sardinia were found to have higher concentrations, due to production methods. Other research shows that the darker the wine, in general, the healthier.

However none of this is meant to suggest you ought to cultivate a wine habit if you don't want to or don't particularly enjoy it. Immoderate alcohol consumption has a greater negative effect than the positive beneficial effects. Dr. Schwimmer takes cautionary advice a step further, warning that people at risk for alcohol abuse or alcoholism (for example, those with a personal or family history) should not consume wine or other alcoholic beverages. Fortunately for teetotalers, there's an excellent alternative—red grape juice and grapes themselves are rich sources of many of the same beneficial compounds as red wine. Other antioxidant-packed options include blueberries, cranberries, elderberries and pomegranates. If you're worried about the consequences of imbibing too much nectar of the Gods, just reach for a bunch of grapes.

The Power of Yogurt

Yogurt reduces risk for bladder cancer. A recent study found that consuming two or more servings of yogurt a day was associated with a 45% reduction in bladder cancer for women and a 36% reduction in men, compared with people who didn't consume yogurt.

Why: The researchers believe that lactic acid bacteria in yogurt may destroy harmful carcinogens that otherwise may form in the bladder.

Susanna C. Larsson, PhD, division of nutritional epidemiology, National Institute of Environmental Medicine, Karolinska Institutet, Stockholm, Sweden.

Onions and Garlic Curb Cancer Risk

In a 13-year study of the diets of about 25,000 people, participants who ate the most onions and/or garlic were 10% to 88% less likely to develop several types of cancer—including colorectal, esophageal, oral and ovarian—than those who ate the least.

Theory: Onions and garlic contain antioxidants, including allicin and quercetin, that prevent cell damage that can lead to cancer.

Self-defense: Aim to eat one-half cup of onions (any type) and/or one to two cloves of garlic (chopped or crushed) several times weekly.

Carlotta Galeone, PhD, researcher, Mario Negri Institute of Pharmacological Research, Milan, Italy.

Ultimate Cancer-Fighting Food...Now in Capsule Form, Too

Mark A. Stengler, NMD, licensed naturopathic medical doctor in private practice, Stengler Center for Integrative Medicine, Encinitas, California...adjunct associate clinical professor at the National College of Natural Medicine, Portland, Oregon...author of many books, including *The Natural Physician's Healing Therapies* and coauthor of *Prescription for Natural Cures* (both from Bottom Line Books)...and author of the *Bottom Line/Natural Healing* newsletter. *www.drstengler.com.*

I do not like broccoli. I haven't liked it since I was a little kid and my mother made me eat it. I'm president of the United States, and I'm not going to eat any more broccoli!" George H.W. Bush spoke these words early in his tenure at the White House. Unfortunately, he is missing out on a potent cancer-fighting food.

If you share the former president's aversion to broccoli, you'll be happy to learn of new alternatives that offer even more health benefits. *First, some background information...*

DEFICIENT DIETS

Researchers have published eye-opening studies on the compound *sulforaphane*, found in broccoli and similar vegetables. Sulforaphane helps prevent cancers of the breast, ovary, prostate, bone, brain, bladder, liver, lung and stomach, and combats other conditions associated with aging and cell death.

It is no secret that the average American fails to consume the seven to nine daily servings of fruits and vegetables recommended to provide dietary protection against cancer and other diseases. And for many people, the produce they do eat seldom includes the recommended one to two daily servings of cruciferous vegetables (so called because the plants' flowers have four petals arranged like a crucifix), such as cauliflower, kale, bok choy, rutabagas, radishes, turnips, brussels sprouts and, of course, broccoli. An analysis published in *The Journal of Nutrition*, which looked at dietary data on 4,806 men and women ages 25 to 75, revealed that just 3% of the group consumed broccoli during either of two typical days. Consumption of dark green vegetables averaged just one-fifth of a serving per day.

Cruciferous vegetables are a rich source of healthful plant chemicals called phytochemicals or phytonutrients. These include cancer-fighting *thiols* (such as the sulfur-containing glucosinolates) and *indoles* (which bind chemical carcinogens and activate detoxifying enzymes). Yet even veggie lovers may find it difficult to ingest therapeutic amounts of cruciferous vegetables on a regular basis. This problem is compounded by the fact that cooking can destroy phytonutrients, so health benefits are diminished unless the vegetables are consumed raw or lightly steamed.

SGS DISCOVERED

Scientists at the Johns Hopkins University School of Medicine identified the compound *sulforaphane glucosinolate* (SGS)—a naturally occurring precursor to sulforaphane—in 1992 and began to research its cancer-fighting potential. Leading this effort was Paul Talalay, MD, a professor of pharmacology and director of the university's Laboratory for Molecular Sciences.

His strategy: To support the body's natural detoxification capacity to fight cancer-causing chemicals and cell-damaging free radicals. It is well accepted that cell DNA controls replication of cells and that damage to cell DNA is an important factor in the development of cancer.

In 1994, Dr. Talalay looked at the impact of SGS on mammary (breast) tumors in rats exposed to a potent carcinogen. Results were astounding. The number of rats that developed tumors was reduced by as much as 60%...the number of tumors in each animal was reduced by 80%...and the size of the tumors that did develop was reduced by 75%. Subsequently, hundreds of other test tube and animal studies have confirmed the anticancer properties of sulforaphane.

Toxins (natural and man-made) go through phases of breakdown in the cells of the body, particularly the liver. *Sulforaphane promotes detoxification by...*

• **Supporting enzymes that destroy carcinogens.**

• **Stimulating longer-lasting protective antioxidant effects than other nutrients do.**

• **Replenishing the cells' levels of the amino acid glutathione, strengthening the immune system.**

• **Inhibiting COX-2, an inflammatory enzyme that contributes to cancerous changes in cells.**

• **Limiting DNA damage and abnormal cell growth.**

SUPER SPROUTS

Dr. Talalay discovered that various types of fresh and frozen broccoli differed significantly in the amounts of SGS they contained—and that the older the broccoli was, the lower its SGS. Painstaking research uncovered certain varieties of three-day-old broccoli sprouts—which look like a cross between alfalfa sprouts and bean sprouts—that contained up to 50 times more SGS than mature, cooked broccoli. One ounce of these sprouts could provide as much SGS as three pounds of cooked broccoli.

This set the stage for a fascinating study, published in *Cancer Epidemiology Biomarkers & Prevention*. The study was conducted in a rural area near Shanghai where liver cancer is common because local grain is contaminated with *aflatoxin*, a carcinogen produced by mold.

In the study, broccoli sprouts with known levels of SGS were grown at the site in China. Three days after the shoots emerged from the soil, the sprouts were picked and used to prepare a liquid extract to ensure standard dosages. One hundred local residents drank five ounces of diluted extract in tea form (equal to eating two ounces of sprouts) daily for two weeks. A control group drank a tea indistinguishable in taste and appearance but containing no SGS.

Great results: Analysis of the participants' urine showed that in people who drank the SGS extract, carcinogens were being removed from the body—providing the first direct evidence that broccoli sprouts can enhance the human body's detoxifying system, reducing the risk of cancer.

NEW WAYS TO GET GREENS

Broccoli sprouts and SGS are safe for everyone. (If you have thyroid problems, check with your doctor—there is a slight risk that broccoli sprouts may suppress thyroid function. There is no concern with the SGS supplement.) Because the SGS content of broccoli sprouts can vary greatly depending on seed type and growing methods, I recommend the sprouts developed by the Johns Hopkins team. These are now available under the brand name BroccoSprouts, from Brassica Protection Products LLC (877-747-1277, *www.brassica.com*). Sold in health-food and grocery stores nationwide, these broccoli sprouts contain standardized and therapeutic amounts of sulforaphane.

Alternatively, you can grow your own broccoli sprouts. Order the seeds from the Mail Order Catalog for Healthy Eating (800-695-2241).

For optimal health, eat one-half cup (one ounce) of BroccoSprouts every other day. Each serving contains 73 mg of SGS. They are most beneficial when eaten raw, so sprinkle them on salads and sandwiches. The taste is similar to that of a radish, with a spicy flavor that results from the release of sulforaphane as you chew. Even people who hate broccoli usually enjoy the tangy taste of broccoli sprouts.

Miracles Do Happen— True Stories of Spontaneous Healing

Joan Borysenko, PhD, cofounder and former director of the mind-body clinical programs at two Harvard Medical School hospitals, now merged as Boston's Beth Israel Deaconess Medical Center. Based in Boulder, Colorado, she runs workshops and conducts lectures on mind-body healing. *Minding the Body, Mending the Mind* (Da Capo). *joanborysenko.com*. She is also founding partner of Mind/Body Health Sciences, LLC in Boulder.

O n occasion, a health problem that was expected to be permanent or fatal instead disappears without medical intervention. The limited research that has been done suggests that the reason why one person recovers when most others do not might have as much to do with the mind as the body.

We interviewed Joan Borysenko, PhD, a former Harvard medical scientist who is a renowned expert in the field of mind/body healing. *She relayed these true stories of spontaneous healing…*

MIND/BODY CURE

In 1985, Alice Epstein, a sociology doctoral student at the University of Massachusetts, was diagnosed with kidney cancer. One of her kidneys was removed, but it was no use—the cancer had spread to her lungs, and treatment was impossible. Epstein was told she had only a few more months to live.

With no way to treat the physical problem, Epstein and her psychology-professor husband decided to treat her mind. Epstein used meditation to reduce her stress, and psychotherapy to deal with the angry, unhappy com-

ponent of her personality. Within six weeks, tests showed that her cancer was going into remission. Her progress slowed when she took time off from the intensive psychotherapy but resumed once the psychotherapy resumed. The cancer eventually disappeared. Epstein earned her PhD and is still alive today, more than 20 years later.

What may have happened. Eliminating stress and anger will not cure every disease, but it can trigger a host of biochemical changes in the body—including providing a boost to the immune system. It is possible that Epstein's aggressive mental treatments played a role in her return to physical health.

A VISION IN LOURDES

Nearly 150 years ago, a teenage girl in Lourdes, France, reported seeing a vision of the Virgin Mary. Ever since, the waters in that area have been credited with healing powers. Most of these incidents involve cancer, multiple sclerosis and other diseases that occasionally go into remission, even without a visit to Lourdes.

The 1908 case of Marie Bire is more interesting. The 41-year-old French woman was blind as a result of optic atrophy—the degeneration of her optic nerve. According to medical science, it should not have been possible for optic nerves to recover from such a condition.

At Lourdes, the blind Bire attended Mass and received Holy Communion. Then, as the Blessed Sacrament in procession was passing the place where she sat, she suddenly regained her sight. Ten doctors examined Bire. They all found that her optic nerves were still withered but that she could see.

What may have happened. We do not have to believe in divine miracles to believe that Bire's faith might have played a role in her recovery. Studies have found that depending upon the medical condition, between 30% and 50% of people respond to placebos. If you tell these people that you have given them painkillers, their brain activity will show that they actually feel less pain.

CONFIDENCE DESPITE THE ODDS

In 1975, Ian Gawler, a 24-year-old Australian veterinarian and decathlete, learned that he

113

had bone cancer in his right leg. The leg was amputated, but the cancer reappeared later that year and spread throughout his body. In 1976, Gawler was given two weeks to live. No one had ever been known to recover from such an advanced case of this form of cancer. As a doctor, Gawler knew that the reasonable response was to prepare for death. Instead, he remained certain that he would recover. He focused on meditation, positive thinking and a natural diet.

Gawler did recover. He now runs The Gawler Foundation (*www.gawler.org*), which provides support for others suffering from serious illnesses. The foundation stresses healthy food, meditation and belief in recovery.

What may have happened. We cannot simply imagine cancer away, but there is reason to think that believing in the desired health outcome might improve the odds that it will occur.

SURROUNDED BY LOVE

Fifty years ago, the outlook was bleak for those suffering psychotic hallucinations. Today's pharmaceuticals and cognitive behavior therapy were not yet available. Recovery was very rare.

That was bad news for one previously healthy 10-year-old girl growing up in the 1950s. Her nightmares had entered her waking life—she saw snakes, scorpions and headhunters. The girl believed that these tormentors were going to kill her family and that the only way she could stop them was to repeat obsessive-compulsive behaviors, such as scraping the inside of her mouth with her fingernails, reading books only upside down and backward, rereading each sentence three times and erasing everything she wrote three times before continuing. The girl eventually was pulled from school and lived each day in a landscape of terror.

For months, she prayed intensely for a cure. One day during these prayers, she suddenly felt surrounded by love and wisdom, as though she were being held in the arms of God. Her fear instantly disappeared, and she stopped her obsessive-compulsive behavior cold turkey. Within days, all of her symptoms were gone, never to return.

I was that little girl. The experience sparked my lifelong interest in psychology and in spirituality.

What may have happened. Most people with mental disorders cannot just pray their way to recovery. Still, it is worth noting that many people who experience spontaneous healing also experience a transformative spiritual episode similar to mine—a single moment when they feel aided by a loving, powerful outside force.

HOW TO USE YOUR MIND TO HEAL

Some things we can do when we are seriously ill that will benefit our overall health...

Do not let your mind be pulled into worry or into the past or the future. Spend time each day doing something that makes you feel good and keeps you in the present, whether it is gardening, meditating or walking in nature.

Forgive any wrongs that have been done to you. Letting go of anger and regrets can reduce stress and boost your immune system.

Have gratitude. Before going to bed, be truly grateful for something that happened that day. Wasn't it wonderful when someone smiled at you? Soak up these positive feelings.

Imagine the health outcome that you desire. Picture the disease disappearing from your body. If you have trouble visualizing a positive health outcome, begin by picturing other things that make you happy.

Sweet Cancer Prevention

The sweet-tasting compound in licorice, *glycyrrhizic acid*, has been shown in animal studies to help stop the progression of colon cancer. The finding may lead to new approaches to preventing malignancies of the colon.

Vanderbilt University Medical Center.

Heat Is Good

Heat may kill some cancer cells directly and render others more responsive to radiation treatment.

Recent finding: Treating superficial (or "contained") tumors in tissue of the breast, cervix, head, neck and skin with hyperthermia—gradually increasing the temperature of the cancerous tissue to between 105°F and 113°F—reduced the risk of recurrence by 68%.

Ellen Jones, MD, PhD, associate professor, department of radiation oncology, Duke University School of Medicine, Durham, North Carolina, and leader of a study of 109 patients with recurrent, superficial cancers, published in *Journal of Clinical Oncology*.

Breast Cancers That Disappear Without Treatment

Susan Love, MD, adjunct professor of surgery, David Geffen School of Medicine, UCLA, Los Angeles, California. Dr. Love is founder, president and medical director of the Dr. Susan Love Research Foundation (*www.dslrf.org*) and author of *Dr. Susan Love's Breast Book* (Da Capo).

Mammograms save many lives, but screening for breast cancer also produces many false positive results—leading to unnecessary, invasive testing, not to mention untold anxiety for women and their loved ones. A recent study has identified yet another concern. In Norway, investigators found that women who underwent screening mammography were significantly more likely to be diagnosed with breast cancer than those who did not get screened, leading to the possibility that some breast cancers disappear spontaneously on their own without treatment. It's an intriguing finding, given how much time, cost and anxiety is associated with diagnosing breast cancer—even more

so when you consider how many women might not require aggressive treatment, including potent drugs, powerful radiation and painful, disfiguring surgery, for cancers that might disappear on their own.

We spoke with one of the country's leading breast cancer authorities, Susan Love, MD, a clinical professor of surgery at UCLA's David Geffen School of Medicine, founder of the Dr. Susan Love Research Foundation (*www.dslrf.org*) and author of *Dr. Susan Love's Breast Book*. She called the study "extremely encouraging," noting it might someday enable researchers to identify which types of breast cancers require treatment and which can simply be monitored...but she cautions that we're not there yet. At present, women should continue to get their regularly scheduled mammograms.

MORE SCREENING = MORE POSITIVE DIAGNOSES

In the study, investigators compared the number of breast cancers detected in two groups of Norwegian women, ages 50 to 64 (over 100,000 participants), who underwent mammography screening. One group received three mammograms between 1996 and 2001 as part of a new national screening program. The other group had just a single screening in 1997.

Theoretically, these comparable groups should have the same number of cancers, says Dr. Love. Yet that did not prove to be the case. Researchers found 22% more breast cancers in the women who underwent more frequent mammograms. This raises the possibility that left untreated, these tumors might have spontaneously regressed. It's not such a far-fetched theory, given that scientists already know of at least one other cancer—a rare childhood cancer called a *neuroblastoma*—that is known to regress without treatment in as many as 7% of cases that are detected through screening.

These results were published in the *Archives of Internal Medicine*. Though the study results raised a hubbub, Dr. Love didn't find them surprising and said she suspects the type that disappears on its own might be one called "almost normal" breast cancer because it is so non-aggressive. "It's just a hunch though," she

115

notes—agreeing with the researchers that further study is required.

"WATCH AND WAIT" A POSSIBLE NEW APPROACH?

Just as "watch and wait" is a treatment strategy for some prostate cancers, perhaps research will identify certain types of breast cancers that can safely be approached in the same way, says Dr. Love. Looking ahead, she notes that this and similar studies may even lead to changes in what's considered "cancer." It may be that in some people, some groups of abnormal cells may appear that will never develop into a life-threatening tumor and should not be referred to—or more importantly treated as—cancer.

As things now stand, though, it's impossible to predict whether a tumor will spontaneously regress, nor will that likely be possible anytime soon. For now, the American Cancer Society (*www.cancer.org*) recommends that women get an annual mammogram beginning at age 40. Women at high risk—those with a family history of breast cancer or who test positive for a genetic mutation in BRCA 1 or BRCA 2 genes—should also get an MRI. If you are uncertain, consult your physician to determine your risk level.

Raspberries May Prevent Oral Cancer

The pulp of black raspberries contains antioxidants and anti-inflammatory acids that may slow the growth of—or even eliminate—cancerous lesions in the mouth. Researchers now are testing a raspberry-based gel for treatment of lesions. Oral cancer, generally associated with alcohol and tobacco use, causes 8,000 deaths in the US each year.

Russell J. Mumper, PhD, vice chair and associate professor of pharmaceutical sciences, University of Kentucky, Lexington.

Vitamin C...A Natural Form of Chemotherapy

Mark A. Stengler, NMD, licensed naturopathic medical doctor in private practice, Stengler Center for Integrative Medicine, Encinitas, California...adjunct associate clinical professor at the National College of Natural Medicine, Portland, Oregon...author of many books, including *The Natural Physician's Healing Therapies* and coauthor of *Prescription for Natural Cures* (both from Bottom Line Books)...and author of the *Bottom Line/Natural Healing* newsletter. *www.drstengler.com*

Most people have never heard of intravenous (IV) vitamin C, and yet it is one of the best alternative therapies to fight cancer. As most people know, vitamin C is an antioxidant with an immune-boosting effect. But when I—and a host of other natural physicians—administer it at very high doses, it plays an altogether different role, acting like a type of natural chemotherapy and killing cancer cells. When used in conjunction with regular chemotherapy, IV vitamin C works right alongside it, helping to kill cancer cells while also boosting the immune system and helping the body to rid itself of unwanted waste products.

At my clinic, I use IV vitamin C treatment for patients at all stages of cancer. All of these patients are also under the care of an oncologist. I give IV vitamin C to cancer patients at the outset of their treatment, to those who have tried conventional treatments to no avail and to those in remission who want an immune system boost. For patients with terminal disease, it helps to improve quality of life by increasing their energy and reducing nausea.

The use of vitamins in the treatment of cancer is controversial, extending back 40 years to when Nobel Laureate Linus Pauling, PhD, first proposed the use of high-dose vitamin C in the treatment of cancer. Many oncologists today remain skeptical about using any type of vitamin therapy in the treatment of cancer. Cancer specialists maintain that some types of chemotherapy and radiation kill cancer cells by generating large numbers of destructive free radicals. Because vitamin C is an antioxidant, they believe that it will neutralize these free radicals and reduce the effectiveness of chemotherapy and radiation.

I think this view is simplistic. At low doses (under 25 grams, or 25,000 milligrams), vitamin C's antioxidant properties do help to neutralize disease-causing free radicals. But at doses higher than 25 grams, vitamin C has a pro-oxidant effect that exploits a weakness in the biochemistry of cancer cells and increases production of hydrogen peroxide, an acid that has been shown to kill cancer cells without harming healthy cells.

It's impossible to achieve the required high concentrations of vitamin C through oral supplements alone. The body regulates the amount of vitamin C that can be absorbed through the gut, and very large amounts of the vitamin will cause diarrhea. Intravenous vitamin C bypasses this problem because it goes directly into the bloodstream. I provide my patients with IV vitamin C in the office. They lie comfortably in a reclining chair during a one- to two-hour treatment session, at which time they receive doses of 30 grams to 75 grams of vitamin C.

PROMISING RESEARCH

The benefits of IV vitamin C for cancer patients has been demonstrated in studies, including those by researchers at the National Institutes of Health. Laboratory studies have shown that IV vitamin C kills cancer cells but not normal cells. Studies by physicians at University of Kansas Medical Center in Kansas City, for example, described two cases in which patients suffering from advanced ovarian cancer underwent surgery and then received chemotherapy and IV vitamin C. Three years after treatment, both women had no sign of disease, which is quite unusual, because the prognosis for ovarian cancer typically is quite poor. Other research has shown the benefit of this treatment for terminally ill patients. A Korean study found that a combination of IV and oral vitamin C improved quality of life, reducing nausea and increasing energy in terminally ill patients.

Most researchers agree that data from large clinical trials is needed. Several clinical trials currently are under way to assess the effect of IV vitamin C and other antioxidants on different types of cancers.

WHAT TO DO

Many oncologists will not advocate vitamin therapy in any form.

My advice: While you're undergoing conventional therapy, look for a medical doctor or naturopathic physician experienced in IV therapies to work with your oncologist. You and your doctors can decide whether to administer IV vitamins during or immediately after receiving conventional therapies. Your doctor will determine the number of treatments you need. Some patients get one or two IV vitamin C infusions weekly for the first year after diagnosis and initial treatment for cancer, and then every other week for a few years to help prevent cancer cells from returning and to boost the immune system.

Large amounts of vitamin C are nontoxic and generally safe for everyone except those with kidney failure, who can't tolerate large amounts. In addition, a small percentage of people are deficient in the enzyme *glucose-6-phosphate dehydrogenase* (G6PD), which is needed to maintain normal red blood cells. Without this enzyme, large amounts of vitamin C can cause *hemolytic anemia*, a type of anemia that involves the abnormal breakdown of red blood cells. Before receiving IV vitamin C, ask your doctor to test you for this deficiency. If you have it, you should not have IV vitamin C.

Note that patients' response to cancer treatment of any kind varies, and no physician can ever know for certain how a tumor will respond to a specific treatment.

Red Chili Pepper Fights Cancer

It contains *capsaicin*, an anti-inflammatory that is effective against cancer cells. In tests, capsaicin caused cancer cells to die without damaging normal ones. Though clinical trials are needed before a recommendation to eat chili pepper can be made, it can be enjoyed as part of your regular diet.

Sanjay K. Srivastava, PhD, associate professor of biomedical sciences Texas Tech University Health Sciences Center School of Pharmacy, Amarillo, Texas.

Exercise: Rx for Cancer

Melinda Irwin, PhD, associate professor, Yale School of Public Health.

Claudio Battaglini, PhD, assistant professor, Department of Exercise and Sport Science, University of North Carolina.

Julie Goodale, personal trainer and certified cancer exercise trainer in New York. *www.life-cise.com*

Keith Block, MD, medical director of the Block Center for Integrative Cancer Treatment in Chicago, and author of Life Over Cancer (Bantam). *www.blockmd.com*

The oncologists have finally taken a lesson from the fitness instructors.

"Oncologists should recommend exercise to their patients, because of the accumulating scientific evidence that exercise can improve both the quality of life and the prognosis for cancer patients," says Melinda Irwin, PhD, of Yale University, at a recent annual meeting of the American Association for Cancer Research. As one standout example of that evidence, Dr. Irwin cited a study showing that regular physical activity can reduce the death rate by 67% in breast cancer patients—a reduction, she says, that matches "standard medical treatments" for the disease.

However, continues Dr. Irwin, only half of cancer patients say that their oncologists even mention exercise.

It's well worth their mentioning it—and you hearing about it. Because if you're in the midst of a cancer treatment such as chemotherapy or radiation and want to reduce side effects such as fatigue...or if you're a cancer survivor who wants to prevent the recurrence of cancer...or if you've never set foot in an oncologist's office, but want to prevent cancer from happening in the first place—recent studies show there's probably no stronger Rx than exercise.

NEWEST RESEARCH

Dozens of new studies show that exercise can help you walk (or run or bike or swim) away from cancer.

•**Preventing cancer.** In a 17-year study of more than 2,600 men, Finnish researchers found that men who exercised an average of 30 minutes a day had a 37% lower risk of developing and dying from any cancer. The findings were in the *British Journal of Sports Medicine.*

•**Preventing prostate cancer.** Researchers at the Duke University Medical Center studied 190 men who had a prostate biopsy (removal of tissue to test for cancer). Those who had been exercising regularly had a 35% lower risk of having the disease. And among those who had prostate cancer, exercise was linked to a 14% lower risk of developing an aggressive, faster-growing form of the disease. The findings were in the *Journal of Urology.*

In another study, researchers at the National Cancer Institute found that four or more hours of exercise a week decreased the risk of prostate cancer in African-American men by 41%. (Black men have a 30 to 50% higher risk for prostate cancer, and often develop a more aggressive form of the disease, with a death rate twice as high as white men.)

•**Preventing endometrial cancer.** Researchers at the National Cancer Institute analyzed health data from more than 109,000 women and found that those who exercised five or more times a week had a 23% lower risk of developing endometrial cancer, compared with those who rarely exercised. When they focused their analysis on overweight women, they found those who exercised lowered their risk by 39%.

•**Preventing breast cancer.** In a study of more than 110,000 postmenopausal women, those who engaged in more than seven hours per week of moderate or vigorous exercise for the previous 10 years had a 16% lower risk of developing breast cancer, compared with inactive women. The findings were in *BMC Cancer.*

•**Preventing the recurrence of breast cancer.** Researchers in Canada analyzed health data from more than 1,200 breast cancer survivors and found that those who exercised the most had a 56% lower risk of dying from breast cancer (or any other cause), compared with those who exercised the least. The findings were in the *International Journal of Cancer.*

And in a Chinese study on more than 1,800 breast cancer survivors, those who engaged in any type of regular exercise—such as taking a brisk, 45-minute walk three days a week—reported less emotional distress, better body image, better relationships and a greater ability to engage in the daily activities of work or school.

• **Surviving colon cancer.** Researchers at the Harvard School of Public Health studied 668 men with colon cancer—and found that those who exercised the most had a 53% lower risk of dying from the disease, compared with men who exercised the least. The findings were in *Annals of Internal Medicine.*

• **Help for leukemia fatigue.** Researchers at the UNC Lineberger Comprehensive Cancer Center at the University of North Carolina at Chapel Hill found that regular exercise (a customized program that could include stretching, aerobic exercise, strength training, and "core" exercises such as Pilates) can dramatically relieve fatigue and depression in people with leukemia, with fatigue decreasing by 64% and depression by 40%.

"This result is important because of the numerous side effects related to cancer treatment for leukemia, which requires confinement to a hospital room for four to six weeks to avoid the risk of infection," says Claudio Battaglini, PhD, the study leader.

"We have demonstrated that these patients not only can complete an exercise program in the hospital, but that they receive both physical and psychological benefits that could assist in their recovery." The findings were published in *Integrative Cancer Therapies.*

• **Cancer survivors—exercise, and survive longer.** Researchers in England found that cancer survivors who engaged in at least three, 20-minute sessions of vigorous exercise a week were 53% less likely to die, compared with people who didn't exercise. The findings were in *Cancer Causes and Control.*

WHOLE BODY FITNESS PROGRAM

"It used to be that oncologists told cancer patients to go home and rest—they were treated as if they were fragile, like china," says Keith Block, MD, Medical Director of the Block Center for Integrative Cancer Treatment in Chicago, Director of Integrative Medical Education at the University of Illinois College of Medicine, and author of *Life Over Cancer* (Bantam). "But the most recent research shows the more exercise you get, the better your odds of surviving cancer and reducing the debilitating side effects of cancer treatment."

Dr. Block's treatment for his cancer patients includes a "whole-body fitness program" that consists of…

• **Muscle strengthening** (through resistance training, using either weights or resistance bands such as Thera-bands),

• **Muscle lengthening** (through stretching or yoga),

• **Cardiovascular endurance** (through an aerobic exercise such as walking) and

• **Cardiovascular recovery** (also called "interval training," or short, intense bursts of aerobic exercise).

"Individualize your exercise program to your needs and capabilities," says Dr. Block. For those who have been sedentary, he says the ideal fitness program consists of regular, short bouts of low-to-moderate exercise that increases in intensity and duration as your fitness improves.

Start slow, increase gradually. That opinion is seconded by Julie Goodale, a personal trainer and certified cancer exercise trainer in New York.

"In spite of feeling exhausted from cancer treatments or being really out of shape, find an activity you enjoy and try exercising at an appropriate level," says Goodale.

But a fairly common mistake at this point is ramping up your workout too quickly, she says. "And if you increase too much, too quickly, you're risking injury, because your muscles might not be strong enough."

Better: "Stick with your workout for a week or two before increasing," she advises. "When you're ready to begin increasing, do it gradually, giving your muscles a chance to adjust to the new level.

"You can increase the duration, intention or frequency of your workout—but only increase one element at a time. If you started out with a short amount of time, try increasing the duration first. For example, you walked slowly for 20 minutes—next time you walk, increase the time by 10%, to 22 minutes. After you adjust to that, keep the time the same, but increase the intensity, walking a little faster. After that, add another day of walking into your week—if you started out walking three days, walk four. The same gradual approach holds true for strength training."

To recover from cancer, try interval training. "During cancer treatment, you will undergo events that are emotionally and physically draining, such as surgery and chemotherapy," says Dr. Block. "One of the few ways to improve your recovery capacity is by placing yourself in an exercise-induced stressful situation, over and over, and then training your body to tackle the stress and return to its healthy baseline—for instance, returning your heart rate to normal after strenuous physical activity."

That type of repetitive strenuous activity is called "interval training"—and you can do it for 15 to 30 seconds, 40 or 50 times a day, gradually building up to one minute, two minutes or three-minute sessions of high-intensity exercise, says Dr. Block.

Interval exercises can include running up and down stairs, running in place or jumping jacks—any exercise that quickly boosts your heart rate.

"With interval training, it's amazing how the body is very quickly trained to bounce back—and impressive to see cancer patients shift rapidly into a stronger state," says Dr. Block.

120

Marijuana Compound May Stop Metastatic Breast Cancer

Sean D. McAllister, PhD, Basic Science Researcher, California Pacific Medical Center Research Institute, San Francisco.

Pierre-Yves Desprez, PhD, Basic Science Researcher, California Pacific Medical Center Research Institute, San Francisco.

Manuel Guzman, PhD, professor, biochemistry and molecular biology, Complutense University, Madrid, Spain.

Molecular Cancer Therapeutics.

A nontoxic, nonpsychoactive compound in marijuana may block the progress of metastatic breast cancer, according to a new study by researchers in California.

"This is a new way to treat a patient that is not toxic like chemotherapy or radiotherapy. It is a new approach for metastatic cancer," said lead researcher Sean D. McAllister, PhD, an associate scientist at the California Pacific Medical Center Research Institute in San Francisco.

HOW IT WORKS

The compound found in cannabis, called *cannabidiol* (CBD), inhibits a gene, Id-1, that researchers believe is responsible for the metastatic process that spreads cells from the original tumor throughout the body.

Opting for a musical metaphor, senior researcher Pierre-Yves Desprez, PhD, likened Id-1 to "an (orchestra) conductor. In this case, you shoot the conductor, and the whole orchestra is going to stop. If you shoot the violinist, the orchestra just continues to play."

In humans, the Id-1 gene is found only in metastatic cancer cells, said Dr. Desprez, a staff scientist at the institute. Before birth, they are present and involved in the development of human embryos, but after birth, they go silent—and should stay that way, he said.

But in metastatic cancer "when (the genes) wake up, they are very bad," he said. "They push the cells to behave like embryonic cells and grow. They go crazy, they proliferate, they migrate." Dr. Desprez said, "We need to be able to turn them off."

NEW FINDINGS

According to the new study, CBD does exactly that.

"We are focusing on the latest stages of cancer," Dr. Desprez added. The cancer cell itself is not the problem, because a tumor can be "removed easily by surgery," he said. The problem is the development of metastatic cells, which is "conducted" by Id-1.

Drs. McAllister and Desprez said they are not suggesting that patients with hormone-independent metastatic breast cancer smoke marijuana. For one thing, a sufficient amount of CBD could never be obtained in that way, they said.

The research that has been done on marijuana and its compounds, however, is helpful, Dr. McAllister, said. CBD has been around for a long time, and researchers have found it is not psychoactive, and its "toxicity is very low," he added.

If Drs. McAllister and Desprez's work results in the development of a cancer treatment, someone with metastatic cancer might be placed on CBD for several years. That means low toxicity is important, Dr. McAllister explained.

Dr. McAllister also suggested that Id-1 is "so important in providing the [metastatic] mechanism in these cells in so many types of cancers" that they "provide us an opportunity potentially to target other types of cancers."

TREATMENT WITH CBD

Further study is needed before CBD can be conclusively identified as a treatment option, Drs. McAllister and Desprez said. "We need to involve a team of physicians, because we are bench (basic) scientists," Dr. McAllister noted.

One expert called the findings intriguing but preliminary.

"This is the first evidence that a cannabinoid can target the expression of an important breast cancer metastasis gene," noted Manuel Guzman, PhD, a Spanish expert on cannabinoids and cancer. He described the California study as giving "preliminary insight into the question of whether CBD could be used clinically to treat metastatic breast cancer."

However, "all the experiments in the paper have been conducted in cultured cells and none of them in any animal model of breast cancer, which would be one of the steps for further research," added Dr. Guzman, who is a professor of biochemistry and molecular biology at Complutense University in Madrid.

For more on breast cancer, go to the National Breast Cancer Foundation Web site at *www. nationalbreastcancer.org*.

Broccoli Gets Cancer-Fighting Boost

When you eat broccoli with certain other vegetables, such as broccoli sprouts, arugula or radishes, you get twice the cancer-fighting power of broccoli consumed on its own, say University of Illinois researchers. These additional vegetables contain the enzyme *myrosinase*, which boosts the effectiveness of broccoli's cancer-preventive component, *sulforaphane*. To protect the nutrients and the enzyme, steam broccoli and vegetables for only two to four minutes.

Mark A. Stengler, NMD, licensed naturopathic medical doctor in private practice, Stengler Center for Integrative Medicine, Encinitas, California...adjunct associate clinical professor at the National College of Natural Medicine, Portland, Oregon...author of many books and of the *Bottom Line/Natural Healing* newsletter. *www.drstengler.com*

Breast Cancer Patients Benefit From Vitamin D

Researchers from the University of Rochester Medical Center in New York have found that women with aggressive, difficult-to-treat breast cancer often are deficient in vitamin D. The study is one of the first to assess vitamin D deficiency and poor prognosis. It's a good idea to have your doctor check your vitamin D level—especially if you are a cancer patient—and supplement accordingly.

Mark A. Stengler, NMD, licensed naturopathic medical doctor in private practice, Stengler Center for Integrative Medicine, Encinitas, California...adjunct associate clinical professor at the National College of Natural Medicine, Portland, Oregon...author of many books and of the *Bottom Line/Natural Healing* newsletter. *www.drstengler.com*

Brisk Walking May Reduce Prostate Cancer Progression

Researchers from the University of California, San Francisco, and Harvard School of Public Health found that men diagnosed with early-stage prostate cancer who walked briskly—at least three miles per hour—for three hours or more weekly were 57% less likely to need a second round of treatment (treatment type was not specified in this study) or show any progression of the disease than those who walked more slowly or for less time. To benefit, the exercise needed to be vigorous enough to elevate the heart rate—another example of physical activity having a positive effect on disease.

Mark A. Stengler, NMD, licensed naturopathic medical doctor in private practice, Stengler Center for Integrative Medicine, Encinitas, California...adjunct associate clinical professor at the National College of Natural Medicine, Portland, Oregon...author of many books and of the *Bottom Line/Natural Healing* newsletter. *www.drstengler.com*

8

Cholesterol and Heart Cures

The Food that Lowers Cholesterol 24%...In Just Five Weeks

If you're one of the millions of Americans with high cholesterol, chances are your doctor has told you what not to eat—high-fat meats and dairy, for example. But certain foods actually can lower your cholesterol and, in some cases, eliminate the need for cholesterol-lowering drugs. Regularly including these foods can have a particularly powerful effect on reducing LDL—the "bad" cholesterol that damages arteries and other blood vessels. High LDL levels are associated with an increased risk for heart attack and stroke.

OAT BRAN, BARLEY AND MORE

Soluble fiber is present in plant-based foods in the form of gums and pectins. The National Cholesterol Education Program Adult Treatment Panel states that five to 10 grams (g) of

soluble fiber daily can help to lower LDL by as much as 5%.

A specific type of soluble fiber—*beta-glucan* (found in oat bran and barley)—has an even more potent cholesterol-lowering effect...

• **In a study, men eating 6g of soluble fiber from barley per day** lowered their LDL cholesterol by an average of 24% in five weeks.

• **In a study, men given 6g of beta-glucan in a fortified bread**—who also were following a low-fat diet and walking 60 minutes per day—experienced an average reduction in LDL cholesterol of 28%.

How it works: In the intestines, soluble fiber attaches itself to cholesterol and bile acids. Bile acids help with fat digestion. They are made from cholesterol, so when the body

Andrea Chernus, MS, RD, registered dietician, certified diabetes educator and exercise physiologist who maintains a private practice in New York City. She counsels patients on high cholesterol, diabetes, weight management and sports nutrition. She was formerly the clinical nutritionist for Columbia University, New York City. *http://achernus.mydiabeteseducator.org*

123

needs to make more bile acids, it pulls cholesterol from the bloodstream. The process of binding soluble fiber to bile acids forces the body to make more bile and use up cholesterol from the body's supply. Because fiber is not digested, it carries the cholesterol and bile acids out of the body, lowering the body's cholesterol.

Best sources of soluble fiber: Oat bran, oatmeal, barley, apples, citrus fruits, pears, kidney and lima beans, carrots, broccoli and brussels sprouts. Psyllium seed husks also are a good source and are found in some cereals, such as Kellogg's All-Bran Buds cereal.

Hot cereal made of 100% oat bran has about 3g of soluble fiber per serving...plain oatmeal has about 2g. Most cold oat-based cereals have one gram. Fruits and vegetables have 0.5g to 1g of soluble fiber per serving.

Beware: Commercially prepared muffins, pretzels and breads made with oat bran may not contain much soluble fiber. Also, some may be high in saturated or trans fats, sugars and sodium. As a rough guide, check the label to make sure oat bran is one of the first ingredients listed on the food label. (Soluble fiber does not have to be listed separately from total fiber.)

PLANT STEROLS AND STANOLS

Plant sterols (phytosterols) and plant stanols (phytostanols) are substances that block absorption of cholesterol. They are particularly high in vegetable oils and, to a lesser degree, in fruits, vegetables, nuts and seeds. More than 25 studies have proved their effectiveness in cholesterol reduction. *Examples...*

• **In a study, 155 adults with high cholesterol took in 1.5g per day of plant sterols from margarine.** After six months, they had an average reduction in LDL cholesterol of 11% (and 9% reduction in total cholesterol).

• **In another study, 72 adults with high cholesterol took in 2g per day of plant sterols from phytosterol-fortified orange juice.** After eight weeks, their average reduction in LDL cholesterol was 12% (7% reduction in total cholesterol).

How they work: Plant sterols and stanols help block the absorption of dietary cholesterol

and the reabsorption of cholesterol back into our intestinal tract. They compete with cholesterol for incorporation into mixed micelles, which are composite molecules that contain both water- and fat-soluble substances. In the body, micelles are used to carry fats through the bloodstream. When cholesterol is blocked from being absorbed and incorporated into these molecules, it is excreted from the body.

Best sources: To get a cholesterol-lowering dose from ordinary food, you would have to eat hundreds of calories worth of oils per day or bushels of fruits and vegetables. But researchers have isolated plant sterols and stanols, and food companies have incorporated them into "functional foods."

Until recently, only certain margarines contained these cholesterol-lowering ingredients, but food companies now have put them into lower-fat foods, such as yogurts, juices, breads and more. A dose of 2g to 3g of plant sterols and stanols per day has the greatest impact on lowering LDL cholesterol, reducing it by 6% to 15%. Higher doses of sterols and stanols are not more effective.

Foods containing effective amounts of plant sterols and stanols include Promise Benecol and Take Control margarines...Minute Maid Heartwise Orange Juice...Nature Valley Healthy Heart Granola Bars...Hain Celestial Rice Dream beverage...Lifetime low-fat cheese...Oroweat whole-grain bread...and VitaMuffins.

The FDA allows foods containing sterols and stanols that meet certain criteria to put a health claim on the label that they can help reduce the risk of coronary heart disease.

Beware: Margarines and juices are dense in calories. Check food labels to see how much you need to eat to obtain 2g to 3g of sterols and stanols.

If you're worried about calories, you can take sterol/stanol supplements. Generally, they are called beta-sitosterol or sitostanol. It is safe to use these supplements along with statin drugs for an additional cholesterol-lowering effect.

NUTS

People who are trying to lower cholesterol levels often eliminate nuts from their diets because nuts are high in fat and calories. But nuts contain mostly monounsaturated fats, which, when substituted for the saturated fats found in high-fat meats and dairy, not only can lower LDL levels but also boost HDL "good" cholesterol levels.

Studies have shown the greatest effect when nuts comprise 20% of one's total calories, which typically amounts to 1.5 to 3.5 ounces of nuts daily (about one-quarter to one-half cup).

On average, LDL cholesterol levels fall 8% to 12% when walnuts or almonds are substituted for saturated fats. HDL levels may increase by 9% to 20%. Other nuts, such as peanuts (technically a legume), pistachios and pecans, have been shown to lower cholesterol, but fewer studies are available on these varieties.

How they work: The exact mechanism of nuts' healthful effects hasn't been discovered yet, but nuts contain a combination of plant sterols, fiber and healthy fats.

Beware: Because nuts are high in calories, the trick is to substitute nuts for less healthful, high-fat foods, including cheese and meat.

Pets May Prevent Heart Attacks

Adnan I. Qureshi, MD, executive director, Minnesota Stroke Initiative, and professor of neurology, neurosurgery and radiology, University of Minnesota, Minneapolis.

Kathie Cole, RN, clinical nurse, UCLA Medical Center/School of Nursing, Los Angeles.

American Stroke Association International Stroke Conference, New Orleans.

Whether it's a frisky kitten or a tubby tabby, a cat at home could cut your heart attack risk by almost a third, according to recent research. The 10-year study of more than 4,300 Americans, suggests that the stress relief pets provide humans is heart-healthy.

Bonus: Dog lovers shouldn't feel left out. Although the study found no such benefit from "man's best friend," that's probably because there simply weren't enough dog own-

ers in the study to draw firm conclusions, the researchers said.

"For years we have known that psychological stress and anxiety are related to cardiovascular events, particularly heart attacks," noted study senior author Dr. Adnan Qureshi, executive director of the Stroke Center at the University of Minnesota in Minneapolis. According to Qureshi, the research shows that "essentially there is a benefit in relieving those inciting factors from pets."

The findings were presented during the American Stroke Association's International Stroke Conference in New Orleans.

The stress-cardiovascular disease link is very well-documented in scientific literature, and the affection and pleasure pets give humans is a known stress-buster. In fact, an earlier study presented at an American Heart Association meeting found that a single 12-minute visit with a dog improved the heart and lung function of people with heart failure.

In Qureshi's study, the team analyzed data on 4,435 Americans, aged 30 to 75, who took part in the federal government's second National Health and Nutrition Examination Study, which ran from 1976-1980. According to the data in the survey, 2,435 of the participants either owned a cat or had owned a cat in the past, while the remaining 2,000 had never done so.

Qureshi's team then tracked rates of death from all causes, including heart and stroke. Cat owners "appeared to have a lower rate of dying from heart attacks" over 10 years of follow-up compared to feline-free folk, Qureshi said.

The magnitude of the effect—a 30 percent reduction in heart attack risk—"was a little bit surprising," he added. "We certainly expected an effect, because we thought that there was a biologically plausible mechanism at work, but the magnitude of the effect was hard to predict."

Qureshi—proud owner of his own feline, Ninja—stressed that dogs probably would bring people the same kind of benefit, but the numbers of dog owners in the study wasn't big enough to count statistically.

Kathie Cole, a clinical nurse at the UCLA Medical Center and School of Nursing and the lead author of the dog-and-heart-failure study, said she wasn't surprised by the Minnesota findings.

"I would be inclined to think that any animal that is perceived as meaningful to a person in a positive way would have health benefits," Cole said. She pointed to multiple studies that have found that animal companions "have a calming effect in regard to mental stressors."

Both researchers believe pet ownership should be perceived as a low-cost, low-risk medical intervention that can potentially save or extend lives, especially for the elderly. "The problem right now is that so many apartment buildings or nursing homes aren't allowing animals in," Cole said. "That's the problem I see from a community standpoint."

Qureshi agreed that cats, dogs or other pets may bring tangible medical benefits to owners. "This opens a whole new avenue or intervention that we hadn't looked at before, one that can be made at the public level," he said. And unlike drugs or surgery, pet ownership "doesn't appear to have any risks to it," he added.

Helpful: If you are considering adopting a pet, contact the American Veterinary Medical Association (800-248-2862, *www.avma.org*) for information on responsible pet ownership.

Tomatoes Are Good For You

When 21 healthy people ate a tomato-free diet for three weeks, followed by a three-week diet that included about two tablespoons of ketchup and nearly two cups of tomato juice daily, participants' LDL "bad" cholesterol levels decreased, on average, by 12.9%.

Theory: Antioxidants in tomatoes inhibit oxidation of fats.

For heart health: Add tomato products (such as low-sodium tomato juice) to your daily diet.

Sohvi Hörkkö, MD, PhD, researchers, Institute of Diagnotics, Department of Medical Microbiology, University of Oulu, Finland.

You Don't Need Drugs to Control Your Cholesterol

Allan Magaziner, DO, clinical instructor in the department of family practice at the Robert Wood Johnson University of Medicine and Dentistry in New Brunswick, New Jersey, and founder and medical director of the Magaziner Center for Wellness in Cherry Hill, New Jersey (*www.drmagaziner.com*). A past president of the American College for Advancement in Medicine, he is the author of *The All-Natural Cardio Cure* (Avery).

It's widely known that low cholesterol levels help prevent heart attack and stroke. But that's only part of the story. Levels of HDL "good" cholesterol must be high enough to carry harmful forms of cholesterol to the liver to be excreted.

Recent finding: Research has shown that decreasing LDL "bad" cholesterol by 40% and increasing HDL by 30% lowers the risk for heart attack or stroke by 70%—a much greater reduction of risk than occurs from lowering either total cholesterol or LDL levels.

The pharmaceutical industry has worked feverishly to develop a prescription medication that significantly increases HDL levels, to be used as a complement to cholesterol-lowering statins that focus primarily on lowering LDL levels.

Examples: The drug *torcetrapib* was pegged as a blockbuster that increases HDL levels by 60%—that is, until late-stage clinical trials showed that torcetrapib actually increased heart problems and death rates.

What you may not know: Therapeutic doses of niacin (vitamin B-3) effectively boost HDL levels—and lower LDL and total cholesterol.

THE "CHOLESTEROL VITAMIN"

Over fifty years ago, Canadian scientists discovered that high doses of *nicotinic acid*—a form of niacin—could lower total cholesterol. In a 1975 study of men with heart disease, niacin was shown to reduce the rate of second heart attacks. Later, niacin was found to boost heart-protective HDL levels.

Although niacin alone cannot help everyone with abnormal cholesterol levels—often it is best used in combination with a statin—the vitamin is one of the most effective nondrug therapies available.

Ask your doctor about taking niacin if after trying cholesterol-lowering medication you have suffered side effects or your cholesterol levels have not improved within three months of getting a cholesterol test. Or consider trying niacin with the nondrug therapies described below.

How to use: Start with 100 mg of niacin daily and build up over one week to 500 mg a day. Every week, increase the dose by 500 mg until you reach 2,000 mg a day, taken in three divided doses, with meals. Be certain to use nicotinic acid, not *niacinamide*, a form of B vitamin that does not improve cholesterol levels. Consult your doctor before taking niacin.

The most common side effect of niacin is flushing—a warm, itchy, rash-like reddening of the face, neck and chest, which lasts about 10 minutes. Flushing is caused by niacin's ability to trigger vasodilation (widening of blood vessels).

To lessen this side effect, choose a form of niacin known as *inositol hexanicotinate*. It helps prevent the flush without reducing niacin's effectiveness.

Caution: Niacin should be avoided by people with a history of liver disease or stomach ulcers and used with caution by patients with diabetes and/or gallbladder disease. In addition, high-dose niacin (2,000 mg or more) may interact with certain medications, including alpha-blockers, such as *doxazosin* (Cardura), and the diabetes drug *metformin* (Glucophage).

OTHER NONDRUG THERAPIES

A diet that keeps sugar and processed food to an absolute minimum and emphasizes fruits and vegetables…whole grains…beans…fish… lean meats…and nuts and seeds can help lower LDL cholesterol and raise HDL levels. So can regular exercise, such as brisk walking, and losing excess weight.

Other nondrug approaches can lower total and LDL cholesterol and boost HDL. *Combine the following nondrug therapies with niacin for maximum effectiveness…*

•**Red yeast rice.** This Chinese medicine—a yeast that is grown on white rice, then fermented—contains *monacolins*, substances that act as naturally occurring statins. Research in China shows that red yeast rice can lower total cholesterol by 11% to 30%. Typical use: Take 1,200 to 2,400 mg a day of red yeast rice, in two to four doses, with meals.

Not recommended: Policosanol—a supplement derived from cane sugar that also contains natural statins—has been widely promoted as effective for lowering cholesterol. However, several recent studies show that policosanol has no significant effect on cholesterol.

•**Fish oil and flaxseed.** Fish oil and flaxseed supply omega-3 fatty acids, which lower total cholesterol and LDL levels and raise HDL levels.

Typical dose: For fish oil, take supplements containing a total of 3 g daily of *eicosapentaenoic acid* (EPA) and *docosahexaenoic acid* (DHA). If you take a blood-thinning drug, such as aspirin or *warfarin* (Coumadin), check with your doctor before taking this dose of fish oil. Or use one to three teaspoons of ground flaxseed a day, sprinkled on food or mixed with water or juice. Flaxseed also can help relieve constipation and ease arthritis pain.

•**Soy.** Many studies show that soy can help lower total and LDL cholesterol.

Typical use: Try to get 20 g of soy protein a day—the equivalent of eight ounces of tofu… or one cup of edamame (soy) beans.

Important: Soy ice cream and other processed soy foods don't deliver enough soy to help reduce cholesterol.

Caution: If you have been diagnosed with a hormone-dependent cancer, such as some breast malignancies, or are at risk for such a condition, check with your doctor before adding soy to your diet.

• **Plant sterols.** These natural substances, which block the absorption of cholesterol in the intestines, are found in fruits, vegetables, beans, grains and other plants. Regular intake can reduce total cholesterol by 10% and LDL by 14%. Products with plant sterols (or a similar form, plant stanols) include spreads, salad dressings, snack bars and dietary supplements.

Typical use: Aim for 1 g to 2 g daily of plant sterols.

• **Walnuts.** A recent study published in the medical journal *Angiology* showed that people who ate a handful of walnuts daily for eight weeks had a 9% increase in HDL. Walnuts contain polyphenol antioxidants, which also inhibit oxidation of LDL cholesterol. Recommended intake: One ounce of raw walnuts three times daily.

The Amazing Power of Aspirin

Randall S. Stafford, MD, PhD, associate professor of medicine, Stanford Prevention Research Center, Stanford University, Palo Alto, California. Dr. Stafford is author or coauthor of more than 110 scientific papers in leading medical journals. He is on the advisory panel of experts of "Aspirin Talks," an educational campaign from the American College of Preventive Medicine.

It costs pennies a pill—but for heart disease and stroke, the number-one and number-three killers of Americans, aspirin can be just as powerfully preventive as more expensive medications, such as cholesterol-lowering statins.

Two-thirds of people at high risk for heart attack and stroke don't take aspirin daily—leading to an estimated yearly death toll of 45,000 people who might have lived if they had taken a low-dose aspirin every day. *And recent evidence shows that aspirin also plays a role in fighting colon cancer and possibly other diseases…*

PROTECTING DISEASED ARTERIES

If you've had a heart attack, taking aspirin daily reduces your risk for a second attack by 23%. If you have angina—chest pain that signals serious heart disease—daily aspirin reduces heart attack risk by 51%. Type 2 diabetes—which damages arteries, increasing risk for heart attack and stroke—is another reason for daily aspirin. Taking aspirin if you have diagnosed heart disease or type 2 diabetes is called secondary prevention—it's too late to prevent the problem, but you're controlling it.

What to do: If you have heart disease or type 2 diabetes, talk to your doctor about aspirin therapy. The recommended dosage for secondary prevention is 81 milligrams (mg) daily, or one "baby aspirin." There continues to be debate about whether 162 mg daily may be more protective for some people with heart disease or diabetes—ask your doctor.

PREVENTING HEART ATTACK

In March 2009, the US Preventive Services Task Force (USPSTF) recommended the daily use of aspirin for primary prevention—preventing heart attack and stroke in people who don't have diagnosed cardiovascular disease.

Because older age is a risk factor for heart attacks and strokes, the recommendation included all men between the ages of 45 and 79 and all women between the ages of 55 and 79.

Among these groups, the USPSTF said to use aspirin for primary prevention only in cases in which the benefits are likely to outweigh the risks. When aspirin blocks the production of blood-clotting *thromboxane*, it increases the risk for internal bleeding.

The benefits of taking aspirin are likely to be greater than the risks in those with an elevated risk for heart attack and stroke. These risk factors include high total cholesterol, lower than normal HDL (good) cholesterol, high blood pressure, smoking and older age.

Factors that may indicate aspirin is too risky for you include…

• **Recent bleeding from a stomach ulcer or hemorrhagic stroke,** caused by a ruptured blood vessel

• **History of gastrointestinal (GI)** bleeding caused by other nonsteroidal anti-inflammatory drugs (NSAIDs)

• **Taking an anti-inflammatory corticosteroid,** such as prednisone

• **Rheumatoid arthritis.**

AGE 80 OR OLDER

The USPSTF didn't include a recommendation for people age 80 or older, because there's not enough scientific evidence to know whether aspirin protects this age group. However, your risk for heart attack and stroke increases with age, so those over 80 are likely to benefit from aspirin, but they also are more likely to have GI or brain bleeding.

What to do: If you're 80 or older, ask your doctor about taking aspirin. You probably shouldn't take it if you have a history of GI bleeding or falls (a head injury is more likely to cause hemorrhagic stroke in someone taking aspirin).

COLON CANCER

A study by researchers at Harvard Medical School, published in *The Journal of the American Medical Association*, showed that people with colorectal cancer who began taking aspirin regularly after diagnosis had a 29% lower risk of dying from the disease than those who never used aspirin. Researchers also found that those who used aspirin regularly before their diagnosis had a 61% lower risk of dying from the disease. Aspirin reduces inflammation, which may play a role in the progress of colon cancer.

What to do: If you've been diagnosed with colorectal cancer, talk to your doctor about taking aspirin. There is not enough scientific evidence to justify taking aspirin to prevent colorectal cancer.

USING ASPIRIN WISELY

• **Don't worry about the formulation.** In most cases, aspirin doesn't cause GI bleeding because it irritates your GI tract—the bleeding is caused by a systemic effect on *cyclooxygenases* (COX). That means enteric-coated tablets don't decrease the risk for GI bleeding.

• **Be cautious of blood-thinning supplements.** Fish oil and the herb ginkgo biloba also affect platelets, increasing the risk for internal bleeding. If you're taking aspirin, talk to your doctor about whether it's safe to take those supplements.

• **Don't take aspirin and another NSAID at the same time.** Recent research shows that NSAIDs, such as *ibuprofen* and *naproxen* (Aleve, Naprosyn), interfere with aspirin's ability to affect COX. If you take another NSAID, take it four to six hours before or after taking aspirin.

• **Think twice about stopping aspirin before surgery.** Surgeons often ask patients to stop taking aspirin about two weeks before surgery. But if you take aspirin for secondary prevention, the risk for a heart attack may outweigh the risk for additional bleeding during surgery. Ask your physician.

• **If you think you're having a heart attack, call 911 immediately and take aspirin.** Chew an uncoated full-strength (325-mg) aspirin right away. Taking aspirin once a day for the next month can reduce the risk for death by 23% and may significantly reduce damage to the heart.

HOW ASPIRIN WORKS

Aspirin is *acetylsalicylic acid*—a compound that blocks the action of COX, enzymes that are found in every cell.

COX help manufacture prostaglandins, hormones that control pain, fever and inflammation. COX also help produce *thromboxane*, which allows cells in the bloodstream called platelets to stick together, forming blood clots.

By impeding prostaglandins, aspirin lowers fever, relieves acute pain such as headache, and eases the soreness that accompanies inflammation. By reducing thromboxane, aspirin helps stop the formation of blood clots, reducing the risk for a heart attack and stroke.

The Truth About Aspirin—It May Not Protect Your Heart...But Natural Solutions Can

Mark A. Stengler, NMD, licensed naturopathic medical doctor in private practice, Stengler Center for Integrative Medicine, Encinitas, California...adjunct associate clinical professor at the National College of Natural Medicine, Portland, Oregon...author of many books, including *The Natural Physician's Healing Therapies* and coauthor of *Prescription for Natural Cures* (both from Bottom Line Books)...and author of the *Bottom Line/Natural Healing* newsletter. *www.drstengler.com*

Every morning, some 50 million Americans pop a low-dose aspirin into their mouths with the hope that it will help prevent a heart attack or stroke. For many, taking a daily aspirin is a habit, a no-brainer—a seemingly simple way to protect against cardiovascular disease.

The problem: Aspirin is overprescribed and causes many uncomfortable and possibly dangerous side effects (see the list at the end of this article). In addition, a little-known phenomenon called aspirin resistance means that, for some people, aspirin provides no protection at all.

Good news: There are several natural alternatives to aspirin that have the potential to help more people without the damaging side effects.

ASPIRIN RESISTANCE

For a number of people, aspirin neither prevents blood clots nor reduces inflammation. Aspirin resistance has no symptoms. Sadly, people find out that the daily aspirin they are taking has no effect only when they suffer a heart attack or stroke.

There currently is no single laboratory test for, or accepted definition of, aspirin resistance. Estimates of how many people are aspirin resistant vary widely, from as low as 5.5% to an astonishing 60%, according to a recent study in *Journal of the American College of Cardiology.*

Aspirin is a mild anticoagulant—it reduces the risk of an abnormal blood clot forming that could cause a heart attack or stroke. Stronger anticlotting medication, such as *warfarin* (Coumadin) or *heparin*, generally is given to people who are at higher risk of developing blood clots. Possible side effects from these stronger medications include hemorrhage and hypersensitivity (characterized by chills, asthma, red marks and itchy skin).

NATURAL ANTICLOTTING PROTECTION

Everyone who is concerned with heart health should follow a Mediterranean-style diet, consisting mainly of whole grains, vegetables and olive oil, as well as cold-water fish, such as salmon. This type of diet has been shown to significantly reduce the risk for heart attack and stroke.

Next: Take steps to reduce your risk for cardiovascular disease. Risk is determined by age, gender, family and medical history, smoking, cholesterol levels and other cardiovascular risk markers, blood pressure, weight and whether you have diabetes.

In addition, holistic physicians often use a blood test to track *fibrinogen*, a protein essential to blood clot formation. High fibrinogen levels can indicate a risk of developing a blood clot. I monitor fibrinogen levels and use a laboratory test to measure the time it takes for a patient's blood to clot. I order these tests every few months until the readings are normal.

If you are already taking any anticoagulant medication, including aspirin, check with your doctor before taking any of the supplements below. People who take an anticoagulant are at greater risk for hemorrhage because the medication reduces the body's ability to form a blood clot and stop internal or external bleeding.

My recommendations: Three natural anticoagulants—and one clot-busting enzyme—that can be used in place of aspirin. *These supplements, which are available at health-food stores, can be used as follows...*

• **For those who don't have heart disease and want to prevent it,** take fish oil, vitamin E and bromelain.

• **For those with atherosclerosis (fatty buildup in the arteries),** take *nattokinase* and fish oil.

•**For those with elevated fibrinogen,** take nattokinase and fish oil, and then add vitamin E and bromelain if lab tests indicate fibrinogen has not decreased after two months.

•**Fish oil.** Omega-3 essential fatty acids are necessary for natural cardiovascular disease prevention and treatment. Research has shown that patients with coronary artery disease (plaque in the arteries of the heart) who were given fish oil supplements had a mild-to-moderate regression of atherosclerosis as measured by angiography. This means that even people with existing plaque have a chance to reduce it with fish oil.

The beneficial omega-3 fatty acids in fish oil are combined *eicosapentaenoic acid* (EPA) and *docosahexaenoic acid* (DHA).

Best fish sources: Oily, cold-water fish (salmon, herring, sardines, mackerel, anchovies), either broiled or baked. (Vegetarians can get their omega-3s from flaxseed or hemp seed.) To prevent coronary disease, consume two to three servings of fish weekly or take 1,500 milligrams (mg) daily of combined EPA and DHA. For those who already have atherosclerosis and high levels of fibrinogen, take 3,000 mg daily of combined EPA and DHA (1,500 mg twice daily with meals). Keeping atherosclerosis under control can be a lifelong battle, so patients can take these amounts indefinitely.

•**Vitamin E.** In moderate doses, this antioxidant has natural blood-thinning properties. Vitamin E is a collection of eight related compounds—*tocopherols* and *tocotrienols*. Look for mixed tocopherol and tocotrienol vitamin E—it is better than any single tocopherol formulation. Take 800 international units (IU) to 1,200 IU daily. Ask your holistic doctor or cardiologist about the amount that is right for you based on your cardiovascular health.

•**Bromelain.** Found in pineapples, this enzyme acts as an anticoagulant by helping to break down excess fibrin (a blood protein made from fibrinogen that forms at the site of a blood clot). Take 500 mg three times daily, not around mealtimes. If you have ulcers, don't take bromelain.

•**Nattokinase.** Extracted from the traditional Japanese food natto, this enzyme is made from fermented soybeans. With its strong fibrin-dissolving effect, nattokinase is a more aggressive approach to treatment than other natural therapies. It is recommended for people with elevated fibrinogen or a history of heart disease. Researchers have found that it can effectively and safely prevent blood clots without any side effects. Some holistic practitioners have even been able to help their patients who are taking medications such as warfarin switch to nattokinase.

For people with atherosclerosis or high fibrinogen, take 2,000 fibrinolytic units (FU) to 4,000 FU of a nattokinase supplement twice daily under the supervision of a health-care professional. Supervision is important with all anticoagulants because there is the danger that too much can lead to hemorrhage and too little to heart attack or stroke. Nattokinase should not be taken with other blood thinners, such as aspirin or warfarin.

WHO SHOULD TAKE ASPIRIN

For some people, aspirin is indeed a lifesaver. With few exceptions, anyone who thinks he/she is having a heart attack should chew and swallow 325 mg of aspirin immediately. (Chewing any of the supplements will not have the same effect.) Most heart attack patients also are advised to continue taking this amount daily for one month under a cardiologist's care—because people who survive a heart attack are especially prone to another one in the weeks afterward. After one month, I believe only one group should continue to take aspirin—those at high risk for cardiovascular disease who are unwilling to take supplements and change their diets and lifestyles.

Caution: Don't take aspirin if you are allergic to it...suspect that you are having a stroke...or have been told by your physician not to take it.

If you are on aspirin therapy, keep in mind that regular use can deplete your body of several nutrients. To protect yourself, take the following daily—folic acid (400 micrograms, or mcg), vitamin C (500 mg), vitamin B-12 (100 mcg), zinc (30 mg). When using zinc long-term, also take copper (1 mg).

Best: Don't take these supplements at the same time of day that you take aspirin.

WHO SHOULD DEFINITELY NOT TAKE ASPIRIN

I disagree with the way many doctors routinely put patients with any risk for cardiovascular disease (or no particular risk at all) on a daily aspirin. This includes a wide swath of people—men over age 40...women over age 50 who have atherosclerosis or high cholesterol...people over age 40 who have diabetes...people who have a parent or sibling with heart disease...and others.

In addition, some people should flat-out avoid aspirin (although after a heart attack, a cardiologist would determine use), including...

•**People with active peptic ulcers.** Aspirin erodes the stomach lining.

•**Those with poor kidney or liver function.** Aspirin can do further damage to these organs.

•**Patients taking anticoagulant medications, such as warfarin.** It can increase the risk of bleeding.

•**Asthma patients.** Aspirin can make breathing difficult in some patients whose asthma is triggered by the chemicals in aspirin.

WHAT IS ASPIRIN?

Aspirin-like substances date back to the ancient Greeks, who used a powder made from willow tree back to relieve fever and pain. Aspirin belongs to a class of drugs called nonsteroidal anti-inflammatory drugs (NSAIDs). They work by inhibiting the enzymes that make prostaglandins, chemicals that promote inflammation, pain and fever, and are necessary for blood clotting.

ASPIRIN'S SERIOUS SIDE EFFECTS

People often think of aspirin as a completely benign substance. *It is not. In fact, its side effects may surprise you...*

•**Gastrointestinal bleeding.** In the US, about 103,000 hospitalizations and about 16,500 deaths occur annually from gastrointestinal bleeding related to NSAIDs, including aspirin.

•**Dyspepsia.** This condition, which is characterized by pain or discomfort in the upper abdomen, is reported by 12% of users of aspirin and other NSAIDs.

•**Gastroduodenal lesions.** In a study of arthritic patients taking NSAIDs for pain, 30% developed painful gastroduodenal lesions or sores in the stomach and/or small intestine.

•**Cataracts.** Prolonged aspirin use can increase risk for cataracts (hardening and clouding of the lens of the eye) by 55%, according to a study in *Ophthalmology*.

Natural Remedies That Work Like Drugs Without the Side Effects And High Cost

Tod Cooperman, MD, founder and president of ConsumerLab.com, the leading independent evaluator of nutritional and vitamin/mineral supplements, White Plains, New York. Reports can be found at *www.consumerlab.com* (subscription required). He also is editor of *ConsumerLab.com's Guide to Buying Vitamins & Supplements* (ConsumerLab.com).

Most people assume that prescription medications are stronger and more effective than supplements. But we have found that some supplements can be just as effective—without the side effects that often accompany prescription drugs.

Also, people with chronic conditions who have no insurance or are under-insured or who have been hit with higher co-pays can save hundreds or even thousands of dollars a year by using supplements in place of drugs.

Caution: Always check with your doctor before stopping a prescription drug or taking a supplement.

Here, natural alternatives to commonly prescribed medications. If there are two alternatives, try one. If that doesn't work, try the other. Dosages are those typically prescribed, but always follow directions on the supplement label or from your health practitioner.

HIGH CHOLESTEROL

Statins, the most popular drugs for lowering cholesterol, can reduce LDL (bad) cholesterol by as much as 60%, depending on the drug and dose. Drawback: Some of these drugs can cause liver problems and/or a type of muscle pain known as *myopathy.*

Alternative 1: Red yeast rice. It contains *monacolins,* chemical compounds that inhibit the body's production of cholesterol. One of these compounds, *lovastatin,* is chemically similar to the active ingredient in some statin drugs.

One study found that people taking red yeast rice supplements had reductions in LDL of 23%. When the supplements were combined with healthy lifestyle changes, LDL dropped by 42%.

Other benefits: Because red yeast rice contains a variety of cholesterol-lowering compounds, it may be effective in patients who don't respond to single-ingredient statins. It also appears to be less likely to cause liver problems and muscle pain.

Dose: 600 milligrams (mg) of red yeast rice extract, taken twice daily.

Alternative 2: Phytosterols. These are naturally occurring plant compounds that come in supplement form as well as in cholesterol-lowering margarines, such as Benecol and Take Control. Plant sterols inhibit the absorption of cholesterol in the intestine and can lower LDL by between 10% and 14%.

Dose: 1.3 grams (g) of a plant sterol supplement daily, divided into two doses. Or two tablespoons of a cholesterol-lowering margarine.

OSTEOARTHRITIS

It's the most common form of arthritis, affecting up to 20 million American adults. Osteoarthritis occurs when cartilage in the joints wears and breaks down, causing pain and stiffness. People with frequent or severe symptoms often depend on prescription-strength anti-inflammatory drugs. These drugs reduce symptoms but don't change the outcome of the disease. They also can cause stomach upset or other gastrointestinal problems.

Alternative 1: Glucosamine. This supplement usually is derived from shellfish, though vegetable-based versions are starting to appear. It helps the body repair and rebuild damaged cartilage. It can help reduce pain as well as subsequent joint damage.

Dose: 1,500 mg, once daily.

Alternative 2: Glucosamine plus chondroitin. This supplement combination is more expensive than glucosamine alone, but it sometimes helps patients who don't respond to glucosamine. Chondroitin, the added ingredient that typically is made from cow or pig cartilage, promotes the absorption of fluids into connective tissue and aids in flexibility and repair.

Dose: 1,500 mg of glucosamine and 1,200 mg of chondroitin, once daily.

Important: Studies have revealed that supplements protect joints better than they relieve pain. Most people who take them still need an occasional anti-inflammatory painkiller.

RHEUMATOID ARTHRITIS

This form of arthritis causes inflammation throughout the body that can damage joints as well as the eyes, lungs and/or heart. Most people with rheumatoid arthritis take prescription drugs, such as *methotrexate* (Rheumatrex) or *hydroxychloroquine* (Plaquenil). Most rheumatoid drugs are expensive, and many have a high risk for side effects, including suppressed immunity.

Supplementation can reduce inflammation and potentially reduce the dosage of prescription drugs.

Alternative: Fish and fish oil. The omega-3 fatty acids in cold-water fish, such as salmon and tuna, have potent anti-inflammatory effects. A study at the University of Pittsburgh School of Medicine found that 59% of patients given supplemental omega-3s had decreased joint pain.

Dose: A total of 1,200 mg to 2,400 mg of EPA and DHA (types of fish oil) daily, or eat three or more fish servings a week. Caution: Fish oil may interact with blood-thinning drugs, such as *warfarin* (Coumadin).

133

DEPRESSION

Antidepressant medications, including *selective serotonin reuptake inhibitors* (SSRIs), such as *paroxetine* (Paxil), *escitalopram* (Lexapro) and *citalopram* (Celexa), have revolutionized the treatment of depression. Many people who take them, however, experience troublesome side effects, including heightened anxiety and reduced libido.

Alternative 1: St. John's wort. It appears to be as effective for mild-to-moderate depression as SSRIs but with milder side effects. It is not effective for patients with major depression and should not be taken with prescription antidepressants. It also may interact with other medications, including blood thinners, such as *warfarin* (Coumadin).

Dose: 300 mg, three times daily. Look for a product that contains 1% to 3% *hypericin*, the active ingredient.

Alternative 2: Fish oil. It improves a number of emotional and mental disorders, including depression and bipolar disorder. A study found that those who combined EPA with an antidepressant medication did better than those using either treatment alone.

Dose: 1 g of EPA, once daily, or eat three or more fish servings a week. (See fish oil caution on page 30.)

ENLARGED PROSTATE

Starting in their 40s, many men experience a rapid growth of the prostate gland. If the inner part of the gland gets too large, it can press against the urethra. This condition, called *benign prostatic hyperplasia* (BPH), can cause irritation or difficulty urinating.

Some drugs, such as *finasteride* (Proscar), reduce the size of the prostate gland. Others, such as *terazosin* (Hytrin) and *doxazosin* (Cardura), relax the prostate and make it easier to urinate but also may cause dizziness.

Alternative: Saw palmetto. This herbal supplement helps prevent testosterone from fueling the growth of prostate cells. In some but not all studies, it has been shown to be as effective as finasteride for men with mild symptoms of BPH.

Dose: 160 mg, twice daily. It can take several months to a year before saw palmetto is fully effective.

9

Stroke Damage Cures

How Brain Scientist Jill Bolte Taylor Came Back from a Stroke

In 1996, Jill Bolte Taylor, PhD, a 37-year-old brain scientist, had a severe hemorrhagic (bleeding) stroke in the left hemisphere of her brain.

Taylor's cognitive abilities degenerated rapidly in the hours following the stroke. Bleeding affected the motor cortex (paralyzing her right arm)...the sensory cortex (making it difficult for her to see or hear)...and the brain's language centers (making it difficult for her to speak).

After struggling to call for help, she was taken to the hospital, where she underwent surgery two-and-a-half weeks later to remove a golf ball–sized blood clot in her brain.

Today, Taylor is completely recovered—all of her physical, cognitive and emotional abilities are intact. Her recovery refutes the widely held belief that if a stroke survivor doesn't regain a particular ability within six months, it will never be regained.

We recently spoke with Taylor, a neuroanatomist (a scientist specializing in the anatomy of the brain) who lectures widely, about her stroke recovery. The strategies she shared also can be used by all those who have had a debilitating ischemic stroke (in which a blood clot stops blood supply to an area of the brain) or any severe brain injury...

STEP 1: MOVE TO RECOVER

People who survive a stroke often experience crushing fatigue due to the damage that occurs to brain cells (neurons)—this affects their energy levels and abilities to process information. Simple tasks, such as changing the position of your body or even opening your

Jill Bolte Taylor, PhD, neuroanatomist affiliated with the Indiana University School of Medicine in Indianapolis. She is a national spokesperson for the Harvard Brain Tissue Resource Center, which collects human brain tissue for research, and author of *My Stroke of Insight: A Brain Scientist's Personal Journey* (Plume).

eyes, are extraordinarily difficult. But the same activities that restore physical strength also force individual neurons to reconnect and communicate with one another—a process that is essential for post-stroke neurological recovery.

Helpful: Any physical activity is beneficial —even basic movements, such as standing up or sitting down.

Important: When you feel rested and capable of expending the necessary energy, you should push yourself to do more and more physically each day. As I gained strength, I progressed to trying more difficult activities, such as standing at the sink and doing dishes.

STEP 2: ESCAPE THE MENTAL NOISE

Neurons that are damaged by a stroke are unable to process normal stimuli, such as bright lights or the sound of a television. As a result, visual or auditory distractions may be interpreted by the brain as mental "noise." Saturating the brain with such stimuli may make it much harder for the neurons to recover and may impede the retention of new information.

Helpful: After any kind of stroke or other brain trauma, alternate periods of sleep with briefer periods (about 20 minutes) of learning and cognitive challenges (such as those described below). Periods of sleep (as much as needed until waking up naturally) allow the brain to assimilate information that is gleaned during periods of wakefulness.

STEP 3: WORK THE MIND

The brain has remarkable "plasticity" (the ability to form new connections between the surviving neurons). After a stroke, if there is damage to the brain areas that control movement, sensory perceptions and cognition, you need to challenge these areas.

Examples…

• **Multiple-choice questions.** My mother, who was my primary caregiver, understood that asking "yes" or "no" questions didn't force me to think hard enough. That's why she asked me multiple-choice questions—for example, did I want minestrone soup or a grilled cheese sandwich? Each question forced me to relearn words.

• **Simple puzzles.** If you've had a serious stroke, putting together a simple jigsaw puzzle may be a huge challenge. You might not recognize shapes or colors. You might not have the dexterity to put the pieces together. But doing such a puzzle is a superb exercise because it forces you to work different parts of the brain at the same time.

• **Reading.** It's among the hardest tasks because, for many stroke patients, the entire concept of letters and words is lost—temporarily for some stroke survivors, but permanently for others. I had to relearn everything from scratch—that the squiggles that make up letters have names…that combinations of letters make sounds…and that combinations of sounds make words.

Helpful: I started with children's picture books, which would be appropriate for most stroke patients who are relearning to read.

STEP 4: THE SIMPLEST STEPS

Healthy people can't begin to comprehend how complicated things seem after a stroke. When I first started walking, for example, I didn't understand the concept of sidewalk cracks. Each time I saw one, I had to stop and analyze whether it was important.

Helpful: Caregivers need to break down tasks to the simplest levels. For example, a stroke patient might not understand how to sit up in bed. He/she might need to spend days just learning how to shift body weight. In my case, I had to learn to simply hold an eating utensil before I could imagine raising it to my mouth.

STEP 5: FOCUS ON ABILITIES

When you've had a stroke, the extent of your disabilities can be overwhelming. It took me eight years before I was fully recovered. Patients can easily get frustrated and quit trying. At that point, if a patient is not aware of what recovery step needs to be taken next, he may never actually take that next step. It's normal for a stroke survivor to reach a recovery plateau, to continue to learn, then hit another plateau. There are many plateaus along the way.

Helpful: Even if progress seems exceptionally slow, remind a person who has had a stroke of the smallest successes—it may be something as simple as once again being able to hold a fork securely.

If you are the stroke survivor, use small triumphs as inspiration. In my case, it was embarrassing to drool in front of strangers, but I reminded myself that I had managed to swallow.

After my stroke, I never imagined that I would regain enough of my abilities to return to a career as a scientist and teacher. I've managed to do both—in fact, at the same level and intensity. My stroke recovery gave me an opportunity to start my life again.

Hyperbaric Medicine... The Oxygen Cure

Mark A. Stengler, NMD, licensed naturopathic medical doctor in private practice, Stengler Center for Integrative Medicine, Encinitas, California...adjunct associate clinical professor at the National College of Natural Medicine, Portland, Oregon...author of many books, including *The Natural Physician's Healing Therapies* and coauthor of *Prescription for Natural Cures* (both from Bottom Line Books)...and author of the *Bottom Line/Natural Healing* newsletter. *www.drstengler.com.*

H yperbaric medicine, the therapeutic use of oxygen at levels higher than are in our atmosphere, has been around for more than a century. It is perhaps best known as a treatment for deep-sea divers who have decompression sickness ("the bends"). This noninvasive therapy, also known as *hyperbaric oxygen therapy* (HBOT), is proving to help a range of other medical conditions, from wound healing to stroke recovery.

To learn more about how HBOT works, we spoke with Robert Lyne-Sands, an engineer and designer of hyperbaric chambers, who is director of Healing Chambers International (*www.hboinfo.com*), a center for hyperbaric therapy in San Diego.

THE SCIENCE OF HYPERBARIC THERAPY

During HBOT, the patient breathes 100% oxygen while in an airtight chamber. This is about five times as much oxygen as we typically breathe at sea level. The increased pressure, combined with the pure oxygen, causes the extra oxygen to permeate the body's cells.

Saturating the body's cells in oxygen, HBOT supercharges the body's repair cells (white blood cells and other immune system cells) so that they work more powerfully and effectively. Typically these repair cells require up to 24 times as much oxygen as ordinary cells do. HBOT also increases the number of circulating stem cells, which are critical to injury repair of tissues and organs. That is why wounds become inflamed and swollen—blood vessels are dilating to rush more oxygen-filled red blood cells to the injured tissue. With HBOT, inflammation is reduced because the cells have the oxygen that they need to heal.

FOR SEVERE INJURIES

The history of HBOT has been marked by debate about its benefits. However, its effectiveness at healing injured tissue is no longer disputed. A study from Doctors Medical Center in San Pablo, California, found that patients with soft-tissue infections treated with HBOT had an 88% survival rate and zero amputations, compared with a 66% survival rate and 50% amputations for those who did not receive HBOT. And a Swedish study found that 76% of patients with diabetic foot ulcers completely recovered after HBOT, compared with 48% of those receiving conventional therapy.

Today HBOT is widely used for severe injuries that don't easily heal with conventional medical treatments. Medicare currently provides reimbursements for 15 HBOT treatments, including for gangrene, crush injuries and severe burns.

BEYOND WOUND HEALING

HBOT has the potential to treat other conditions as well...

•**Stroke and other neurological conditions.** HBOT has been shown to regenerate damaged brain and nerve cells. Stroke occurs when blood doesn't reach brain tissue—but the brain damage is due to that tissue being deprived of oxygen. It is believed that HBOT stimulates formation of new blood vessels and helps damaged tissue survive. Studies have shown that it can reduce damage and long-term effects if given a few days after a stroke.

Even patients treated 10 years after a stroke have improved cognitive and motor function. HBOT also can help improve motor function in patients with cerebral palsy.

HBOT is currently being tested for the following conditions...

• **Lyme disease.** HBOT may be able to treat nerve damage associated with the disease and to kill the bacteria that causes Lyme disease.

• **Lupus and rheumatoid arthritis.** The extra oxygen shuts down the inflammation process, the root of these autoimmune conditions.

• **Cancer.** HBOT even shows potential for shrinking some cancerous tumors, although this is highly controversial, since there is a counteracting concern that the extra oxygen could spur some cancers to grow more rapidly.

• **Autism.** HBOT may improve the symptoms of autism by reducing inflammation.

HOW HBOT IS ADMINISTERED

Today there are about 600 hospital-based or freestanding hyperbaric facilities in the US. Some are large multichamber units that several people can use at the same time, while others are single-person units in which the patient sits or lies down. In the US, HBOT can be given only with a doctor's prescription. While treatment generally is safe, the pressure and oxygen flow must be carefully monitored at all times. HBOT is not recommended for people with respiratory infections or high fever, because the pressure might harm them.

During HBOT, patients may feel sensations similar to those experienced while flying in an airplane. Some feel pressure in their ears, others feel their ears pop.

Cost varies greatly—from $1,500 to $2,000 per treatment at a hospital-based hyperbaric unit to about $150 to $250 per treatment at a freestanding facility, which is just as safe and effective as a hospital-based HBOT. Regardless of the type of facility, insurance pays for only those conditions that have been approved. Inflatable air chambers for home use are not effective and not recommended.

HBOT sessions last about an hour and a half. Some conditions require just two or three sessions, while others require up to five sessions weekly for one to three months. To find a hyperbaric treatment center near you, contact the Undersea and Hyperbaric Medical Society (877-533-8467, *www.uhms.org*).

People Who Drink Tea Are Less Likely to Have a Stroke

A recent analysis of nine studies involving nearly 195,000 adults found that for each additional three cups of black or green tea consumed daily, stroke risk dropped by 21%.

Theory: The antioxidant *epigallocatechin gallate* or the amino acid *theanine*, both found in tea, may have anti-inflammatory effects that protect the heart and brain. (Processing that is done for decaffeinated tea may remove these ingredients.)

Lenore Arab, PhD, professor of medicine and adjunct professor of biological chemistry, David Geffen School of Medicine, University of California, Los Angeles.

Better Stroke Protection

In a study of 673 men and women who suffered ischemic strokes (due to impaired blood flow to the brain), those who performed aerobic exercise (such as brisk walking or swimming) at least four times weekly before their strokes were better able to perform daily tasks (such as bathing) and had fewer functional problems (related to driving, for example) than those who were less active. Theory: Exercise promotes blood flow, building resilience to stroke-related neurological damage. To help protect against the disabling effects of a stroke: After checking with your doctor, aim to exercise briskly (intensely enough to sweat) for at least 30 minutes most days.

James Meschia, MD, director, cerebrovascular division, Mayo Clinic, Jacksonville, Florida.

Coffee Reduces Stroke Risk

Drinking one or more cups of coffee daily was associated with a 22% to 25% reduction in stroke risk.

Theory: Coffee beans contain antioxidants and other disease-fighting chemicals that reduce inflammation and improve insulin activity. Moderate coffee consumption also has been linked to decreased risk for diabetes, colon cancer, heart disease, liver disease and Parkinson's disease.

Susanna Larsson, PhD, is in the division of nutritional epidemiology at Institute of Environmental Medicine, Karolinska Institute, Stockholm, Sweden. She was lead researcher of a study of 34,670 women, published in *Stroke*.

The Benefit of Chocolate

In one study, people who ate one serving of chocolate a week were 22% less likely to have a stroke than those who ate no chocolate. In another study, people who ate 50 grams (1.75 ounces) of chocolate per week were 46% less likely to die following a stroke than those who ate no chocolate.

Possible reason: Chocolate is a rich source of antioxidants that may protect against stroke.

Sarah Sahib, researcher at McMaster University, Hamilton, Ontario, Canada, is lead author of an analysis of studies on chocolate and stroke.

One Man's Ultimate Stroke Recovery

Diane Ackerman, who has written more than 20 books, including works of nonfiction, such as *The Zookeeper's Wife* (W.W. Norton) and *An Alchemy of Mind: The Marvel and Mystery of the Brain* (Scribner), and poetry.

In 2004, at age 75, novelist and poet Paul West suffered a massive stroke that left him unable to walk or speak. In the seven years since then, he has regained most of his speech and mobility and written three new books.

How did he do it?

Much of the credit goes to West's wife of more than 30 years, poet and nonfiction author Diane Ackerman, whose book *One Hundred Names for Love: A Stroke, a Marriage, and the Language of Healing* chronicles his recovery.

We recently spoke with her to learn what advice she would offer to those who are struggling to recover from a stroke or any other serious health challenge—and their caregivers…

• **To what do you attribute Paul's impressive recovery?** Hard work on Paul's part and a kind of offbeat therapy on my part. We both had determination and stayed hopeful that he could improve.

After all sorts of catastrophic illnesses, the body needs time to heal. Despite what many doctors tell people after a stroke, improvement is not necessarily limited to a "window of opportunity" of a few months. Six months later, a year later and so on, Paul continued to make significant progress. Of course, he still struggles at times when speaking, but he can express what he wants to say. And his balance isn't perfect, so he needs someone to keep an eye on him when he walks. But even now, he continues to improve. Just recently, he learned to write checks again—nearly seven years after the stroke.

• **What were some of the unique strategies you used to help your husband improve?** Paul's stroke damaged the part of his brain that controls language. This resulted in aphasia, a disorder that impairs the expression and understanding of language as well as reading and writing. For Paul to relearn language, his brain had to cut new pathways—that is, "rewire" itself.

An hour a day of speech therapy could do only so much. Relearning language is like becoming a great violinist—it requires constant practice and not giving up.

I made up word games for Paul using the names of people we knew and everyday things around him. For example, I made up funny Mad-Lib–type fill-in-the-blank exercises. I also encouraged him to dictate his memories of

what had happened. And when he lament-
ed that he couldn't remember any of his pet
names for me, I suggested that he make up
some new ones. They're wild and wonderful.

Some of my favorites: Spy Elf of the Morning Hallelujahs...My Little Bucket of Hair...
and O Parakeet of the Lissome Star.

•**Was this process frustrating for him?** At
times. But I insisted that he talk even when
the right words didn't come. For example,
when he couldn't retrieve the word for computer, he called it "light-dancing mailbox"—a
great phrase, so poetic.

Bringing fun into the process also helped.
I often tried to get him to talk when we were
cuddling in bed. Aphasics have most trouble
when they're stressed—if they're relaxed, feeling cozy, they do better.

When the words came out "wrong," I kept
my mind open to the inadvertent beauty. As I
say at the end of the book, a bell with a crack in
it may not ring as clearly, but it rings as sweetly.

•**How did you deal with your own emotions?** The most soothing thing was getting
out in nature—it always refreshed my spirit.
I also meditated. But what really helped was
work. It was my sanctuary. I wrote my most
recent book after Paul had his stroke. A home
health aide came in for a few hours each day,
allowing me to write during that time.

People tend to feel guilty. They think, How
can I be having fun when my loved one is
suffering? But it's important to remind yourself that your loved one wouldn't want you to
be a caregiver. So get out of the house and
do something that has nothing to do with illness—whatever you find to be replenishing.

•**How did you enlist the help of others?**
It's important to have loved ones and friends
around and not to lose contact with them during illness. I encouraged friends to come and
talk with Paul, to take it more slowly and give
him time to speak.

People also need to find out what resources
are available. The Web sites of the National
Institute of Neurological Disorders and Stroke,
www.ninds.nih.gov, and the National Aphasia
Association, *www.aphasia.org*, can give all sorts

of tips and leads about groups you can find in
your own community.

•**What was your biggest challenge?** To
keep love alive in the midst of crisis. If you
are to stay married, you have to be able to
embrace the changes as part of your journey
together.

Stroke Rehab Made Much Easier

Yaffa Liebermann, PT, GCS, physical therapist who
is board certified by the American Physical Therapy
Association and a geriatric clinical specialist. Founder and CEO of Prime Rehabilitation Services, Inc., in
Yorktown Heights, New York, she has worked with
stroke survivors for 44 years as a practicing physical
therapist. Liebermann is the author of *Stroke Restora-
tion: Functional Movements for Patients and Caregivers*
(Prime Rehabilitation Services, Inc.).

Until relatively recently, doctors and physical therapists believed that a person
who underwent physical rehabilitation
immediately following a stroke would reach
his/her maximum recovery within six months.

Now: Researchers have discovered that an
intensive program of physical therapy can produce positive results for many stroke survivors
far beyond this time frame.

Even though physical rehabilitation ideally
begins as soon as possible after a stroke (to
stimulate brain-cell function and help prevent
joint stiffness and muscle weakness), the following techniques can be used by most people
who are trying to regain function and mobility—no matter how long ago the stroke was
experienced...*

SURVIVING A STROKE

There are approximately 5.5 million people
in the US who have survived a stroke. About
two-thirds of stroke survivors lose basic functional abilities, such as movement, speech and
balance. Without enough blood, brain cells die
and the abilities controlled by the parts of the
brain affected by the stroke are lost.

*Before starting this regimen, discuss the strategies
with your doctor and/or a physical therapist.

The severity of the disability depends on the size of the stroke. Some people who have a stroke may experience weakness in an arm or leg, but more extreme cases can involve paralysis.

Problem: Stroke rehabilitation (typically administered by a physical therapist) is offered at hundreds of facilities across the US, but many stroke patients stop exercising when they complete their initial rehabilitation program.**

This is an important issue since research shows that repetition is the best way to improve neuroplasticity—the brain's ability to "rewire" itself to promote recovery.

Solution: Stroke survivors can incorporate into their daily activities basic techniques that focus on three key areas that are crucial to continued rehabilitation. Because they are so simple and easy to perform, these strategies don't even feel like formal exercise and can be used with or without the help of a physical therapist.

STRATEGY 1
CHALLENGE THE WEAK SIDE

It's tempting, if you've had a stroke, to use the stronger side of your body. For example, you may prefer to put your weight on your stronger leg when you stand or use your stronger arm to perform tasks. However, you must shift weight to your weak side to regain movement.

What to do: To begin, bear your body weight as evenly as possible on both legs when you stand to improve muscle tone and normalize your movements. Use your stronger hand to support yourself and/or ask someone to stand beside you. You can practice this while standing behind a stable chair, holding on to a table or gripping a counter. Whenever possible, try to stand with equal weight on both feet.

Also helpful: If you have leg weakness, tap your feet whenever possible while standing or sitting. If you have weakness in an arm, use both hands to drum your fingers on a tabletop for several minutes each day. While seated, lean on your weak arm (for one to two minutes—but stop if you feel pain) while keep-

**To locate a stroke rehabilitation center near you, contact the Commission on Accreditation of Rehabilitation Facilities (888-281-6531, *www.carf.org*).

ing your elbow straight. Repeat on your other arm. Do this several times daily.

STRATEGY 2
MASTER TRUNK CONTROL

The trunk—or core—of the body provides strength for virtually all movements. But if one side of the body is weakened, the corresponding side of the trunk is not as strong, which forces the other side to do more. Strengthening the trunk creates more stability, which improves posture and helps facilitate easier movement of the arms and legs.

What to do: If you've had a relatively mild stroke, observe yourself in a standing position in front of a full-length mirror. If you lean to one side, that is generally your stronger side. Even though you may think that you would know whether you have weakness in certain parts of your body, you should look in a mirror because it's common to reposition your body to accommodate an injury without even realizing it.

To strengthen your trunk: Do rotation exercises (on your own, if possible, or with the help of a physical therapist or family member). To begin, lie on your back in bed, bend your knees, then slowly move your legs from side to side. Do this for about 10 minutes or until you feel fatigued first thing in the morning and at bedtime.

Also helpful: Once you can stand from a seated position and distribute your weight evenly on both legs, stand near a waist-high surface, such as a desk or counter. In each hand, roll an object, such as a can or bottle, on the surface. Do this for about 10 minutes or until you feel fatigued.

For the lower body: Hold on to the back of a stable chair and lift one leg backward as high as you comfortably can without leaning forward. Hold the position for a few seconds, then repeat on the other side. Do three sets of 10 repetitions on each leg three times weekly. When this becomes easy, ask your doctor or physical therapist about adding a light ankle weight to each leg.

STRATEGY 3
USE THE POWER OF YOUR BREATH

Many people who suffer a stroke are greatly weakened by the experience and, as a result, may suffer from shortness of breath. But correct breathing techniques practiced in rehabilitation prepare patients to cope with stressful situations (such as stair climbing) and overcome shortness of breath.

What to do: To improve breathing skills, exhale twice as long as you inhale. Example: A few times a day, inhale for a count of three and exhale for a count of six. Since deep inhalations may cause feelings of light-headedness in some stroke survivors, do not repeat the inhalation- exhalation series more than five times in a row. If someone is able to gently massage your shoulders at the same time, this often helps release tension and promotes good airflow.

Make a game: Whenever you bend your trunk, exhale for a count of six, and inhale for a count of three when you straighten up. Also, try exhaling when you reach for a cup or when you stoop down to retrieve an object. Then inhale as you sit back to drink or stand.

Virtual Stroke Rehab

A virtual-reality program makes stroke rehabilitation more fun. Patients wearing goggles see bugs flying nearby. When they successfully "smack" them, the bugs move farther away, improving the patients' range of motion.

University of Central Florida

Magnets May Help Stroke Patients

In a procedure called repetitive transcranial magnetic stimulation, electromagnets are strategically placed on a stroke patient's head. The magnets deliver tiny electric currents to the area of the brain affected by the stroke, reducing muscle weakness and improving overall motor function.

Recent finding: Patients given this treatment in addition to physical therapy showed significant improvement in motor function, compared with those who did not receive brain stimulation. Study participants had strokes between one and 36 months before starting this treatment.

Anwar Etribi, PhD, emeritus professor of neurology, Ain Shams University, Cairo, Egypt, and leader of a study published in *European Journal of Neurology*.

Stroke Patients May Improve Years After Their Strokes

Even two to three years after their strokes, patients still can learn to use undamaged areas of the brain to perform tasks, especially if their physical therapy includes long-term, supervised walking on a treadmill. Physical therapy typically is prescribed for only 30 to 60 days following a stroke because, until recently, it was believed that patients could make significant improvements only within that time frame.

Daniel F. Hanley, MD, department of neurology, Johns Hopkins University School of Medicine, Baltimore, and leader of a study published in *Stroke*.

Music Therapy for Stroke Patients

In a small study of men and women who suffered partial vision loss due to stroke, the patients were better able to identify shapes and lights while listening to music they enjoyed.

Theory: Pleasing music activates brain areas linked to positive emotional responses to stimuli, improving awareness of the visual world.

If you have experienced vision loss due to stroke: Ask your doctor whether music therapy might benefit you.

David Soto, PhD, research fellow, division of neuroscience and mental health, Imperial College, London.

Better Stroke Recovery

Seventy-one patients who had suffered a stroke an average of four years earlier walked on a treadmill three times weekly for up to 40 minutes each session or did stretching exercises (with the assistance of a therapist) for the same amount of time.

Result: The treadmill group's walking speed rose by 51%, on average, compared with an average increase of 19% for the stretching group.

Theory: The brain "recruits" other regions to take over functions (such as walking) normally controlled by brain areas damaged by stroke.

If you have had a stroke: Ask your doctor whether supervised walking would benefit you.

Daniel F. Hanley, MD, Jeffrey and Harriet Legum professor of neurology, Johns Hopkins University School of Medicine, Baltimore.

10

Blood Pressure Cures

What You're Not Being Told About Hypertension

Getting your blood pressure checked is a routine part of most physical exams. But how the measurement is taken and the treatment your doctor recommends if you have high blood pressure (hypertension) can have a profound effect on your health.

High blood pressure occurs when the force with which blood travels through the arteries is higher than it needs to be. Blood pressure readings consist of two measurements—*systolic pressure* (top number) measures the force as the heart contracts…*diastolic* (bottom number) represents the pressure between beats. Hypertension typically is defined as 140/90 mmHg or above, although readings above 120/80 mmHg are considered higher than optimal.

It's well-known that hypertension is often "silent" (causing no symptoms) and that it can lead to death or disability due to heart attack…stroke…and kidney damage.

What you may not know: One-third to one-half of all patients who take medication for hypertension lower their blood pressure insufficiently…take the wrong drugs…or suffer unnecessary side effects.

Samuel J. Mann, MD, a renowned hypertension specialist at New York-Presbyterian Hospital in New York City shares his insights about these and other dangerous traps…

Trap: Getting inaccurate blood pressure readings. The equipment in doctors' offices and home arm-cuff blood pressure monitors are usually accurate, but how they're used can greatly affect readings. *Three common mistakes…*

Mistake 1: Rushing the test. It takes five to 10 minutes of sitting quietly for blood pressure

---

Samuel J. Mann, MD, hypertension specialist and attending physician at New York–Presbyterian Hospital and professor of clinical medicine at Weill-Cornell Medical College, both in New York City. He is the author of *Healing Hypertension: A Revolutionary New Approach* (Wiley).

to stabilize. Testing too quickly can produce a reading that's considerably higher than your usual resting blood pressure.

Mistake 2: Using a cuff that's too small. Doctors often use the same blood pressure cuff on all patients—but if you have a large arm, the reading can be artificially high. Ask your doctor whether the blood pressure cuff size is right for you.

Mistake 3: Talking while blood pressure is being measured. It can add 10 millimeters or even more to the systolic (top number) reading.

Trap: Ignoring "white-coat hypertension." Up to 20% of people exhibit elevations in blood pressure in the doctor's office even though their pressure at home is normal. This phenomenon, known as white-coat hypertension, sometimes is due to the anxiety many people experience when they go to the doctor.

We used to think that white-coat hypertension was insignificant. Now, a study published in the *Journal of Human Hypertension* shows that people who exhibit this trait do face higher risks—for both heart attack and true hypertension at some point in their lives—than those whose office blood pressure is normal.

It's not yet clear why these patients have higher risks. Studies of patients who perform home monitoring suggest that their pressure tends to be slightly higher than what's considered optimal even if it's not high enough to be classified as hypertension.

Warning: Some people with white-coat hypertension are undertreated because their doctors tend to ignore elevated office readings while not paying attention to a gradual rise in home readings. Others are overtreated based on the elevated office readings, even though home readings are normal.

Helpful: Patients who have hypertension—or those at risk of getting it (due to such factors as family history and being overweight)—should use a home monitor to check their blood pressure two or three times a week. Take three readings each time, waiting about one to two minutes between each measurement.

Trap: Overtreating hypertension because of high readings obtained at times of stress. It's clear that blood pressure rises sharply at moments when people are angry, anxious or stressed. Many people have their blood pressure checked—or check it themselves—at such times, and their doctors increase medication based on these readings.

Helpful: Blood pressure elevation during emotional moments is normal. If your blood pressure is otherwise normal, an increase in medication usually is not necessary.

Trap: Taking the wrong drug. Up to 25% of patients with hypertension take a beta-blocker to lower blood pressure. This type of drug inhibits the kidneys' secretion of the enzyme renin, which results in lower levels of angiotensin II, a peptide that constricts blood vessels.

Beta-blockers also reduce the rate and force of heart contractions. However, most beta-blockers, including the widely prescribed *metoprolol* (Lopressor) and *atenolol* (Tenormin), have the undesirable effect of reducing blood flow.

These effects often result in fatigue. Many patients don't even realize how fatigued they are until they stop taking the beta-blocker and experience a sudden boost in energy.

Fact: The majority of patients with hypertension who suffer from fatigue due to a beta-blocker don't even need to take this drug. For most patients, it's best to start with other drugs or drug combinations, such as a diuretic (sodium-excreting pill) and/or an *angiotensin-converting enzyme* (ACE) inhibitor or an *angiotensin receptor blocker* (ARB).

Exception: Beta-blockers are usually a good choice for patients with hypertension who also have underlying coronary artery disease or who have had a heart attack.

If you need a beta-blocker: Ask your doctor about newer versions, such as *nebivolol* (Bystolic), that dilate arteries. Nebivolol is less likely to cause fatigue.

Trap: Switching to a newer drug—without good reason. Even if people are getting good results with the blood pressure medication they are taking, there's often a temptation to switch to a newer drug. Some newer drugs may have features that are an improvement over older medications, but others may offer little advantage and are not worth the extra cost.

Example: Aliskiren (Tekturna) is the first FDA-approved medication in a new class of blood pressure drugs known as direct renin inhibitors. Aliskiren inhibits the blood pressure–raising effects of the renin-angiotensin system. However, it is no more effective at lowering blood pressure than older treatments, such as ACE inhibitors or ARBs.

Switching drugs does make sense if you're not achieving optimal control—or if your current treatment is causing side effects. But for most patients, the older drugs are both effective and well-tolerated—and much less expensive.

Trap: Taking medication unnecessarily. It's estimated that only about 40% of patients with hypertension achieve optimal control by taking a single drug (monotherapy). Most patients will eventually need multiple drugs—but monotherapy is effective for some patients, particularly those with mild (stage 1) hypertension (defined as systolic pressure of 140 mmHg to 159 mmHg and/or diastolic pressure of 90 mmHg to 99 mmHg).

Adding drugs invariably increases both the cost of treatment and the risk for side effects. If a drug doesn't work within a few weeks, then switching drugs is an alternative to simply adding drugs. Or if a second drug is added and it normalizes your blood pressure, your doctor may consider reducing the dose of—or stopping—the first drug.

Skim Milk Lowers Hypertension

A two-year study of 5,880 people found that those who consumed more than two to three servings of skim milk and other low-fat dairy products daily had half the risk of developing high blood pressure of those who rarely or never consumed such foods.

Whole milk products were not found to reduce hypertension risk.

Theory: The calcium, which is highly absorbable in skim dairy products, may decrease blood pressure.

Alvaro Alonso, MD, PhD, assistant professor, division of Epidemiology and Community Health, School of Public Health, University of Minnesota, Minneapolis, Minnesota.

Hibiscus Tea Curbs Blood Pressure

In a study of 65 adults with prehypertension or mild hypertension, those who drank hibiscus tea had a 7.2-point drop, on average, in systolic (top number) blood pressure, compared with a one-point drop, on average, in the placebo group.

Theory: Antioxidant flavonoids in hibiscus help lower blood pressure.

If you have been diagnosed with prehypertension or hypertension: Three cups daily of hibiscus tea may benefit you.

Diane L. McKay, PhD, assistant professor of nutrition, science and policy, Tufts University, Boston.

Beet Juice Lowers Blood Pressure

Mark A. Stengler, NMD, licensed naturopathic medical doctor in private practice, Stengler Center for Integrative Medicine, Encinitas, California...adjunct associate clinical professor at the National College of Natural Medicine, Portland, Oregon...author of many books, including *The Natural Physician's Healing Therapies* and coauthor of *Prescription for Natural Cures* (both from Bottom Line Books)...and author of the *Bottom Line/Natural Healing* newsletter. *www.drstengler.com*

In a British study, 14 healthy participants drank 17 ounces of either water or beetroot (beet) juice. Blood pressure was measured every 15 minutes for one hour before, and three hours after, the beverages were consumed, and again after 24 hours.

Results: Among beet juice drinkers, the maximum decreases in blood pressure—10.4 points systolic (top number) and 8.1 points diastolic (bottom number)—occurred two-and-a-half to three hours after ingestion, when blood levels of nitrite, a key element in the juice, peaked. After 24 hours, blood pressure still was somewhat lowered. Water drinkers experienced no significant changes.

My view: Nitrite is converted in the stomach into nitric oxide, which dilates blood vessels, reduces inflammation and combats clotting—improving circulation and lowering blood pressure. Though this study was small, I find it encouraging.

Recommended: If you have high blood pressure, drink four to eight ounces (17 ounces is unrealistic) of beet juice daily. Mix with carrot or celery juice if you desire.

Sleep More to Lower Blood Pressure

People who get five hours or less of sleep a night were more than twice as likely to develop high blood pressure as people who slept seven to eight hours, according to a recent study.

Theory: Blood pressure drops by 10% to 20% during sleep, so a sleep deficit raises average 24-hour blood pressure and increases the workload on the cardiovascular system. Lack of sleep also boosts stress, which increases appetite for salt and decreases salt excretion—further raising hypertension risk in some people.

James E. Gangwisch, PhD, assistant professor, department of psychiatry, College of Physicians and Surgeons, Columbia University, New York City, and leader of a study of 4,810 people, published in *Hypertension*.

Put Away those Dangerous Drugs… And Try these Natural Alternatives

Mark A. Stengler, NMD, licensed naturopathic medical doctor in private practice, Stengler Center for Integrative Medicine, Encinitas, California…adjunct associate clinical professor at the National College of Natural Medicine, Portland, Oregon…author of many books, including *The Natural Physician's Healing Therapies* and coauthor of *Prescription for Natural Cures* (both from Bottom Line Books)…and author of the *Bottom Line/Natural Healing* newsletter. *www.drstengler.com*

Isn't it strange when some wholesome-looking actor appears on a TV commercial to promote a pharmaceutical? The ad tells you how great the drug is, then proceeds with a long, rapid-fire list of potential side effects. What a contradiction!

It's hard to believe, but Americans spend close to $200 billion each year on prescription drugs. Now, many people are concerned about the side effects of these medications—and with good reason. Each year, 2.9% to 3.7% of hospitalizations in the US are due to adverse reactions to medications.

The solution is to get healthy—and stay healthy—using natural methods. Many nutritional supplements can be used safely and effectively in place of prescription medications. Whether you're treating heartburn, high blood pressure, elevated cholesterol, depression or any number of other common ailments, there are excellent natural alternatives.

Caution: Do not stop taking a prescription drug or begin using a supplement unless you are being monitored by a health professional. These natural alternatives work best when combined with diet and lifestyle improvements, particularly regular exercise, stress-reduction techniques and adequate sleep.

STOMACH MEDICATIONS

Up to 18% of Americans experience heartburn at least once weekly. Heartburn that occurs more than twice a week may be *gastroesophageal reflux disease* (GERD), a condition in which stomach contents back up into the esophagus. The most commonly prescribed

147

drugs for heartburn and GERD are *esomeprazole* (Nexium), *lansoprazole* (Prevacid), *rabeprazole* (Aciphex), *omeprazole* (Prilosec) and *pantoprazole* (Protonix). Known as *proton pump inhibitors* (PPIs), these drugs block the production of stomach acid. And they carry a hefty price tag—about $4 per dose. Potential side effects include diarrhea, vomiting, headache, rash, dizziness, abnormal heartbeat, muscle pain, leg cramps and water retention.

Natural alternatives: Try them in this order—each one alone—for two weeks at a time until you find what works effectively for you. You can take more than one at a time.

• **Licorice root** (in chewable wafers or powder form) reduces heartburn and irritation of the digestive tract lining. Take 500 mg to 1,000 mg three times daily 30 minutes before meals. A special type of licorice root, known as *deglycyrrhizinated licorice* (DGL), does not elevate blood pressure, as do some varieties of the herb. DGL is widely available at health-food stores and pharmacies. It should relieve your symptoms within two weeks. Take as needed if symptoms recur.

• **Nux vomica,** a homeopathic remedy derived from the seeds of the poison nut tree, has helped many of my patients reduce or eliminate heartburn. It soothes irritation of the digestive lining and is believed to help the upper esophageal valve close more efficiently, thereby preventing reflux. Take two 30C potency pellets three times daily until your symptoms are eliminated. Improvement should occur within two weeks. Resume treatment if symptoms return. Because nux vomica is also used to treat asthma, it is good for asthmatics who suffer from heartburn.

• **Aloe vera,** a cactus-like member of the lily family, soothes and promotes healing of the lining of the digestive tract. Some people who don't respond to DGL get relief from aloe vera. Drink one-quarter cup of aloe vera juice or take a 500-mg capsule three times daily.

ANTIDEPRESSANTS

• **Sertraline** (Zoloft), *escitalopram* (Lexapro) and *fluoxetine* (Prozac) are the most popular prescription antidepressants sold in the US. They belong to a class of drugs called *selective serotonin reuptake inhibitors* (SSRIs). Serotonin, a neurotransmitter (chemical messenger) produced by nerve cells in the brain, plays an important role in balancing mood. SSRIs temporarily block serotonin from returning to the neuron that released it, boosting the amount of available serotonin.

Potential side effects of SSRIs include drowsiness, nervousness, insomnia, dizziness, nausea, tremors, loss of appetite, headache, diarrhea, dry mouth, irregular heartbeat, skin rash, weight loss or weight gain, and activation of mania in patients with bipolar disorder (also known as manic-depressive illness). These drugs also can cause sexual side effects, including loss of libido and decrease in the intensity of orgasms. The FDA has warned that children and adults taking antidepressants should be monitored for signs of worsening depression or suicidal thoughts.

Natural alternatives: Try them in this order for six to eight weeks. If effective, continue indefinitely. You can take more than one at a time.

• **S-adenosylmethionine (SAMe),** a nutritional supplement derived from the amino acid *methionine*, is excellent for mild to moderate depression. SAMe is thought to work by increasing the production of mood-boosting neurotransmitters. Some studies have shown SAMe to be as effective as pharmaceutical antidepressants—or, in some cases, even more so. Take 400 mg two or three times daily on an empty stomach. Do not use this supplement if you are taking an antidepressant or antianxiety medication—or if you have bipolar disorder. Like SSRIs, SAMe may activate a manic phase in bipolar patients.

• **5-hydroxytryptophan (5-HTP)** is a quick-acting, mood-enhancing amino acid that I recommend for my patients with mild to moderate depression. In the body, 5-HTP is converted into serotonin, helping to raise levels of this mood-balancing neurotransmitter. Take 100 mg two to three times daily on an empty stomach. Do not take 5-HTP in combination with pharmaceutical antidepressant or antianxiety medication.

• **St. John's wort is an herb that is widely used in Europe to treat depression.** In a review of 23 studies, it was found to be as effective as pharmaceutical therapy for mild to moderate depression. I recommend taking 600 mg of a 0.3% hypericin extract in the morning and 300 mg in the afternoon or evening. St. John's wort should not be used by women who take birth control pills or by anyone taking HIV medication or immune-suppressing drugs. Do not take St. John's wort with antidepressant or antianxiety medication.

• **Fish oil has been shown to help mild to moderate depression.** Take a formula that contains 1,000 mg of combined *docosahexaenoic acid* (DHA) and *eicosapentaenoic acid* (EPA) daily. Nordic Naturals and Carlson both make good formulas that are available at health-food stores. Fish oil can be taken indefinitely.

• **B vitamins improve the efficiency of many functions,** including the conversion of glucose to fuel and the synthesis of neurotransmitters. Deficiencies of B vitamins (notably B-3) can lead to anxiety and agitation. Take a 50-mg B complex daily for as long as you like.

CHOLESTEROL-LOWERING DRUGS

An estimated 11 million Americans take cholesterol-lowering statins. *Atorvastatin* (Lipitor), *simvastatin* (Zocor) and *rosuvastatin* (Crestor) are the most commonly prescribed in the US. One month's supply of one of these drugs costs $80 to more than $120.

Such drugs work by inhibiting a liver enzyme that helps produce the "bad" cholesterol, known as *low-density lipoprotein* (LDL) cholesterol. These drugs also decrease fats in the blood known as triglycerides and increase "good" *high-density lipoprotein* (HDL) cholesterol levels. Possible side effects include abdominal pain and digestive upset, joint pain, and muscle weakness and pain. One of the most frightening side effects is *rhabdomyolysis*. This condition affects only one in 100,000 people taking statins each year, but it results in severe pain and may cause kidney failure.

Natural alternatives: Try red yeast rice extract, then retest cholesterol levels in three months. Continue only if effective. If not, try policosanol.

• **Red yeast rice extract** is a supplement that has been shown to reduce total and LDL cholesterol levels by 11% to 32% and triglyceride levels by 12% to 19%. It has been shown to raise HDL by 15% to 30%. Take 2,400 mg of red yeast rice extract (containing 9.6 mg to 13.5 mg total monacolins) daily. Side effects, such as mild gastrointestinal discomfort, are rare. As with many products, red yeast rice extract should be avoided by people with liver disease.

• **Policosanol,** a derivative of sugarcane, is another well-researched cholesterol-lowering supplement. The *American Heart Journal* published a review of placebo-controlled studies, which found that taking 10 mg to 20 mg of policosanol daily lowered total cholesterol by 17% to 21% and LDL cholesterol by 21% to 29%. The supplement raised HDL cholesterol by 8% to 15%. Policosanol does not effectively lower triglyceride levels, so I don't recommend it for people who need to reduce these blood fats. Anyone else with high cholesterol should consider taking 10 mg to 20 mg daily.

Important: If your cholesterol levels are significantly elevated (in the mid-300s or higher), you may need to take a statin before trying these natural alternatives. Statins also may be prescribed to help reduce inflammation following a heart attack.

BLOOD PRESSURE MEDICATION

High blood pressure (hypertension) is estimated to affect one of every four adult Americans. *Tenormin* (Atenolol), *lisinopril* (Zestril) and *furosemide* (Lasix) are the most popular prescription drugs for high blood pressure. These drugs are relatively inexpensive—ranging from $11 to $36 per month.

• **Tenormin** (a so-called beta-blocker) works by blocking nerve impulses of the sympathetic nervous system, a portion of the involuntary nervous system that helps control the body's response to stress (the "fight or flight" reaction). Blood pressure is then lowered by reducing the heart rate and the force of the heart muscle contraction. Possible side effects include digestive upset, fatigue, insomnia, impotence, light-headedness, slow heart rate, low blood pressure (a dangerous condition that can lead to fainting and fatigue), numbness, tingling, sore throat and shortness of breath.

● **Lisinopril is an angiotensin-converting enzyme (ACE) inhibitor.** It triggers the relaxation of blood vessels. Relaxed blood vessels help lower blood pressure. Side effects of lisinopril can include chest pain, cough, diarrhea and low blood pressure.

● **Furosemide is a diuretic that causes water excretion.** By blocking absorption of salt and fluid in the kidneys, the drug causes an increase in urine output. Water excretion helps reduce blood volume, which means less work for your arteries and veins. Potential side effects include irregular heartbeat, dizziness, abdominal pain or diarrhea, low blood pressure and an imbalance of electrolytes (key minerals that are needed for vital body functions), leading to muscle cramps or weakness.

Important: If you have moderate to severe high blood pressure (160/100 and above), you may need prescription medication. You may be able to limit your need for prescription blood pressure drugs if you work with your doctor to incorporate natural therapies.

Natural alternatives: Try the first two extracts below for 30 days. If your blood pressure doesn't improve, try using all of the natural treatments together. You should see improvement within four weeks—and can continue the regimen indefinitely.

● **Hawthorn extract,** derived from the berry of a thorny shrub with white or pink flowers, dilates artery walls, decreasing systolic (top number) and diastolic (bottom number) blood pressure by about 10 points each. Take 250 mg to 500 mg three times daily. Hawthorn extract can have a mild blood-thinning effect, so check with your doctor first if you are taking a blood thinner, such as *warfarin* (Coumadin).

● **Bonito fish extract,** a protein from the muscle tissue of the bonito fish, acts like a natural ACE inhibitor. I recommend a daily dose of 1,500 mg.

● **Coenzyme Q10,** an enzyme found in the energy-producing mitochondria of all cells, has been shown to reduce both systolic and diastolic blood pressure by five to 10 points. You may need to take 200 mg to 300 mg daily for a blood pressure–lowering effect.

Calcium and magnesium relax the nervous system and arteries, lowering blood pressure. I suggest 500 mg of calcium and 250 mg of magnesium twice daily.

Soybean Protein Lowers Blood Pressure

In a study of 302 adults with a median blood pressure of 135/85 mmHg (normal is below 120/80 mmHg), those who ate one cookie containing 40 g of soybean protein a day for 12 weeks had a 4.31-point drop in systolic (top number) pressure and a 2.76-point drop in diastolic (bottom number) pressure compared with those who ate a placebo cookie.

Theory: Soybean protein may influence the sympathetic nervous system, sodium excretion and insulin resistance, all of which affect blood pressure.

Implication: Soybean consumption may be an effective alternative to medication for lowering blood pressure in otherwise healthy people with mild hypertension.

Jiang He, MD, PhD, professor and chair, department of epidemiology, Tulane University School of Public Health and Tropical Medicine, New Orleans.

11

Arthritis Cures

Breakthrough Therapy Helps Heal Joints and Orthopedic Injuries

When pitcher Takashi Saito was with the Los Angeles Dodgers, he suffered a ligament tear in his elbow and was told that he would be sidelined for about a year if he had it surgically repaired. Instead, he underwent an innovative natural treatment called *platelet-rich plasma* (PRP) *therapy*. A few months later, he was pitching pain-free.

PRP is an emerging treatment in the growing field of orthobiologics, which combines cutting-edge technology with therapies that work by stimulating the body's healing processes. In PRP, a patient's own platelets—the blood component that contains major growth factors, naturally occurring substances that stimulate cell growth—are injected into an in-

jured or arthritic area, enhancing the repair response of soft tissue. Until recently, orthopedic applications of PRP were mostly reserved for professional athletes, but now it is available to everyone through some family physicians and orthopedic surgeons.

At my clinic, Bronner Handwerger, ND, uses PRP therapy to treat patients like a professional football player who had a minor knee cartilage tear. He was able to resume training just three days after receiving PRP. Knee injuries such as his usually take weeks to heal. James Baum, DO, of Santa Fe, New Mexico, is one of many orthopedic surgeons around the country who offers PRP therapy for a variety of conditions. He has treated scores of patients, including a woman with debilitating spinal stenosis

Mark A. Stengler, NMD, licensed naturopathic medical doctor in private practice, Stengler Center for Integrative Medicine, Encinitas, California…adjunct associate clinical professor at the National College of Natural Medicine, Portland, Oregon…author of many books, including *The Natural Physician's Healing Therapies* and coauthor of *Prescription for Natural Cures* (both from Bottom Line Books)…and author of the *Bottom Line/Natural Healing* newsletter. *www.drstengler.com*

(narrowing of one or more areas of the spine) who now is symptom-free after four injections. He treated another woman who could barely walk because of an arthritic hip. Now, after receiving several PRP injections, she is walking pain-free.

PRP appears to help many types of injuries. Other applications currently being studied include injecting PRP at the site of bone fractures and using it to help speed healing after connective-tissue surgeries. Although it has not yet been shown definitively whether PRP can regenerate cartilage, Dr. Baum believes that clinical research will mirror his own experience in stimulating cartilage regeneration—and that PRP will be crucial in combating the growing epidemic of osteoarthritis as the American population ages.

HOW IT WORKS

In a doctor's office, a few tablespoons of blood are drawn and run through a machine that separates out the platelets. The resulting fluid contains four to 10 times the blood's normal concentration of growth factors. Along with a local anesthetic, this mixture is injected directly into an injured or arthritic area (ultrasound may be used to guide placement). The procedure takes about an hour.

While there may be some soreness for a few days afterward, patients often have reduced pain and improved movement after just one treatment. Depending on the severity of the condition and an individual's healing response, injections may be repeated up to six times at two- to four-week intervals.

PRP therapy is extremely safe because the patient is injected with parts of his/her own blood. Infection at the injection site is extremely rare. (PRP therapy has not been reviewed by the FDA, which doesn't regulate surgical procedures.) The technique also is safer than many other conventional treatments commonly used to treat joint and connective-tissue injuries, such as cortisone shots, anti-inflammatory medications and surgery. These approaches all have drawbacks—cortisone can weaken tissue over time…anti-inflammatory drugs have potentially dangerous side effects, such as kidney and liver damage…and surgery is expensive and involves a lengthy recovery.

PRP's effectiveness still is being studied, but in one Stanford University study, patients with chronic elbow tendonitis who were given one PRP treatment had a 60% improvement in pain compared to only a 16% improvement in those who received an injection of anesthetic only.

When seeking treatment with PRP, keep these points in mind…

• **Insurance.** Because PRP therapy is new, insurance may not cover it. Check with your insurer before scheduling a procedure. PRP costs about $400 to $600 per injection—based on your injury and the type of equipment used by the doctor—a fraction of what surgery costs.

• **Effectiveness.** This depends in large part on the quality and abundance of the growth factors in a patient's blood. For some people, the results are permanent. Smokers don't respond as well to PRP, because they have reduced platelet activity.

WHAT'S TREATABLE WITH PRP?

PRP therapy can treat the knees, shoulders, elbows, feet, wrist and back for the following…

• **Torn tendons or ligaments**

• **Strained rotator cuff**

• **Arthritic or inflamed joints**

• **Carpal tunnel syndrome**

• **Plantar fasciitis** (an inflammatory condition that affects the tissue under the foot's arch)

• **Torn or strained muscles**

BETTER THAN OTHER NATURAL INJECTIONS

PRP therapy is similar to prolotherapy, another injection technique that stimulates the body's natural healing process and has been found helpful for arthritis and injured cartilage, tendons and ligaments.

The difference: Prolotherapy involves injecting an injured joint or tissue with a harmless but mildly irritating substance, such as a dextrose (sugar) solution. This induces inflammation in the injured area, attracting growth factors that stimulate growth of collagen and other connective tissues. PRP therapy involves injecting growth factors themselves into an area that has a very poor blood supply. Prolotherapy is less expensive (starting at about $125 per treatment) than PRP. Of the two treatments, I recommend PRP because it is more effective.

Natural Remedies for Arthritis Relief

Tod Cooperman, MD, founder and president of ConsumerLab.com, the leading independent evaluator of nutritional and vitamin/mineral supplements, White Plains, New York. Reports can be found at *www.consumerlab.com* (subscription required). He also is editor of *ConsumerLab.com's Guide to Buying Vitamins & Supplements* (ConsumerLab.com).

Most people assume that prescription medications are stronger and more effective than supplements. But some supplements can be just as effective—without the side effects that often accompany prescription drugs.

Also, people with chronic conditions who have no insurance or are under-insured or who have been hit with higher co-pays can save hundreds or even thousands of dollars a year by using supplements in place of drugs.

Caution: Always check with your doctor before stopping a prescription drug or taking a supplement.

Here, natural alternatives to commonly prescribed medications. If there are two alternatives, try one. If that doesn't work, try the other. Dosages are those typically prescribed, but always follow directions on the supplement label or from your health practitioner.

OSTEOARTHRITIS

It's the most common form of arthritis, affecting up to 20 million American adults. Osteoarthritis occurs when cartilage in the joints wears and breaks down, causing pain and stiffness. People with frequent or severe symptoms often depend on prescription-strength anti-inflammatory drugs. These drugs reduce symptoms but don't change the outcome of the disease. They also can cause stomach upset or other gastrointestinal problems.

•**Alternative 1. Glucosamine.** This supplement usually is derived from shellfish, though vegetable-based versions are starting to appear. It helps the body repair and rebuild damaged cartilage. It can help reduce pain as well as subsequent joint damage.

Dose: 1,500 mg, once daily.

•**Alternative 2. Glucosamine plus chondroitin**. This supplement combination is more expensive than glucosamine alone, but it sometimes helps patients who don't respond to glucosamine. Chondroitin, the added ingredient that typically is made from cow or pig cartilage, promotes the absorption of fluids into connective tissue and aids in flexibility and repair.

Dose: 1,500 mg of glucosamine and 1,200 mg of chondroitin, once daily.

Important: Studies reveal that supplements protect joints better than they relieve pain. Most people who take them still need an occasional anti-inflammatory painkiller.

RHEUMATOID ARTHRITIS

This form of arthritis causes inflammation throughout the body that can damage joints as well as the eyes, lungs and/or heart. Most people with rheumatoid arthritis take prescription drugs, such as *methotrexate* (Rheumatrex) or *hydroxychloroquine* (Plaquenil). Most rheumatoid drugs are expensive, and many have a high risk for side effects, including suppressed immunity.

Supplementation can reduce inflammation and potentially reduce the dosage of prescription drugs.

•**Alternative. Fish and fish oil.** The omega-3 fatty acids in cold-water fish, such as salmon and tuna, have potent anti-inflammatory effects. A study at the University of Pittsburgh School of Medicine found that 59% of patients given supplemental omega-3s had decreased joint pain.

Dose: A total of 1,200 mg to 2,400 mg of EPA and DHA (types of fish oil) daily, or eat three or more fish servings a week.

Caution: Fish oil may interact with blood-thinning drugs, such as *warfarin* (Coumadin).

Alignment Technique

Structural Integration (SI) is a bodywork technique that focuses on the fascia, the protective connective tissue that surrounds the muscles. Founded by Ida P. Rolf, the technique also is sometimes known as "rolfing." SI therapists use pressure and stretching to lengthen and manipulate fascia to enhance body alignment and balance. SI is based on the theory that through the force of gravity and injury, the body's structure becomes misaligned...and fascia shortens, resulting in pain and stiffness. I find that SI is helpful for those with muscle or spine pain. You can find out about practitioners near you from the International Association of Structural Integrators at 414-908-4947 or *www.theiasi.org.*

Mark A. Stengler, NMD, licensed naturopathic medical doctor in private practice, Stengler Center for Integrative Medicine, Encinitas, California...adjunct associate clinical professor at the National College of Natural Medicine, Portland, Oregon...author of many books and the *Bottom Line/Natural Healing* newsletter. *www.drstengler.com*

Hyaluronic Acid...Help For Painful Joints and Problem Skin

Mark A. Stengler, NMD, licensed naturopathic medical doctor in private practice, Stengler Center for Integrative Medicine, Encinitas, California...adjunct associate clinical professor at the National College of Natural Medicine, Portland, Oregon...author of many books, including *The Natural Physician's Healing Therapies* and coauthor of *Prescription for Natural Cures* (both from Bottom Line Books)...and author of the *Bottom Line/Natural Healing* newsletter. *www.drstengler.com*

On her first visit to me, 60-year-old Jenny said, "Every time I hear of a supplement that might reduce my arthritis pain, I try it—but I've gotten very little relief. I've almost given up on finding anything that works." I paid close attention as she named nearly a dozen supplements she had taken for the arthritis in her hips and knees. Then

I mentioned one oral supplement that had not been on her list—*hyaluronic acid* (HA). "I've never even heard of it, but it's worth trying," Jenny said. Six weeks later, she walked nimbly into my clinic and reported a dramatic reduction in her pain and stiffness. She was surprised at this success—but I was not.

HA has been so effective for so many of my arthritis patients that I consider it an up-and-coming superstar among nutritional supplements. Bonus: HA also promotes skin health.

WHAT IS HYALURONIC ACID?

A naturally occurring substance in the body, the HA molecule is formed by two sugars strung together in a long chain. HA is an essential component of the joints, skin, eyes and blood vessels (as well as the umbilical cord). HA deficiencies, which develop for reasons that are not well-understood, contribute to premature aging and disease in these tissues. As yet, there is no reliable test to measure HA levels.

HA is a key component of synovial fluid, the lubricating fluid in joint cavities. This fluid, which is secreted by a membrane that forms a capsule around the ends of bones, has two main purposes. First, it helps to minimize friction and prevent breakdown of the joints (like the oil used to lubricate moving car parts). Second, synovial fluid helps with shock absorption within joints. Cartilage is the main shock absorber, but it does not contain blood vessels—so synovial fluid transports the nutrients required for cartilage healing and regeneration, and removes waste products. In addition, HA is an actual component of cartilage and is required for healthy cartilage formation.

•**There are two main types of arthritis.** Osteoarthritis is caused by the normal wear and tear of aging and/or by injury. Rheumatoid arthritis is an autoimmune disease in which the immune system attacks the body's own joint tissue and causes deterioration. As either type of arthritis progresses, the synovial fluid degrades, lessening its lubricating and shock-absorbing abilities...and cartilage breaks down and becomes inflamed. Supplementing with HA helps to counteract both of these effects.

THE FIGHT AGAINST ARTHRITIS

When I mention HA to patients, most say they've never heard of it. I expect this to change as news of HA's effectiveness spreads.

• **HA injections.** In 1997, HA injections were approved by the FDA for patients with osteoarthritis of the knee, and they now are being studied for use in shoulder, hip and ankle joints. Injectable HA products include Hyalgan, Supartz, Orthovisc and Synvisc.

HA injections go directly into the affected joint or joints…are done in a doctor's office using local anesthetic…take just a few minutes… and usually are given three to five times, each one week apart. Side effects include minor swelling, temporary pain, rash and/or bruising at the injection site. While not everyone who receives HA injections finds relief, for many people the painful symptoms of arthritis are noticeably reduced for up to six months (especially in the early stages of the disease), allowing patients to delay or avoid joint-replacement surgery.

For now, only a limited number of rheumatologists and osteopaths provide this therapy. HA shots cost about $230 each and may or may not be covered by insurance, depending on your policy. Fortunately, there is a promising alternative—oral HA.

• **HA oral supplementation.** With regard to HA's use as an oral supplement, the big question is whether it can be absorbed and used by the body when taken in capsule form. Critics of HA supplementation say that its molecular structure is too large to be absorbed in the digestive tract—yet several studies in the past four years have shown otherwise.

One of the first studies to demonstrate that HA is absorbed effectively into the bloodstream and the joints was presented at the Experimental Biology Conference. Researchers gave rats and dogs one oral dose of HA that was radio labeled (chemically joined with a radioactive substance), allowing it to be tracked with diagnostic imaging. Result: HA was absorbed into the animals' bloodstreams and distributed to their joints. Although no similar studies have been done on people, I think it is logical to assume that HA's absorbability in humans may be similar to its action in animals.

Why am I keen on supplemental HA for arthritis? During the past year, several dozens of my patients with osteoarthritis and rheumatoid arthritis have taken nonprescription oral HA with good results. I have found that HA by itself can produce significant results—and in many cases, results are even better when HA is taken in combination with mainstay joint supplements, such as chondroitin, fish oil, glucosamine, methylsulfonylmethane (MSM) and/or S-adenosylmethionine (SAMe).

This is wonderful news, because HA often allows patients to reduce or discontinue the pharmaceutical nonsteroidal anti-inflammatory (NSAID) drugs, such as *ibuprofen* (Motrin) and *naproxen* (Aleve). These drugs are associated with serious adverse side effects, including bleeding stomach ulcers, liver and kidney damage, and increased risk for heart attack and stroke.

HA is an example of a supplement that works well in the real world but has generated limited published data. Existing research mostly involves a patented HA product called BioCell Collagen II (714-632-1231, *www.bio celltechnology.com*), made from the sternal cartilage of chickens and used as an ingredient in various brands of HA oral supplements. One small study included 16 patients with osteoarthritis of the knee or hand who were taking COX-2 inhibitors or other NSAIDs. Eight patients took 1,000 mg of BioCell daily, while the other eight took a placebo. After two months of treatment, the group receiving BioCell reported significant improvement in pain, range of motion and swelling—whereas the placebo group showed no significant changes. One such product, sold at health-food stores, is BioCell Chicken Sternum Collagen Type II, made by Premier Labs LLC (888-678-7145, *www. premierlabsllc.com*).

Other oral products contain a type of HA called *sodium hyaluronate*, which is produced during microbial fermentation. While I am not aware of any human studies on this form of HA, animal studies suggest that it is safe and several of my patients have reported positive effects. One such product available in health-food stores is Now Foods Hyaluronic Acid (888-669-3663, *www.nowfoods.com*). The recommended dosage is 100 mg twice daily. The Now Foods capsules, like brands that contain BioCell, can be used indefinitely, generally are safe and only rarely cause mild digestive upset.

HYALURONIC HELP FOR THE SKIN

Another benefit of HA is that it improves the health of the largest human organ—the skin. Here's how…

One of the most important proteins of the skin is collagen, the "glue" of connective tissue that holds the skin together, thereby maintaining its elasticity and form. HA supports collagen production and also is critical for maintaining moisture in and between skin cells. A lack of HA—typically brought on by illness or aging—may contribute to skin dryness, thinning and wrinkles.

•**HA injections.** Like the better-known collagen injections, HA injections can be used to minimize wrinkles, lines and pitting from acne or scars, and to plump up thin lips. HA and collagen injections both typically need to be repeated after six to nine months—but HA is less likely to provoke an allergic reaction.

FDA-approved HA injectable skin fillers include Hylaform and Restylane. Possible side effects include brief redness, swelling and/or tenderness at the injection site. Health insurance generally does not cover cosmetic treatments.

Caution: Cosmetic HA injections should be administered by an experienced cosmetic surgeon, not a family practitioner.

•**HA oral supplementation.** Recently I spoke with a patient who had thin, easily bruised skin as a result of using oral steroids for several years to treat Crohn's disease (an inflammatory condition of the digestive tract). After various foods and supplements failed to improve her skin condition, I recommended an HA oral supplement called Purity Products Ultimate HA Formula (800-256-6102, *www.purityproducts. com*). Eight weeks after she started to take HA, this patient reported that for the first time in years, she was not covered in bruises. Note: HA oral supplements designed to promote skin health generally contain the same active HA ingredient as those marketed for joint health.

•**HA topical ointment.** Some evidence suggests that HA skin ointment also may reduce wrinkles and skin pitting. One study I obtained from a private research lab showed that topical HA inhibited production of *hyaluronidase*, an enzyme in the skin and connective tissues that degrades the body's own natural wrinkle-fighting HA. In a separate in vitro (test-tube) study from Pennsylvania State University, topical HA was shown to stimulate production of collagen-producing cells called *fibroblasts*, which potentially could further reduce wrinkles and lines.

One commercially available topical skin product that contains BioCell is Skin Eternal Hyaluronic Serum by Source Naturals (800-815-2333, *www.sourcenaturals.com*). Place one to four drops of serum on your finger and gently massage into the skin where desired. It is generally safe for everyone. Rare side effects may include redness and irritation. I suggest trying it for two months to evaluate its effectiveness. If you are satisfied, topical HA can be used indefinitely to optimize the health and appearance of your skin.

While further studies clearly are needed to confirm the benefits of HA, I am optimistic about its potential. After all, it is not often that so promising a therapy arrives on the health-care scene.

FURTHER RELIEF FROM ARTHRITIS

For maximum relief from arthritis pain and inflammation, combine hyaluronic acid (HA) oral supplements or injections with other natural supplements described below. All are available in health-food stores and, unless noted, generally are safe for everyone. Mild arthritis symptoms may respond to the lower end of the dosage range, while severe symptoms may require the higher dosage.

•**Chondroitin,** a substance derived from cow cartilage.

Dosage: 1,200 mg daily. Lower the dosage or discontinue use if you experience digestive upset, such as nausea.

•**Fish oil** in the form of *docosahexaenoic acid* (DHA) and *eicosapentaenoic acid* (EPA), combined.

Dosage: 1,000 mg to 2,000 mg daily.

Caution: Get your doctor's approval first if you take a blood thinner, such as aspirin or *warfarin* (Coumadin).

• **Glucosamine, a substance derived from shellfish.**

Dosage: 1,500 mg daily. Lower the dosage or discontinue use if you experience digestive upset, such as diarrhea.

Caution: Check with your doctor before using if you are allergic to shellfish...or if you have diabetes, because glucosamine may cause blood-sugar fluctuations.

• **Methylsulfonylmethane (MSM),** an organic sulfur compound.

Dosage: 2,000 mg to 6,000 mg daily.

• ***S-adenosylmethionine* (SAMe),** an amino acid-like substance.

Dosage: 600 mg to 1,200 mg daily.

How to use: For rheumatoid arthritis, take fish oil and MSM. For osteoarthritis, start with glucosamine and MSM...and if symptoms are not adequately relieved within two months, also take chondroitin, fish oil and SAMe.

7 Must-Have Healing Herbs

Kathy Abascal, RH, registered herbalist who practices in Vashon, Washington. A member of the American Herbalists Guild, she is coauthor of *Clinical Botanical Medicine* (Mary Ann Liebert).

Until recently, if you peeked inside the medicine cabinet of a typical American household, you were likely to find such items as aspirin for headaches...an anti-inflammatory ointment for sore muscles and joints...an antihistamine for colds—and perhaps even a prescription sedative for sleep problems and/or an antidepressant.

Latest development: With the recent economic downturn and rising drug costs, many Americans are turning to medicinal alternatives. Recently, nationwide sales of herbal supplements totaled $4.8 billion, up more than 4% from the previous year. Perhaps due to the recession, Americans now appear to be trying many of the same herb-based products that have been used for generations in other parts of the world as the front-line treatments for many common conditions.

How herbs can help you: Compared with many medications widely used in the US, herbal therapies tend to have fewer side effects, are generally just as effective—if not more so— and are often less expensive.*

Seven of the most useful herbs to have on hand in your home...

ECHINACEA FOR COLDS

A recent study reported that echinacea is not effective for the common cold. Then, another study, found that it does help. Does it or doesn't it?

Echinacea stimulates both white blood cells (which attack viruses) and natural killer cells (which destroy virus-infected cells). Most scientific studies of echinacea involve dosing patients every four to six hours. That's not enough.

How to use: Add about one teaspoon of echinacea tincture to one-half cup of water. Drink it once every waking hour at the first signs of a cold until symptoms subside.

Helpful: Add to the mixture one-half teaspoon of elderberry tincture—which also helps boost immunity—for additional antiviral effects.

EUCALYPTUS FOR CONGESTION

Used as an essential oil, eucalyptus penetrates the mucous membranes and promotes drainage—helpful for relieving symptoms caused by the common cold and/or sinusitis (inflammation of the sinuses). The oil also has antimicrobial properties that can inhibit viruses and bacteria.

How to use: At the first signs of a cold or sinusitis, put five to 10 drops of eucalyptus essential oil in a large bowl. Add one to two cups of steaming hot water. (The dose is correct if you can smell the eucalyptus.) Put a towel over your head, and lean over the bowl (with your eyes closed) and breathe in the steam for about

---

*If you have a chronic condition and/or take prescription medication, consult your doctor before taking herbs.

10 minutes. Repeat as needed, using fresh eucalyptus oil each time.

Caution: Keep your head far enough from the steaming water to avoid burning yourself.

TURMERIC
FOR JOINT PAIN

Studies show that this extremely potent anti-inflammatory herb is about as effective as nonsteroidal anti-inflammatory drugs—such as aspirin and *ibuprofen* (Advil)—for easing joint pain. Unlike these and similar drugs, turmeric (taken at the doses recommended below) rarely causes stomach upset or other side effects.

How to use: Take 400 mg to 500 mg, three times daily. For additional benefits, use powdered turmeric when cooking. As little as one-quarter teaspoon per recipe will have anti-inflammatory effects over time.

Important: When cooking, use turmeric and black pepper. This greatly increases absorption of turmeric into the bloodstream.

Also helpful: Look for a turmeric supplement formula that includes black pepper.

VALERIAN
FOR INSOMNIA

Compounds in valerian act on brain receptors to induce drowsiness and relaxation.

How to use: Take one-half teaspoon of valerian tincture, diluted in water according to the instructions on the label, one hour before bedtime and one-half teaspoon at bedtime, as needed. In small doses—about one-quarter to one-half of the insomnia dose—valerian also can help reduce mild anxiety. Most people avoid valerian tea due to its unpleasant odor.

WHITE WILLOW BARK
FOR HEADACHES

It contains salicin, a chemical that's converted in the body into salicylic acid, an aspirin-like substance. Some studies indicate that white willow bark works as well as aspirin (minus the side effects, such as gastrointestinal upset) for headaches and other types of pain, such as osteoarthritis pain and low-back pain.

How to use: Take 200 mg, twice daily with food for headache and other types of pain (described above).

Caution: If you take a blood thinner, such as *warfarin* (Coumadin), consult your physician before using white willow bark, which also has blood-thinning effects.

ST. JOHN'S WORT
TO LIFT YOUR MOOD

It's thought to inhibit the activity of enzymes that break down serotonin, a neurotransmitter that plays a key role in regulating mood.

Studies have shown that St. John's wort is as effective for mild to moderate depression as some prescription antidepressants.

St. John's wort also is one of the most effective herbs for treating seasonal affective disorder (SAD), a form of depression that tends to occur in winter.

Caution: Consult your doctor before trying St. John's wort if you take a prescription antidepressant or other medication—or drink alcohol.

How to use: The recommended dose is usually 300 mg, three times daily (standardized to 0.3% hypericin). Consult your doctor for advice on treatment duration.

Helpful: If you suffer from SAD, take 1,000 international units (IU) to 2,000 IU of vitamin D along with St. John's wort. A lack of sun and low levels of vitamin D (also associated with infrequent sun exposure) can cause depression.

ALOE VERA FOR BURNS

Like an antibiotic cream, the gel from aloe leaves has antimicrobial properties. It soothes painful burns.

How to use: Keep an aloe plant in your home. For minor burns, slice open an aloe leaf and squeeze the gel over the affected area. Store-bought aloe gel also is effective.

Helpful: Keep several aloe leaves in the freezer. The cold gel will act as a mild anesthetic.

Looking for Pain Relief? Try Prolotherapy

Allan Magaziner, DO, director of Magaziner Center for Wellness in Cherry Hill, New Jersey, and a clinical instructor at University of Medicine and Dentistry of New Jersey in New Brunswick. His Web site is *www. drmagaziner.com.*

A medical procedure that "tricks" the body into healing itself, prolotherapy treats acute or chronic pain from damaged ligaments, tendons and cartilage. Some studies show significant improvement in patients with injuries or arthritis, especially in the joints, back, neck or jaw. Prolotherapy is used as a first-line therapy or when other treatments fail.

• **How it works.** A physician injects a solution, typically of dextrose (a sugar) and lidocaine (an anesthetic), into the painful area. This provokes minor, temporary inflammation… causing the body to send more blood and nutrients to the spot…which hastens healing.

• **What to expect.** Each session lasts 15 to 30 minutes and includes from one to 20 injections, depending on the areas treated. Patients experience slight discomfort during injection and mild soreness for several days after. Minor pain might need one session…severe pain might require 10 sessions spread over several months.

• **Cautions.** Your doctor may advise you to temporarily reduce or discontinue anti-inflammatory drugs—aspirin, *ibuprofen* (Motrin), *naproxen* (Aleve)—while undergoing prolotherapy. *Acetaminophen* (Tylenol) is okay. If you take blood thinners or other drugs, tell your doctor—extra precautions may be warranted.

• **Finding a practitioner.** Prolotherapy should be administered by a physician trained in the procedure—preferably through the American Association of Orthopaedic Medicine (800-992-2063, *www.aaomed.org*) or Hackett Hemwall Foundation (*www.hacketthemwall.org*). Visit these Web sites for referrals.

Cost: $100 to $400 per session. Because prolotherapy is considered experimental, insurance seldom covers it.

Sitz Baths…A Water Remedy for Many Ailments

Mark A. Stengler, NMD, licensed naturopathic medical doctor in private practice, Stengler Center for Integrative Medicine, Encinitas, California…adjunct associate clinical professor at the National College of Natural Medicine, Portland, Oregon…author of many books, including *The Natural Physician's Healing Therapies* and coauthor of *Prescription for Natural Cures* (both from Bottom Line Books)…and author of the *Bottom Line/Natural Healing* newsletter. *www.drstengler.com*

S itz baths—sitting so that your bottom is in water—can be an easy, at-home way to help many health problems, including urinary tract infections, insomnia, even headaches.

Sitz baths promote healing by changing blood flow to the area, reducing pain and inflammation. Warm water increases blood flow to the area, while cold water helps blood move to other body parts.

What you'll need: Purchase a plastic sitz-bath tub that is placed on the toilet (available at drugstores). These are contoured to focus circulation on the buttocks.

Next best: The bathtub. Fill the tub with water high enough to reach just under the navel while you are seated.

How to do it: Use a thermometer to determine water temperature. To alternate between warm and cold water, have two buckets of water ready or use both the purchased sitz bath and the bathtub.

Conditions: Abdominal or uterine pain, low-back pain, insomnia, hemorrhoids, muscle spasms (add 2 cups of Epsom salts).

Warm treatment: Water 106°F – 110°F, 5 to 8 minutes, one to two times daily.

Conditions: Acute bladder infection, itchy rectum, acute urinary tract infection.

Lukewarm treatment: Water 92°F – 97°F, 15 minutes to one hour (depending on your comfort level), one to two times daily.

Conditions: Constipation, prostate enlargement, uterus or rectum prolapse.

Cold treatment: Water 55°F – 75°F, 5 to 8 minutes, one to two times daily.

Conditions: Vaginal infections, prostatitis, headache, postpartum recovery, chronic urinary tract infection.

Alternating treatment: Warm water for 3 to 5 minutes, followed by 30 to 60 seconds in cold. Repeat three times daily.

If you have diabetes, heart disease or high blood pressure, speak to your doctor before taking a sitz bath because it can cause changes in blood pressure, pulse and glucose levels.

Natural Cures for an Ailing Immune System

Jamison Starbuck, ND, naturopathic physician in family practice in Missoula, Montana. She is past president of the American Association of Naturopathic Physicians and a contributing editor to *The Alternative Advisor: The Complete Guide to Natural Therapies and Alternative Treatments* (Time-Life).

The immune system is remarkable in its ability to help fight off infections and a wide variety of serious illnesses ranging from flu to staph infections. When our defenses go awry, however, our health can be threatened in a number of ways. For unknown reasons, the body's immune system can attack a part of itself, resulting in autoimmune disease.

Examples: *Systemic lupus erythematosus* (commonly known as lupus) can affect the kidneys, skin and blood vessels. With Crohn's disease, the immune system strikes the bowel. In patients who have rheumatoid arthritis, the joints are assaulted.

When a patient is diagnosed with an autoimmune disease, conventional doctors generally begin their treatment with medication. For lupus and Crohn's disease, *prednisone* (a steroid drug) is commonly used. For rheumatoid arthritis, medications typically include nonsteroidal anti-inflammatory drugs (NSAIDs), corticosteroids and, most recently, drugs called *tumor necrosis factor inhibitors*, such as *etanercept* (Enbrel) and *infliximab* (Remicade).

While these medications reduce symptoms, they can cause potentially serious side effects, such as liver damage and hypertension. That's why I prefer to treat symptoms naturally whenever possible, reserving strong medications for flare-ups. *My advice for people with autoimmune disease...*

• **Eat an anti-inflammatory diet.** Limit animal food (meat and poultry) to two meals per day and no more than three to four ounces per meal. Also consume at least five one-half cup servings of vegetables daily...one cup of a whole grain, such as brown rice or millet, and/or legumes, such as lentils or split peas... a small handful of nuts...and two or more pieces of fruit.

• **Take an omega-3 supplement.** For most of my patients with an autoimmune disease, I recommend a daily dose of 2,800 mg of inflammation-fighting omega-3 oils from fish oil, 50% of which should be *eicosapentaenoic acid* (EPA), a fatty acid shown to have strong immune-supportive effects. Omega-3 oils should always be taken with food because they are more readily digested. Check the label to be sure your fish oil source has been tested for heavy metal contamination.

• **Limit your exposure to environmental pollutants and drugs.** Both appear to trigger autoimmune disease in sensitive individuals. Substances that are known to cause this reaction in some people include mercury, cadmium, pesticides, anticonvulsant medications, beta-blockers (taken for heart disease) and estrogens (taken for menopausal symptoms). Talk to your doctor about getting tested for heavy metal toxicity and about taking only those prescription medications that he/she feels are absolutely necessary.

Take a vitamin D supplement daily. An increasing body of scientific evidence links vitamin D deficiency with autoimmune disease. Researchers theorize that vitamin D helps regulate immune cell activity in the body. My recommendation: A supplement containing 800 international units (IU) to 1,200 IU of vitamin D daily.

Leeches—A Suprisingly Effective Therapy

From *Bottom Line's Breakthroughs in Drug-Free Healing* by Bill Gottlieb (Bottom Line Books). *www.bottomlinepublications.com.*

Don't expect your doctor to prescribe them anytime soon (or your local pharmacy to stock them), but European physicians are finding out that leeches*—yes, leeches, the animals detested by Humphrey Bogart in the African Queen but prized by natural healers since antiquity for their power to cure blood clots and disinfect wounds—are adept at reducing arthritis pain…

New study: Doctors in Germany studied 51 people with osteoarthritis of the knee, treating 24 with leech therapy ("a single treatment of four to six locally applied leeches"), and

*www.leechesusa.com, Leeches U.S.A. LTD., 300 Shames Drive, Westbury, New York 11590 (800-645-3569).

27 with four weeks of daily topical application of the NSAID *diclofenac* (Solaraze Gel, Voltaren Topical). After seven days, those receiving leech therapy had a 64% decrease in pain, while those using *diclofenac* had a 16% decrease. The people receiving leech therapy also had less stiffness and more ease performing the tasks of daily living, such as getting dressed—benefits that continued for the next three months, until the end of the study.

"Traditional leech therapy seems to be an effective symptomatic treatment for osteoarthritis of the knee," says Andreas Michalsen, MD, in the *Annals of Internal Medicine*. He also notes that it was "safe and well-tolerated."

Theory: Leech saliva contains anti-inflammatory and other active compounds—factors that reduce blood clotting, improve circulation, anesthetize and cut the production of tissue-damaging proteins.

Latest development: The FDA has formally approved the medical leech—*Hirudo medicinalis*—as a "medical device."

12

Headache and Pain Cures

The Wilen Sisters' Home Remedies that Work Better than Drugs

The Wilen sisters have been using home remedies all their lives, and for the last quarter of a century, they've been researching and writing about them as well.

We asked the Wilens to share the remedies they use most often for a variety of health challenges. The sisters may not always be able to explain why the remedies work—but they work. All use ingredients readily available in most kitchens, supermarkets or health-food stores. Of course, always check with your doctor before taking any dietary supplement or herb.

SORE THROAT

At the first sign of a sore or scratchy throat, mix two teaspoons of apple cider vinegar in six-to-eight ounces of warm water. Take a mouthful, gargle with it and spit it out—then swallow a mouthful. Repeat the gargle/swallow pattern until there's nothing left in the glass. Do this every hour until your throat is better. We usually feel better within two or three hours.

COLDS

We eat chicken soup when we feel a cold coming on. Aside from being a comfort food, it helps prevent a cold from becoming full-blown and/or it shortens the duration of one. We either prepare the soup from scratch, adding lots of veggies (carrots, onions, parsnip, celery, string beans), or we do the next best thing—buy packaged soup found in the supermarket's frozen food section, then add vegetables. In either case, we add the most potent and health-restoring ingredient—garlic. To derive the full healing powers of garlic, add

Lydia Wilen and Joan Wilen, folk-remedy experts based in New York City. The sisters are coauthors of many books, including *Bottom Line's Healing Remedies: Over 1,000 Astounding Ways to Heal Arthritis, Asthma, High Blood Pressure, Varicose Veins, Warts and More!* (Bottom Line Books). *www.bottomlinepublications.com.*

one or two finely minced raw cloves after the warmed soup is in the bowl.

STOP BLEEDING

A simple first-aid procedure to stop a minor cut or gash from bleeding is to cover the cut with cayenne pepper from your spice cabinet. Gently pour on the pepper. Yes, it will sting. And yes, the bleeding will stop quickly.

DIARRHEA

If you must be away from a restroom, prepare slippery elm tea (we use the inner bark powder available at health-food stores). Pour eight ounces of just-boiled water over a heaping teaspoon of the powder. Let it steep for about eight minutes, then strain the liquid into a mug and drink it. It works quickly. For severe cases, do not strain it—just drink this soothing, gloppy tea.

HEARTBURN

We use our mother's remedy. As soon as the burning starts, eat a palmful of almonds—that's about one ounce—and the heartburn stops immediately. Our mom used dry-roasted almonds. We buy raw almond slivers.

STY

A sty is an inflamed swelling on the eyelid. This classic folk remedy sounds ridiculous but has worked for us many times. The minute you feel as though you're getting a sty, take a 14-carat gold ring (wash it first) and rub it several times across your eyelid every 15 minutes or so, until that "sty-ish" feeling disappears… along with the sty. In our experience, it works right away.

BURNED FINGERTIPS

Ever reach for a pot handle that's surprisingly hot? How about grabbing the wrong side of a plugged-in iron? We have a unique way of treating these minor first-degree burns, where the skin is painful and red but unbroken. It's a form of acupressure. Place your thumb on the back side of your earlobe, and the burned fingertips on the front side of the same earlobe. Press firmly. After a minute, the pain is gone.

INSOMNIA

Our new best friends are nuts—in this case, walnuts. They're rich in serotonin, the brain chemical that calms anxiety and allows us to turn off the pressures of the day to get a good night's sleep. Eat a palmful (one ounce) of raw walnuts before going to bed. It's important to chew each mouthful thoroughly, until the nut pieces are ground down.

Optimism Helps Whiplash Recovery

Whiplash patients were interviewed 23 days after being injured and again six months later. Compared with the most optimistic patients, those who'd had similar injuries yet had the lowest expectations for recovery were four times as likely to suffer serious disability. Optimism may help patients stay active, which aids recovery…a mind/body interaction may promote healing.

Best: If you feel pessimistic after an injury, see a mental-health professional.

Lena Holm, DrMedSc, Institute of Environmental Medicine, Stockholm, Sweden, and leader of a study of 1,032 whiplash patients, published in *Public Library of Science* (PLoS) *Medicine* journal.

Drug-Free Pain Relief With New Patch Technology

Mark A. Stengler, NMD, licensed naturopathic medical doctor in private practice, Stengler Center for Integrative Medicine, Encinitas, California…adjunct associate clinical professor at the National College of Natural Medicine, Portland, Oregon…author of many books, including *The Natural Physician's Healing Therapies* and coauthor of *Prescription for Natural Cures* (both from Bottom Line Books)…and author of the *Bottom Line/Natural Healing* newsletter. *www.drstengler.com*

A few months ago, 70-year-old Louise, one of my patients, was in an automobile accident. She wasn't seriously injured, but her back hurt, so her husband took her to a hospital emergency room. She waited for an hour and a half to see a doctor, then gave up and went home. She called me to tell me what had happened. At length, we discussed the nature of her back pain, which sounded like muscle strain. We agreed that her injury was minor and there was no need for immediate medical attention. Relieved that her injury was not severe, Louise went on to mention a new kind of pain patch that she had heard about and recently purchased to ease the occasional ache or pain.

Louise and I had already had several discussions about these pain patches. Called IceWave patches, they were created by a company called LifeWave (*www.LifeWave.com*) for drug-free pain relief.

Patients always are bringing new and interesting products into my office for me to look over. Louise had brought the patches to me, as had several of my other patients, many of whom reported good results after using them.

Louise and I agreed that she should try the patches for her back pain. She called me a few days later—and reported that when she applied the patches to her back, she felt much better in 30 minutes. She continued using the patches during the next several days and went on to make a full recovery without flooding her body with pain medication.

Louise had a phenomenal response to the pain patches. I also have seen a very high percentage of people with arthritis and musculoskeletal problems who respond well to these patches. The patches seem most helpful when used by patients for pain and stiffness related to muscle trauma and for problems such as back spasms or a stiff neck.

INSIDE THE PATCH

There are many types of pain patches on the market. Most release a type of anesthetic into the skin that numbs the area. The IceWave patch is not a medicated patch that contains pain-relieving drugs. It contains no medication, and its ingredients never cross the skin or enter the body. According to the manufacturer, the IceWave patches work by emitting energy frequencies that are stimulated by the body's heat. These frequencies affect the electromagnetic field of nearby cells, reducing pain and inflammation in much the same way that acupressure or acupuncture needles do when applied to various body parts. When the IceWave patches are placed over a painful body part, the area around the patches becomes several degrees cooler as measured by thermography, a type of infrared imaging technique. This indicates that the inflammatory response in that area is being inhibited.

I believe that there is more to learn about how these noninvasive nonmedicinal patches do the job—but there's no question about the good results that my patients have seen.

WHERE TO PLACE THEM

IceWave patches are used in pairs. One patch is placed on the point where the pain is most noticeable. The other is placed a few inches away from it—and is held in place for about 10 seconds to see if there is any noticeable relief. If not, the second patch is moved in a clockwise circle around the other patch (repeating the 10-second test) until the spot that brings maximum pain relief is located.

Some people don't experience any pain relief at all from IceWave patches.

Helpful: Drink plenty of water because being dehydrated seems to prevent the patches from working properly.

There are other ways to place the patches, depending on the nature of the pain. Knee pain, for example, can be treated by placing one patch on the left side of the knee and one on the right. If that doesn't work, the patches can be placed on the same side of the knee, a few inches apart from one another. If you have pain in two different parts of the body, four patches (two sets) can be used at the same time.

LifeWave recommends leaving the patches on for 12 hours, after which they should be discarded. It's generally recommended that users apply the patches in the morning and remove them before going to bed.

Some patients experience immediate relief, while others feel less pain after three to five days of using the patches. The manufacturer claims that the patches can be used safely for longer than five days, but if at any time you feel discomfort, remove them. The patches are nontoxic, and there are no reports of safety issues or side effects from them. The patches are not recommended for use by children or pregnant women, because they have not been tested in these populations.

The IceWave patches are sold through regional distributors and cannot be purchased from LifeWave directly. Prices begin at $19.95 for six patches (three sets). To find a distributor in your area, call 866-420-6288 or go to *www.LifeWave.com* (click on "Customer Service" at the bottom of the page).

I have no financial interest in this company or its products.

Natural Cures for Back Pain

Jamison Starbuck, ND, naturopathic physician in family practice in Missoula, Montana. She is past president of the American Association of Naturopathic Physicians and a contributing editor to *The Alternative Advisor: The Complete Guide to Natural Therapies and Alernative Treatments* (Time-Life).

Low back pain is a common complaint—especially after age 60, when one of every two people is affected. In a recent issue of the *Journal of the American Medical Association* (JAMA), new research concluded that back surgery and nonsurgical treatment provide similar relief for back pain in patients with lumbar disk herniation (protrusion of a disk out of the normal vertebral space).

Whenever possible, I have always urged my patients to opt for nonsurgical treatment of back pain, so it's nice to see that the study results published in JAMA confirm the wisdom of this approach. Nonsurgical treatment, which helps heal back pain in part by improving circulation, is far less expensive than back surgery and avoids its risks, such as infection.* *My advice...*

*Seek medical attention if your back pain is not improving or is getting worse or if you experience numbness in the legs or paralysis.

• **Walk.** Regular walking is by far the best medicine for back pain. Walking uphill is particularly useful because it strengthens muscles that support the low back. Start with very short distances (one-eighth of a block, or about 25 steps). It's fine to start walking at a slow pace. Just keep moving and do the distance three times a day, every day. Wear comfortable, supportive shoes, such as running shoes. Use a walking stick initially, if it helps. As soon as you are able to walk your starting distance without pain, increase the distance.

• **Practice deep breathing.** As you walk, take deep breaths to increase oxygen intake and help relax back muscles. Imagine your back muscles relaxing with each inhalation, strengthening and healing with each exhalation.

• **Try Thai massage.** This ancient, interactive type of massage—which involves "assisted" stretching, yoga, reflexology (massage of pressure points on the feet that correspond to other parts of the body) and acupressure (massage of points on the body that correspond to energy pathways known as "meridians")—reduces back pain. Thai massage increases muscle relaxation, mobility and overall energy. A 60-minute Thai massage, once a week for a month, can significantly improve back health. To find a practitioner, consult Thai Healing Alliance International, *www.thaihealingalliance.com*.

• **Consider trying homeopathic remedies.** *Cuprum metallicum* and *Rhus toxicodendron*, both available at health-food stores, are most widely used for back pain. Cuprum is indicated when the pain is sharp, and the muscles are tight and in spasm. Rhus is useful for stiffness and soreness that improves when you limber up with movement. Take two pellets of the 30-C potency of either remedy, under the tongue, two times a day for no more than two weeks.

• **Soak in Epsom salts.** Add two cups of Epsom salts to a tub of hot water and soak for 20 minutes. Epsom salts reduce back pain by relaxing your muscles. To supplement your pain relief, burn a lavender-scented candle in the bathroom. The aroma of lavender oil helps relax your body and your mind.

The Buzz About Apis

Mark A. Stengler, NMD, licensed naturopathic medical doctor in private practice, Stengler Center for Integrative Medicine, Encinitas, California...adjunct associate clinical professor at the National College of Natural Medicine, Portland, Oregon...author of many books, including *The Natural Physician's Healing Therapies* and coauthor of *Prescription for Natural Cures* (both from Bottom Line Books)...and author of the *Bottom Line/Natural Healing* newsletter. *www.drstengler.com*

*A*pis (pronounced aye-pis) is a remedy that is derived from the honeybee—the stinger as well as the whole bee. Think of the symptoms that a bee sting causes such as stinging, burning, swelling and itching. These are all the symptoms for which apis is beneficial. So a homeopathic doctor may recommend it for bee stings, allergic reactions including hives, arthritis, urinary-tract infections, kidney disease, herpes, sore throat and ovarian pain.

Apis is indicated when symptoms include a lack of thirst, a negative response to heat, and a positive response to cold applications.

Recommendations for...

• **Allergic reactions.** Allergic reactions that cause hives or burning and stinging pains that move around the body can be improved quickly with apis. Apis also improves other symptoms of allergic reaction such as swelling of the throat and eyes. These could be allergic reactions to food or to drugs.

Note: Seek emergency medical treatment for allergic reactions, especially if you start to have trouble catching your breath.

• **Arthritis.** If you have swollen joints that burn or sting—and if your joints feel better after applying cold compresses—then the condition can probably be alleviated with apis.

• **Bee stings.** Apis quickly relieves the pain of a bee sting. This is proof of the homeopathic principle that "like cures like." Take it as soon as possible after getting stung to prevent swelling and other symptoms from getting severe. It is a remedy that should be in your home first-aid kit.

• **Herpes.** Apis is a common remedy for herpes infections. Herpes of the mouth—cold

sores that sting and burn and that have a vesicle formation—improves quickly with apis. This also applies to the acute treatment of genital herpes.

• **Kidney disease.** Apis is used in acute kidney disease such as *glomerulonephritis* or *nephritic syndrome* where there is protein loss in the urine and edema of the body.

• **Meningitis.** Symptoms include a stiff neck, high fever and dilated pupils. Homeopathic apis is most effective in patients whose symptoms are made worse when heat is applied. This remedy can be used in conjunction with conventional treatment.

• **Ovarian pain.** Apis is specific for right-sided ovarian cysts where there is burning and stinging pain. It not only reduces the pain, but also stimulates dissolving of the cysts.

• **Shingles.** Apis is one of the primary homeopathic medicines for shingles, especially when there is stinging or burning. Apis helps to relieve the pain and heal the shingles.

• **Sore throat.** Apis is very effective for relieving a sore and swollen throat, especially when the sore throat has specific characteristics. Those characteristics include a burning pain (that feels better when you have a cold drink) and a bright red, swollen uvula (the flap of tissue in the middle of the mouth).

• **Toxemia in pregnancy.** Apis is a good remedy for toxemia in pregnancy where there is protein in the urine, high blood pressure and lots of body swelling.

• **Urinary-tract infections.** Urinary-tract infections can be helped by apis. This is particularly true for bladder infections that cause scalding pain during urination. If you have a right-sided kidney infection, it's another indication that this remedy will probably work well.

Dosage: For acute conditions such as a bee sting or allergic reaction, I recommend taking the homeopathic formulation with a 30C potency every 15 minutes for two doses. Then wait and see if the remedy is helping. The other option is to take one dose of a higher potency such as a 200C.

For skin rashes, sore throats and other conditions that are not so acute, I recommend taking a 6C, 12C, or 30C potency twice daily for three to five days, or as needed for continued improvement.

What are the side effects?: Side effects are not an issue with apis. It either helps or there is no effect at all. It is also safe to use for children.

What Relief! Natural Ways to Curb Your Pain

Mark A. Stengler, NMD, licensed naturopathic medical doctor in private practice, Stengler Center for Integrative Medicine, Encinitas, California…adjunct associate clinical professor at the National College of Natural Medicine, Portland, Oregon…author of many books, including *The Natural Physician's Healing Therapies* and coauthor of *Prescription for Natural Cures* (both from Bottom Line Books)…and author of the *Bottom Line/Natural Healing* newsletter. *www.drstengler.com*

Not long ago, a 60-year-old woman came to my office suffering from severe arthritis pain in both hands. I gave her a bean-sized dab of a homeopathic gel that she applied directly to the skin on her hands. After a few applications in the span of 30 minutes, her pain was reduced by 90%. She did not need to apply the gel again for two weeks.

I witnessed a similar result with a retired National Football League player. He had severe chronic hip pain from past injuries. With one application of the gel, his pain was relieved by 70% for two full days.

The relief that these people experienced has given them each a new lease on life. But here's the best news—unlike pharmaceutical pain relievers, which often cause gastrointestinal upset or damage to internal organs, natural therapies can reduce pain without adverse effects.

WHAT ARE YOU TAKING FOR PAIN?

Most Americans take too many pharmaceutical pain relievers. An estimated 175 million American adults take over-the-counter (OTC) pain relievers regularly. About one-fifth of Americans in their 60s take at least one painkiller for chronic pain on a regular basis.

The life-threatening risks of anti-inflammatory medications such as *rofecoxib* (Vioxx) and *celecoxib* (Celebrex), two pain relievers that had been heavily prescribed by conventional doctors to treat the chronic pain of arthritis and similar conditions have been revealed. Vioxx was pulled off the market by its manufacturer, Merck, following research that linked it to increased risk of heart attack and stroke. Celebrex carries warnings that it may increase the chance of heat attack or stroke, which can lead to death.

Of course, pain-relieving drugs can be a blessing in the event of injury, severe acute migraines or diseases, such as terminal cancer. A number of years ago, when I had a wisdom tooth extracted, I received a local anesthetic. Afterward, I went to an acupuncturist for pain relief so I wouldn't need any painkillers. For about one hour after the acupuncture, I was fine—but then the pain-relieving endorphins wore off. I tried a few natural remedies, but when the pain became excruciating, I resorted to the OTC pain reliever *acetaminophen* (Tylenol). That did the trick.

But many people use painkillers on a regular basis for several months or even years, which increases the risk of dangerous side effects. For instance, people who rely on acetaminophen increase their risk of developing stomach ulcers, liver disease and kidney disease. If you regularly take Celebrex or an OTC nonsteroidal anti-inflammatory drug (NSAID), such as aspirin or *naproxen* (Aleve), you run the risk of kidney and stomach damage. Regular use of NSAIDs also increases risk of heart attack, according to the FDA.

BETTER RESULTS, FEWER RISKS

Before you take any remedy, it's important for your doctor to identify what is causing your pain. Remember, pain is your body's distress signal that something is being irritated or damaged. Sometimes we protect ourselves by reacting instinctively. If you touch something hot, for example, you eliminate the pain by quickly pulling back your hand.

But what if your back hurts? You may need a pain reliever—but back pain also can be a signal that you're harming your body by bending or sitting the wrong way. You may need to address the underlying cause to prevent further injury. Pain receptors are found in the skin, around bones and joints—even in the walls of arteries. If a muscle is torn, for example, a pain signal is released from fibers in the shredded tissue.

In light of the dangers from prescription and OTC drugs, what safe alternatives are available to you? There are many natural supplements that I recommend.

NATURE'S PAIN RELIEVERS

If you take prescription or OTC pain medication, work with a naturopathic physician, holistic medical doctor or chiropractor who will incorporate natural pain fighters into your treatment regimen. With his/her help, you may be able to reduce your dosage of pain medication (natural pain relievers can be used safely with prescription or OTC painkillers)—or even eliminate the drugs altogether.

Natural pain-fighting supplements are even more effective when combined with physical therapies, such as acupuncture, chiropractic, magnet therapy or osteopathic manipulation (a technique in which an osteopathic physician uses his hands to move a patient's muscles and joints with stretching, gentle pressure and resistance). Physiotherapy (treatment that uses physical agents, such as exercise and massage, to develop, maintain and restore movement and functional ability) also is helpful.

Here are—in no special order—the best natural pain relievers, which can be taken alone or in combination...

• **White willow bark extract is great for headaches, arthritis, muscle aches and fever.** In Europe, doctors prescribe this herbal remedy for back pain, and recent research supports this use. One study conducted in Haifa, Israel, involved 191 patients with chronic low-back pain who took one of two doses of willow bark extract or a placebo daily for four weeks. Researchers found that 39% of patients taking the higher dose of willow bark extract had complete pain relief, compared with only 6% of those taking a placebo. The participants who benefited the most took willow bark extract that contained 240 mg of the compound salicin, the active constituent in this herbal remedy. (Aspirin is made from *acetylsalicylic acid*, which has many of the chemical properties of salicin.) However, aspirin can cause gastrointestinal ulceration and other side effects, including kidney damage. Willow bark extract is believed to work by inhibiting naturally occurring enzymes that cause inflammation and pain.

I recommend taking willow bark extract that contains 240 mg of salicin daily. In rare cases, willow bark extract can cause mild stomach upset. Don't take willow bark if you have a history of ulcers, gastritis or kidney disease. It also should not be taken by anyone who is allergic to aspirin. As with aspirin, willow bark extract should never be given to children under age 12 who have a fever—in rare instances, it can cause a fatal disease called Reye's syndrome. Willow bark extract has blood-thinning properties, so avoid it if you take a blood thinner, such as *warfarin* (Coumadin). For low-back pain, you may need to take willow bark extract for a week or more before you get results.

• **Methylsulfonylmethane (MSM) is a popular nutritional supplement that relieves muscle and joint pain.** According to Stanley Jacob, MD, former professor at Oregon Health & Science University who has conducted much of the original research on MSM, this supplement reduces inflammation by improving blood flow. Your cells have receptors that send out pain signals when they're deprived of blood. That's why increased blood flow diminishes pain.

MSM, a natural compound found in green vegetables, fruits and grains, reduces muscle spasms and softens painful scar tissue from previous injuries. A double-blind study of 50 people with osteoarthritis of the knee found that MSM helps relieve arthritis pain.

Start with a daily dose of 3,000 mg to 5,000 mg of MSM. If your pain and/or inflammation doesn't improve within five days, increase the dose up to 8,000 mg daily, taken in several doses throughout the day. If you develop digestive upset or loose stools, reduce the dosage. If you prefer, you can apply MSM cream (per the label instructions) to your skin at the painful area. This product is available at health-food stores and works well for localized pain. MSM has a mild blood-thinning effect, so check with your doctor if you take a blood thinner.

• **S-adenosylmethionine (SAMe) is a natural compound found in the body.** The supplement is an effective treatment for people who have osteoarthritis accompanied by cartilage degeneration. SAMe's ability to reduce pain, stiffness and swelling is similar to that of NSAIDs such as ibuprofen and naproxen, and the anti-inflammatory medication Celebrex. There's also evidence that SAMe stimulates cartilage repair, which helps prevent bones from rubbing against one another. A 16-week study conducted at the University of California, Irvine, compared two groups of people who were being treated for knee pain caused by osteoarthritis. Some took 1,200 mg of SAMe daily, while others took 200 mg of Celebrex. It took longer for people to get relief from SAMe, but by the second month, SAMe proved to be just as effective as Celebrex.

Most patients with osteoarthritis and fibromyalgia (a disorder characterized by widespread pain in muscles, tendons and ligaments) who take SAMe notice improvement within four to eight weeks. Many studies use 1,200 mg of SAMe daily in divided doses. In my experience, taking 400 mg twice daily works well. It's a good idea to take a multivitamin or 50-mg B-complex supplement daily while you're taking SAMe. The vitamin B-12 and folic acid contained in either supplement help your body metabolize SAMe, which means that the remedy goes to work faster.

• **Kaprex is effective for mild pain caused by injury or osteoarthritis.** It is a blend of hops, rosemary extract and oleanic acid, which is derived from olive leaf extract. Rather than blocking the body's pain-causing enzymes, these natural substances inhibit pain-causing chemicals called prostaglandins.

In a study sponsored by the Institute for Functional Medicine, the research arm of the supplement manufacturer Metagenics, taking Kaprex for six weeks reduced minor pain by as much as 72%. I recommend taking one 440-mg tablet three times daily. Kaprex is manufactured by Metagenics (800-692-9400, *www.metagenics.com*), the institute's product branch. The product is sold only in doctors' offices. To find a practitioner in your area who sells Kaprex, call the toll-free number. Kaprex has no known side effects and does not interact with other medications.

• **Proteolytic enzymes,** including bromelain, trypsin, chymotrypsin, pancreatin, papain and a range of protein-digesting enzymes derived from the fermentation of fungus, reduce pain and inflammation by improving blood flow. You can find these natural pain fighters at health-food stores in products labeled "proteolytic enzymes." Take as directed on the label. Bromelain, a favorite of athletes, is available on its own. Extracted from pineapple stems, bromelain reduces swelling by breaking down blood clots that can form as a result of trauma and impede circulation. It works well for bruises, sprains and surgical recovery. If you use bromelain, take 500 mg three times daily between meals.

Repair is a high-potency formula of proteolytic enzymes that I often recommend. It is manufactured by Enzymedica (to find a retailer, call 888-918-1118 or go to *www.enzymedica.com*). Take two capsules two to three times daily between meals. Don't take Repair or any proteolytic enzyme formula if you have an active ulcer or gastritis. Any enzyme product can have a mild blood-thinning effect, so check with your doctor if you take a blood thinner.

PainMed is the homeopathic gel that gave such quick relief to the patients I described at the beginning of this article. It is remarkably effective for relieving the pain of arthritis, muscle soreness and spasms, sprains, strains, stiffness, headaches (especially due to tension) as well as injuries, including bruises.

PainMed is a combination of nine highly diluted plant and flower materials, including arnica, bryonia, hypericum and ledum. Like other homeopathic remedies, it promotes the body's ability to heal itself. A bean-sized dab works well for anyone who has pain. It should be spread on the skin around the affected area. Following an injury, use it every 15 minutes, for a total of up to four applications. As the pain starts to diminish, apply less often. Do not reapply the gel once the pain is gone. PainMed does not sting, burn or irritate the skin. It is clear, has no odor, does not stain and dries quickly.

Because it has so many uses and works so rapidly, PainMed is a good first-aid remedy to have on hand. To order, contact the manufacturer, GM International, Inc., at 800-228-9850, *www.gmipainmed.com*.

Most Back Pain Has Emotional Roots

John E. Sarno, MD, professor of clinical rehabilitation medicine at New York University School of Medicine and attending physician at the Howard A. Rusk Institute of Rehabilitation Medicine, NYU Medical Center, New York City. He is the author of *Mind Over Back Pain* (Berkley Trade) and *Healing Back Pain: The Mind/Body Connection* (Warner Books).

As anyone who routinely gets migraine or tension headaches or upset stomachs will confirm, real pain can originate in the mind.

When tension mounts, any of a wide range of uncomfortable conditions can develop, from spastic colon—to asthma—to eczema. In fact, the mind can use practically any body organ or system as a defense mechanism to sidetrack itself from the awareness of undesirable, negative emotions.

Currently the most popular distraction is pain in the back, neck or shoulders. It has not always been so. Forty years ago no one took these pains seriously.

Now they are costing the American economy somewhere between $60 billion and $70 billion a year.

Forty or 50 years ago ulcers, colitis and tension headache were the best distractors. But people knew they were caused by tension and doctors learned to clear them up with medication so the brain had to look around for a better hiding place.

The back was perfect because no one suspected it and it gradually took over the number-one spot.

What the brain created was something I call the *tension myositis syndrome*, or TMS, in which pain is caused simply by reducing the blood flow a little. I have found it to be the commonest cause of back pain by far. Fortunately—understanding what's going on usually stops the pain.

WHO CAN GET TMS

It is fair to say that everybody is susceptible. I used to think that it was only the "nervous" types who got it but we now realize that anyone who has pressure in his/her life can get TMS. And strangely, the greatest pressure comes from our own personalities because we pressure ourselves to be perfect and to be good. Since the middle years of life (30 to 60) have the greatest pressures, TMS is most common during these years. This is why persistent pain in the back, neck or shoulders is usually due to TMS.

Caution: Never assume you have TMS unless you have seen a doctor and ruled out serious disorders like tumors, cancer, bone disease and the like.

Each person with TMS develops a pattern of what time of the day or night the pain will appear, what part of the body will be involved, what activities will make it better or worse and how severe the pain will be.

One patient may say, "I'm fine when I get up, but as the day goes on, it gets worse. By late afternoon, I can't sit for more than five minutes at a time."

Another patient may have pain-racked nights followed by increasing relief through the day. They both have TMS.

SEEKING TREATMENT

People with back pain understandably want to know what is wrong and how to get better. They go from practitioner to practitioner, often getting a different diagnosis with each visit.

Surgery is commonly done but since structural abnormalities are rarely responsible for the pain, in my experience, this does not solve the problem—the pain returns to the same or another place, or the problem switches to another organ or system.

A very common misconception is that recurrent back pain is due to an old injury.

Example: "I was ice skating 10 years ago and fell on my tailbone, and my back has hurt on and off ever since."

This makes no sense for the body tends to heal itself, quickly and completely. Recurrent attacks are due to TMS.

Another mistaken idea is that if the pain is excruciating there must be a structural abnormality. In fact, such severe pain is due to muscle spasm, a powerful contraction of muscle when it is suddenly deprived of its full complement of oxygen, as occurs with TMS.

Instead of attributing their pain to psychological factors, most people would rather believe it is the result of some structural abnormality that can be treated surgically, with medication or some other kind of therapy. It is my impression that eight out of 10 people are unable to accept the diagnosis of TMS.

Unfortunate: People who would benefit most from a pyschological diagnosis tend to be the least able to accept it.

Am I saying that people consciously induce their own pain? Of course not. It is the stress and pressures of life that bring on the pain because they lead to internal bad feelings, like anger, which the brain then avoids by turning our attention to the pain.

Patients are often told in pain clinics that they are unconsciously making their pain worse in order to gain certain benefits like sympathy, attention, money, etc. I don't believe that is a significant factor in chronic pain.

Why don't more doctors diagnose TMS? Unfortunately, medical teaching still tends to view the body as a magnificent machine and the doctor as an engineer to that machine. There is still very little awareness in the ranks of medicine of the intimate connection of the mind and body. This is a tragedy for the average patient.

How can you prove that TMS exists? It doesn't show up on an X ray or blood test, but if a large number of patients (thousands) get better when treated for that diagnosis, it must exist.

The cure: Repudiate the structural explanation for the pain and acknowledge that it is due to pressure and tension. This is accomplished through teaching and group meetings. In about 10% of cases it is also necessary to work with a psychotherapist who is familiar with the disorder.

Through the years many people have written to me and described how they were cured by carefully studying my book, *Healing Back Pain.* This is logical because information is the primary therapeutic ingredient. It's what I give my patients.

But remember, one must never consider this diagnosis unless all serious disorders have first been ruled out.

Natural Pain Busters

Mark A. Stengler, NMD, licensed naturopathic medical doctor in private practice, Stengler Center for Integrative Medicine, Encinitas, California...adjunct associate clinical professor at the National College of Natural Medicine, Portland, Oregon...author of many books, including *The Natural Physician's Healing Therapies* and coauthor of *Prescription for Natural Cures* (both from Bottom Line Books)...and author of the *Bottom Line/Natural Healing* newsletter. *www.drstengler.com*

When something hurts, you want to feel better quickly. Often that means reaching for an over-the-counter or prescription drug. But there are natural pain stoppers that offer the same relief—without the risks.

Aspirin and *ibuprofen* (Advil) can both cause intestinal bleeding...*acetaminophen* (Tylenol) can lead to liver damage...powerful prescription pain relievers, such as *acetaminophen-hydrocodone* (Vicodin) and acetaminophen with codeine, may make you drowsy and can be addictive.

Despite the dangers, these medications are valuable for treating occasional severe (long-lasting) or acute (sudden, but stopping abruptly) pain. But for many chronic conditions that need ongoing relief, such as osteoarthritis, natural pain stoppers work just as well with a much lower risk for side effects.

Caution: Severe pain, or mild pain that gets suddenly worse, can be a sign of a serious injury or other medical problem.

Best: Seek medical attention immediately.

HOW TO USE NATURAL REMEDIES

For each common pain problem discussed here, I give more than one treatment. You may have more success with, or simply prefer, a particular treatment. If something has worked for you in the past, start there. If you don't get much relief from a treatment, try another option. If you get only partial improvement, try adding another supplement. Because natural remedies have a very low risk for serious side effects, it's usually safe to use them in combination with prescription or nonprescription medications, such as for high blood pressure—and over the long run, they can help reduce the need for these drugs entirely. Check with your doctor before starting a natural regimen or changing your drug regimen.

Natural remedies also work well in combination with pain-relieving "body work," such as chiropractic, physical therapy as well as acupuncture.

HELP A HEADACHE

Migraines and other headaches are often set off by food sensitivities—most commonly, to red wine, caffeine, chocolate and food additives, such as *monosodium glutamate*. Other triggers, such as lack of sleep or hormonal fluctuations, can also leave you with headache pain.

Best: Pay attention to patterns and avoid your triggers.

Fortunately, headaches are usually very responsive to natural remedies…

• **Mild (tension) headaches.** First, try acupressure. This ancient Chinese technique uses gentle pressure and light massage on specific points.

In traditional Chinese medicine, *chi* (chee) is the vital energy of all living things. Your chi flows along 12 meridians that run through your body and nourish your tissues. Each meridian is associated with a particular organ, such as the liver or gallbladder. Along each meridian are specific points, designated by numbers, that are the spots where the flow of

chi can be affected. For headaches, the standard acupressure points are…

• **Gallbladder 20**—the small indentation below the base of the skull, in the space between the two vertical neck muscles. Push gently for 10 to 15 seconds, wait 10 seconds, then repeat five to 10 times.

• **Large intestine 4**—located in the webbing between the thumb and index finger. Push gently for 10 to 15 seconds (as described above). Do this on one hand, then switch to the other.

• **Yuyao**—the indentation in the middle of each eyebrow (straight up from the pupil). Push gently for 10 to 15 seconds (as described above) on both points simultaneously.

If you don't feel relief within several minutes after trying a particular pressure point, move on to a different one.

Another option for mild headaches: A cup of peppermint tea, or a dab of peppermint oil on the temples, can banish a mild headache quickly.

Note: Peppermint essential oil is highly concentrated—don't take it internally.

To brew peppermint tea, make an infusion using one to two teaspoons dried peppermint leaf in eight ounces of boiling water. Let steep for five minutes. You may find relief after one cup. Drink as much and as often as necessary.

• **Migraine headaches.** The herb feverfew has been used effectively for centuries to treat migraines. Take a feverfew capsule standardized to contain 300 micrograms (mcg) of the active ingredient *parthenolide* every 30 minutes, starting at the onset of symptoms.

Maximum: Four doses daily or until you feel relief.

Prevention: Take a feverfew capsule standardized to contain 300 to 400 mcg of parthenolide—or 30 drops of a standardized tincture, either in a few ounces of water or directly on your tongue, every day. In about three months, you should notice dramatically fewer migraines, and/or less severe symptoms.

Note: Feverfew may thin blood, so consult your doctor if you are taking a blood thinner, such as *warfarin* (Coumadin).

SOOTHE SORE MUSCLES

Natural remedies can help an aching back or sore, cramped muscles. Here, too, acupressure is valuable. Zero in on the points that are most tender and then gently press on them and release, or massage for 10 to 15 seconds, at 10-second intervals, five to 10 times. If you can't reach a spot, have someone do it for you.

For some people, an ice pack on the affected area helps. Others prefer warmth from a hot compress or heating pad. For acute injuries, use cold (within 24 hours). Otherwise, use warmth or alternate warmth and cold. Other remedies that help sore muscles...

• **Herbal arnica cream or tincture** can soothe sore muscles and is also great for bruises. It reduces swelling, which helps lessen pain. Rub a small amount on the affected area. Repeat as needed.

Caution: Don't use on broken skin because it is not intended for internal use.

• **Homeopathic Rhus toxicodendron** is especially helpful in relieving low back pain. Take two pellets of 30C potency twice daily for two or three days.

EASE ARTHRITIC JOINTS

The stiff, swollen joints of osteoarthritis are a major cause of doctors' visits for people over age 45. *But with natural remedies, the pain and joint damage can be kept to a minimum...*

• **Glucosamine sulfate** helps rebuild damaged cartilage in arthritic joints and works as well as or better than many of the drugs doctors recommend. It can take several weeks to feel the benefits. Begin by taking 1,500 to 2,000 mg daily for three months. After that, cut back to 500 to 1,000 mg daily. If symptoms worsen, go back to the higher dose. It's okay to continue with anti-inflammatory drugs, but be sure to tell your doctor if you're using glucosamine.

• **Boswellia,** an herb used in Ayurveda, traditional medicine from India, is a powerful anti-inflammatory that's very helpful for arthritis. Take 1,200 to 1,500 mg of a standardized extract containing 60% to 65% boswellic acids, two to three times daily.

• **Bromelain,** an enzyme derived from pineapple stems, is very effective at reducing pain and swelling. Bromelain supplements come in two designations—MCU (milk-clotting units) and GDU (gelatin-dissolving units). Use either formula, choosing a product that's standardized to either 2,000 MCU per 1,000 mg or 1,200 GDU per 1,000 mg. Take 500 mg three times daily between meals.

Caution: If you take a blood-thinning medication such as warfarin, skip the bromelain—it could thin your blood too much.

Any of these supplements can be used alone or in combination. Natural pain stoppers can be effective alternatives to drugs, but pain is also your body's way of telling you that something is wrong. If your pain is very sudden or severe, and/or accompanied by other symptoms—such as weakness, nausea, redness and swelling in the painful area, shortness of breath or fever—get medical attention immediately.

Quick Cure for Headaches

Put your feet in a bucket of warm water and put an ice pack around your neck. The strategic use of heat and cold causes blood to move away from your head and toward your feet, relieving headache pain. It takes about five to 10 minutes for the pain to recede. This technique might not help people with poorly controlled diabetes or vascular disease who have diminished blood flow to the feet.

Mark A. Stengler, NMD, licensed naturopathic medical doctor in private practice, Stengler Center for Integrative Medicine, Encinitas, California...adjunct associate clinical professor at the National College of Natural Medicine, Portland, Oregon...author of many books and of the *Bottom Line/Natural Healing* newsletter.

13

Ulcer and Digestive Cures

Natural Cures for Heartburn and Ulcers

Doctor, I have heartburn, but I don't want to take a prescription drug. What can I do?" Many people have asked me for such advice—especially since the media have publicized risks associated with popular heartburn and ulcer medications called *proton pump inhibitors* (PPIs). These drugs, including *omeprazole* (Prilosec), *lansoprazole* (Prevacid) and *esomeprazole* (Nexium), offer short-term relief by reducing stomach acid, but they do not cure the underlying problem. Even worse, long-term use (more than a year) of PPIs increases risks for hip fracture (because of decreased mineral absorption)…and the bacterial intestinal infection *Clostridium difficile* (because stomach acid is needed to fight bacteria). For my patients, I use a different approach that focuses on improving digestion and healing the lining of the stomach and the esophagus. *My advice…*

If you suffer from heartburn and/or have an ulcer, avoid any foods that may irritate your condition, such as fried foods, citrus, tomato-based foods and spicy meals. Don't overeat. Large meals increase the demand for stomach acid. Chew thoroughly and eat nothing within two hours of going to bed. Avoid smoking and pain relievers, such as aspirin or *ibuprofen* (Advil), that can cause gastrointestinal irritation.

Herbal tea also can be surprisingly effective for heartburn and ulcers. Chamomile and licorice root are two herbs with a long medicinal history for treating the digestive tract lining.* Drink three cups of either tea daily, on an empty stomach. Use two teaspoons of dried plant or one teabag per eight ounces of water.

*If you have high blood pressure, avoid licorice tea.

Philip M. Tierno, Jr., PhD, director of clinical microbiology and immunology at New York University Medical Center, and associate professor, department of microbiology and pathology at New York University School of Medicine, both in New York City. He is author of *The Secret Life of Germs* (Atria).

174

For heartburn (without ulcer), I suggest that you add stomach acid—which is necessary for good digestion—rather than reduce it with an acid blocker. At the end of your meal, sip on a four-ounce glass of water to which you have added one teaspoon of either apple cider vinegar or fresh lemon juice.

Caution: Do not drink vinegar or lemon water if you have an ulcer or gastritis (inflammation of the lining of the stomach). Discontinue this practice if it causes pain or worsens symptoms.

If you have an ulcer (with or without heartburn), I recommend adding other botanical medicines. The antiseptic herbs echinacea, cranesbill root and Oregon grape root (50 mg each) help reduce bacteria associated with ulcers. The herbs cabbage leaf, marshmallow root and slippery elm bark (200 mg each) help restore the gut's protective lining. Take these herbs three times daily on an empty stomach until the ulcer symptoms have eased, usually for two to eight weeks.

If you take a PPI but want to stop using it, gradually wean yourself off the drug while you add this protocol. Consult your doctor about your plan and schedule a follow-up visit in a month. You can review your condition and discuss what I hope will be good news about your progress.

Difficult-to-Treat GERD

Mark A. Stengler, NMD, licensed naturopathic medical doctor in private practice, Stengler Center for Integrative Medicine, Encinitas, California...adjunct associate clinical professor at the National College of Natural Medicine, Portland, Oregon...author of many books, including *The Natural Physician's Healing Therapies* and coauthor of *Prescription for Natural Cures* (both from Bottom Line Books)...and author of the *Bottom Line/Natural Healing* newsletter. *www.drstengler.com*

I have tried every therapy you can think of," said my new patient Esther, who had suffered from heartburn and bad breath since high school. "I hope you have something that can help me!" This 59-year-old financial adviser had tried pharmaceutical medications and natural remedies—but nothing seemed to stop the constant burning in her chest.

In high school, Esther had been diagnosed with both *gastroesophageal reflux disease* (GERD), a condition in which stomach acids back up into the esophagus, and *irritable bowel syndrome* (IBS), a condition that causes diarrhea, constipation and digestive discomfort. Over the next 40 years, she had taken various acid-blocking medications, such as *esomeprazole* (Nexium) and *omeprazole* (Prilosec). While these medications helped the reflux symptoms (the burning or pressure in her chest), they worsened her IBS symptoms, including diarrhea and abdominal pain.

Esther was especially concerned about the potential long-term side effects of these medications. Her concerns had inspired her to try alternative medicine remedies.

She had already taken many of the classic dietary supplement remedies for GERD that I always first recommend to patients with the condition. These included calcium (which neutralizes stomach acid), *deglycyrrhizinated licorice root* (DGL), probiotics, aloe vera juice and digestive enzymes. Esther was not overweight (which can be a risk factor for GERD) and found that what she ate did not have much impact on her reflux.

For Esther's difficult-to-treat GERD, I suggested a new, less commonly known supplement that has been shown to be effective—orange peel extract. I am using it with more and more patients, and it may become a first-line treatment. Heartburn Free (800-783-2286, *www. enzymatictherapy.com*) contains orange peel extract that is standardized to contain a high concentration of *d-limonene*, a phytochemical found in citrus. The supplement is believed to help the lower esophageal sphincter close more efficiently so that acid doesn't rise up as easily from the stomach. Heartburn Free has no reported side effects. It is safe for all adults except those with gastric ulcers and women who are pregnant or nursing (for whom it has not yet been tested).

I had Esther take one capsule every other day for 10 days. When she followed up with me a month later, she reported that her GERD was 80% better overall and that she had not taken a citrus peel extract capsule in two weeks. Her bad breath, a symptom of GERD, had subsided, as had her IBS, which is not uncommon, because these conditions frequently overlap. This was the best result that she had ever gotten from any treatment. If she experienced any increase in her symptoms, she could start taking the capsules again.

Natural Therapies for Ulcers

James N. Dillard, MD, DC, in private practice, Manhattan and East Hampton, New York. He is a former assistant clinical professor at Columbia University College of Physicians and Surgeons and former clinical director of Columbia's Rosenthal Center for Complementary and Alternative Medicine, both in New York City.

If you've got an ulcer, chances are you're taking an over-the-counter (OTC) antacid and/or prescription medication to neutralize gastric acid or inhibit its production. These medications include *proton pump inhibitors* (PPIs), such as *esomeprazole* (Nexium) and *lansoprazole* (Prevacid), and H2-blocking drugs, such as *cimetidine* (Tagamet) and *ranitidine* (Zantac).

What most people don't realize: There are several natural, complementary remedies that help reduce ulcer symptoms and promote healing while conventional treatment is under way. Some of these treatments also can help prevent ulcers in some patients.

WHAT CAUSES ULCERS

It's been more than 20 years since doctors learned that an infectious disease—rather than emotional stress—was the primary cause of most ulcers.

A screw-shaped bacterium, *Helicobacter pylori*, or H. pylori, burrows through the protective mucous lining in the small intestine and/or stomach, allowing harsh digestive fluids to accumulate and ulcerate the lining. About 50% of Americans over age 60 are infected with H. pylori. The bacterium doesn't always cause ul-

cers—but about 60% of patients with ulcers harbor H. pylori.

The remainder of ulcers are caused by regular use of stomach-damaging nonsteroidal anti-inflammatory drugs (NSAIDs), such as aspirin, *ibuprofen* (Advil) and *naproxen* (Aleve)…alcohol…and/or smoking. Excessive alcohol wears down the lining of the stomach and intestines. Nicotine causes the stomach to produce more acid.

Best complementary treatments…*

NONDRUG THERAPIES

• **Probiotics.** The intestine contains up to four pounds of "friendly" bacteria, which aid digestion. There's some evidence that maintaining adequate levels of beneficial bacteria helps create an inhospitable environment for H. pylori and makes it harder for this ulcer-causing bacterium to thrive.

Self-defense: Take a probiotic supplement that contains *Lactobacillus acidophilus* and *Bifidobacterium bifidus*. These organisms create a healthful mix of bacteria and can inhibit the growth of harmful organisms. Probiotics are helpful if you've taken antibiotics, which can kill off some beneficial bacteria.

The optimal dose for probiotics hasn't been determined. Preliminary research cites a daily dose of up to 10 billion organisms—the amount usually included in one to two capsules. Probiotics are available at health-food stores.

• **Cabbage juice.** This folk remedy has some evidence to support it. Cabbage is high in vitamin C, which seems to inhibit growth of H. pylori. It also contains *glutamine*, an amino acid that may strengthen the protective lining in the stomach.

A small Stanford University School of Medicine study found that ulcer patients who drank about a quart of cabbage juice daily healed significantly faster than those who didn't drink it.

Self-defense: If you have an active ulcer, consider drinking a quart of cabbage juice (about the amount in half a head of cabbage) once daily for up to two weeks.

*Check with your doctor before taking supplements. They can interact with prescription medications.

• **Deglycyrrhizinated licorice (DGL).** Herbalists often recommend fresh licorice root to heal ulcers. Licorice contains *mucin*, a substance that protects the stomach lining, as well as antioxidants that may inhibit H. pylori growth.

However, natural licorice can increase the effects of *aldosterone*, a hormone that promotes water retention and can increase blood pressure in some people. DGL supplements (available at health-food stores) are a better option, because the substances that increase blood pressure have been removed.

Self-defense: Take one DGL tablet before meals, and another before bed. DGL may be effective for people with ulcers whose H. pylori has been successfully treated with antibiotics but who still have some stomach irritation.

• **Vitamin A.** Vitamin A helps repair damaged mucous membranes. A report in the British medical journal *The Lancet* suggests that ulcers heal more quickly in patients given supplemental vitamin A.

Caution: High-dose vitamin A therapy can be toxic, so get your vitamin A from dietary sources along with a daily multivitamin—not from a separate vitamin A supplement.

Self-defense: Get 10,000 international units (IU) of vitamin A daily if you're undergoing ulcer treatment. (A multivitamin typically contains 3,500 IU to 5,000 IU of vitamin A.)

Good food sources: Beef liver (one-and-one-half ounces contains 13,593 IU)...carrots (one raw carrot contains 8,666 IU)...and spinach (one cup of raw spinach contains 2,813 IU).

• **Zinc.** Like vitamin A, zinc is involved in tissue healing. In Europe, a drug compound made with zinc plus an anti-inflammatory is often used for treating ulcers. Early studies indicate that zinc alone can speed ulcer healing and possibly even help prevent some ulcers.

Self-defense: Don't exceed the recommended daily intake (15 mg) of zinc. Take a daily multivitamin that includes zinc...and get adequate intake from dietary sources (five medium fried oysters, 13 mg...3/4 cup fortified breakfast cereal, 15 mg...three-ounces lean beef tenderloin, 5 mg).

ANOTHER WAY TO FIGHT ULCERS

NSAIDs alleviate pain by inhibiting the production of pain-causing chemicals called *prostaglandins*. However, the body produces several kinds of prostaglandins, including some that protect the stomach lining. That's why NSAIDs, which block the production of pain-causing and stomach-protecting prostaglandins, make people who regularly use the drugs more susceptible to ulcers.

Self-defense: If you require regular pain relief, start with *acetaminophen* (Tylenol). It relieves pain without depleting stomach-protecting prostaglandins.

Caution: Taking more than the recommended dosage or drinking alcohol with acetaminophen can cause liver damage.

Also helpful: Ask your doctor about taking *Arthrotec*, a prescription drug combination that includes the NSAID *diclofenac* along with *misoprostol*, which protects the stomach and intestinal lining. One study found that patients taking Arthrotec experienced up to 80% fewer ulcers than those taking an NSAID alone.

Treatment for Colitis

Mark A. Stengler, NMD, licensed naturopathic medical doctor in private practice, Stengler Center for Integrative Medicine, Encinitas, California...adjunct associate clinical professor at the National College of Natural Medicine, Portland, Oregon...author of many books, including *The Natural Physician's Healing Therapies* and coauthor of *Prescription for Natural Cures* (both from Bottom Line Books)...and author of the *Bottom Line/Natural Healing* newsletter. *www.drstengler.com*

A fter five years of suffering, 31-year-old Ann was at her wit's end. She experienced constant severe nausea, intermittent vomiting and diarrhea, and frequent bloody stools. She was down to a skeletal 88 pounds... she hadn't menstruated in almost two years... and her hair and nails had basically stopped growing. Digestive tract bleeding had necessitated two blood transfusions. "The pain is unbearable," she told me tearfully, "and most days, I'm too weak to even get out of bed."

Unable to tolerate solid food, Ann largely subsisted on juice. Her medical doctor had prescribed numerous pills, plus injections of morphine and the steroid prednisone. She had become depressed, anxious and prone to panic attacks.

While taking her medical history, I learned that Ann had been infected five years earlier with *Clostridium difficile*. This bacterium has emerged in recent years in especially virulent forms and is a known cause of colitis (inflammation and ulcers in the lining of the large intestine). Ann had been treated first with a standard antibiotic and then with the more potent antibiotic *metronidazole* (Flagyl). Afterward her stool had tested negative for C. difficile—yet her symptoms had continued to worsen.

I repeated a comprehensive stool test and found no C. difficile infection. However, I did find that Ann had very low levels of beneficial digestive bacteria, such as *Lactobacillus acidophilus* and *Bifidobacterium*. To make her more comfortable, I prescribed the homeopathic remedy *Arsenicum album* (sold in health-food stores), which eases nausea and abdominal pain and also reduces anxiety. In addition, I prescribed a powdered herbal formula that contained turmeric, ginger, quercetin and other anti-inflammatory nutrients...plus the amino acid glutamine, which promotes healing of the digestive tract...and suggested she mix it with almond milk and drink it twice daily. I also recommended that Ann increase her nutrient intake by adding soups and stews to her diet, and I added a probiotic supplement to replenish her beneficial digestive bacteria.

With these changes, Ann slowly improved, day by day. After one month, she reported that her abdominal pain was greatly reduced and that she required less morphine. She had diarrhea far less often and was no longer vomiting. In addition, Ann was sleeping better and her emotional state had improved.

In about four months, Ann's hair and nails started to grow again and she got her period. Her bowel movements normalized, and she could eat most foods without trouble. Her weight increased to a healthy 128 pounds, and she felt strong and energized. "This is the first

time in five years that I haven't been in the hospital during Thanksgiving and Christmas," she told me with obvious delight. Now, a year and half later, Ann takes a lesser dose of the almond-milk herbal formula, plus my high-potency probiotic, and continues to do well.

My Natural Cure for Constipation

Jamison Starbuck, ND, naturopathic physician in family practice in Missoula, Montana. She is past president of the American Association of Naturopathic Physicians and a contributing editor to *The Alternative Advisor: The Complete Guide to Natural Therapies and Alternative Treatments* (Time-Life).

So-called herbal "bowel cleansers" are touted as a healthy and effective treatment for chronic constipation. In my clinical experience, this claim simply is not true. Bowel-cleansing formulas typically contain strong laxative herbs, such as aloe resin (sometimes listed as "aloe leaf"), buckthorn, cascara, rhubarb and senna. These herbs increase peristalsis, the wave-like movement of the bowel that facilitates elimination of stool, but they also irritate the gut wall. Like any good laxative, these herbs will promote a bowel movement, but repeated or large doses create cramping, diarrhea and blood in the stool.

I define constipation as having less than one bowel movement per day. Common causes of constipation include irregular bowel habits (ignoring the urge to go or not allowing enough time)...inadequate fiber and/or water...lack of exercise...and poor digestive function (due to low secretion of digestive enzymes). Medications such as antihypertensives, tricyclic antidepressants, antacids and opiate pain relievers (such as codeine) can cause constipation. Unless your constipation is temporary (caused, for example, by the use of opiate medication following surgery), avoid strong laxatives—even if they are natural or herbal products. The bowel becomes reliant on laxatives, which can worsen your constipation and create inflammation and irritation in your intestinal tract.

Rather than seeking a temporary solution, people who are constipated should slowly retrain their bowels to work correctly. This process usually takes about four weeks. *Here's how...*

1. Eat fiber. Fiber helps retain water in the colon, which promotes softer and larger stool. While a healthy, toned bowel will respond to a moderate amount of fiber, a bowel that has become slack and weak (due to the effects of insufficient fiber) will need much more fiber.

Start with five half-cup servings of vegetables and four half-cup servings of fruit per day. Have at least one cup daily of a whole grain, such as brown rice, oatmeal, quinoa or millet.

2. Exercise. Physical activity improves peristalsis. Get at least 20 minutes each day. My favorite exercises are yoga and aerobic activity, such as brisk walking, cycling or swimming.

3. Drink lemon water. To expand stool size and encourage elimination, drink 64 ounces of water daily.

Twice a day, before meals, drink 16 ounces of water that contains the juice from half a fresh lemon (bottled lemon juice also can be used, but it is not as healthful).

Lemon water encourages the secretion of bile, a digestive fluid that acts as a laxative.

4. Use small doses of herbs. A tea made with equal parts dandelion, yellow dock, burdock and licorice root has a mild laxative effect.

What to do: Mix one-half ounce of each dried herb. Use two teaspoons of the mix per eight ounces of water, simmer for eight minutes, strain and drink.

Start with one cup four times daily during the first week of bowel retraining. Reduce by one cup per week until you are able to eliminate regularly without the tea.

Wormwood: This Controversial Herb Deserves Another Look

Mark A. Stengler, NMD, licensed naturopathic medical doctor in private practice, Stengler Center for Integrative Medicine, Encinitas, California...adjunct associate clinical professor at the National College of Natural Medicine, Portland, Oregon...author of many books, including *The Natural Physician's Healing Therapies* and coauthor of *Prescription for Natural Cures* (both from Bottom Line Books)...and author of the *Bottom Line/Natural Healing* newsletter. *www.drstengler.com*

The herb *wormwood* (*Artemisia absinthium*) has a long history of use in Europe and China as a remedy for digestive disorders. But wormwood has been dogged by controversy. That's because it is a flavoring and color agent in *absinthe*, an alcoholic beverage that was banned in the US and Europe in the early 1900s because it was thought to cause hallucinations and even insanity. A component of wormwood—the chemical *thujone*—was believed to have these mind-altering properties. But some experts have since questioned the science behind this belief, and in the 1990s, Europe lifted the ban on the manufacture and consumption of absinthe...without any related increase in mental illness. In 2007, the US government began allowing *thujone-free absinthe* to be imported into the country, and herbal wormwood is widely available in health-food stores. *Recent research shows that this controversial herb may be helpful in fighting some insidious health conditions...*

•**Crohn's disease.** A study published recently by doctors at Yale University School of Medicine found that wormwood significantly reduced symptoms of Crohn's disease, a form of inflammatory bowel disease that is difficult to treat. Forty patients were given either 750 mg of wormwood extract (*brand name:* Seda-Crohn) or placebos twice daily for 10 weeks. After eight weeks, 13 of the 20 patients (65%) taking wormwood had almost a full remission of symptoms. As a result, they were able to reduce their use of corticosteroid drugs. For most of the patients taking placebos, symptoms worsened.

•**Malaria.** A very close relative of wormwood called sweet wormwood (*Artemisia annua*) has been found beneficial in treating malaria, which is caused by a mosquito-borne parasite.

Although most Americans are not likely to contract malaria, the disease is still a major problem in Africa and throughout the developing world.

The World Health Organization has approved the use of wormwood-based compounds in the treatment of malaria—a sign of the herb's efficacy and safety.

•**Parasitic infections.** Wormwood has a long history of use in traditional Chinese medicine and in Western naturopathic medicine for treating a variety of parasitic infections.

I have found that a wormwood tincture (10 drops three times daily) or capsule (200 mg) helps rid the body of parasites in the digestive tract.

•**Cancer.** Some research suggests that extracts of wormwood might have anticancer benefits. However, the research has been limited to small-scale cell and mouse studies.

Some companies are hyping wormwood as a potential cancer fighter, but at this point, I do not believe there is enough evidence to justify its use in treating cancer.

What about the risk? The amount of thujone in herbal preparations is extremely small—I have never found a problem with its use.

In fact, thujone also is found in the culinary herb sage, commonly used as a rub for Thanksgiving turkeys.

Important: Work with a physician if you suspect that you have any of the conditions mentioned here, and ask about wormwood as a possible treatment.

My patients have not experienced any hallucinations or other side effects as a result of the doses I prescribe.

The All-Purpose Remedy—Licorice Root

Mark A. Stengler, NMD, licensed naturopathic medical doctor in private practice, Stengler Center for Integrative Medicine, Encinitas, California...adjunct associate clinical professor at the National College of Natural Medicine, Portland, Oregon...author of many books, including *The Natural Physician's Healing Therapies* and coauthor of *Prescription for Natural Cures* (both from Bottom Line Books)...and author of the *Bottom Line/Natural Healing* newsletter. *www.drstengler.com*

In my experience, licorice root is the most versatile of all the herbs. Native to both Asia and the Mediterranean, it has been used by practitioners of Ayurvedic and Chinese medicine for over 5,000 years.

In fact, close to 50% of all Chinese herbal formulas contain licorice root. The ancient Chinese texts say it can suppress coughs and moisten the lungs, relieve spasms, and soothe the digestive tract. It is also called a "harmonizing" herb. This means that it helps other herbs to work more effectively to reduce their toxicity when used in a formula.

Licorice also helps detoxify the liver, supports the adrenal glands (your body's major guardians against stress), balances the hormones and has powerful anti-inflammatory effects.

IMMUNITY BOOSTER

Licorice contains two substances, *glycyrrhizin* (pronounced gle-sir-heh-zin) and *glycyrrhetinic* (pronounced gle-sir-heh-ti-nic) acid, that have been shown in animal studies to increase the body's supply of one of nature's most powerful antiviral agents—interferon. Interferon helps to keep viruses from reproducing and stimulates the activity of other beneficial immune cells, as well. That's probably why licorice root is found in so many Western, Chinese, Japanese and Ayurvedic formulas for treating infectious disease.

Licorice root is highly regarded among European physicians as one of the top herbal medicines for combating viral hepatitis. They use the intravenous form for the treatment of both Hepatitis B and C.

DELICIOUS DETOXIFIER

The Chinese have found through many centuries of using licorice that it reduces the toxicity of other herbs, so they add it to many of their remedies. For example, traditional Chinese herbal formulas containing Ma Huang (containing the chemical ephedrine, which helps open respiratory passageways but can also cause stimulant effects, such as fast heartbeat, sweating, and anxiety), almost always contain licorice root, which helps to prevent these unwanted side effects.

Note: The Chinese species of licorice root is *Glycyrrhiza uralensis.* I find it works very similar in action to the kind used in North America—*Glycyrrhiza glabra.*

Dosage: For most conditions, I recommend taking licorice in tincture, capsule, or tablet form. As a tincture, take 10 to 30 drops two to three times daily. As a capsule, take 1,000 to 3,000 milligrams daily.

DGL extract comes in tablet form. Chew one or two tablets (380 milligrams per tablet) 20 minutes before meals or take between meals.

What are the side effects?: High dosages of licorice root (3,000 milligrams daily of the powdered extract or more than 100 milligrams of the constituent glycyrrhizin) taken over many days can have effects similar to those associated with the hormone aldosterone. These include sodium and water retention, and potassium loss, which can lead to high blood pressure. We saw this problem occur when practitioners began recommending very high dosages of licorice root for adrenal burnout and chronic fatigue (which it can help).

Overall, I feel the risk of developing high blood pressure from using licorice is greatly exaggerated. Historically, herbalists have used this root in formulas for thousands of years. The trick is to use it in small amounts.

I do hear the occasional story of someone who feels that taking small amounts of licorice root has caused an increase in his or her blood pressure. This is possible for people who are very sensitive to licorice root or who have low levels of potassium. As a matter of fact, anyone concerned about high blood pressure should increase his or her intake of potassium-rich foods (bananas, orange juice, vegetables, etc.)

and decrease the intake of sodium-containing foods (table salt, canned foods and restaurant foods). Using table-salt substitutes, which usually contain potassium, can help reduce sodium intake. Multivitamins also contain potassium.

Unless instructed to do so by a natural health-care practitioner, people who have kidney failure and hypokalemia (low potassium blood levels) should avoid using licorice root. Likewise, pregnant women and people with high blood pressure should use it with caution and under medical supervision. Whole licorice extract should not be combined with digitalis and diuretic medications. Taking only the DGL extract (for ulcers) eliminates most of the potential risk for high blood pressure.

Recommendations for…

• **Coughs.** Licorice is an excellent herb to use for coughs, both wet and dry. Licorice has a moistening and soothing effect for dry coughs. It also has a direct cough suppressant effect and is a common ingredient in throat lozenges.

• **Detoxification.** Licorice is one of the herbs to consider when undergoing a detoxification program. As I mentioned, it helps support the liver and should be considered along with herbs like milk thistle and dandelion root. It also works well to heal a damaged digestive tract, which is key to long-term detoxification success.

• **Eczema and psoriasis.** Creams containing glycyrrhetinic acid are used to treat inflammatory skin conditions such as eczema and psoriasis. Its effect is similar to that of topical cortisone, and some studies have found it more effective. However, I do not recommend topical treatments (whether natural or pharmaceutical) as the main therapy for skin conditions, as they can simply mask a symptom without treating its underlying cause (e.g., food sensitivities, poor digestion, nutritional deficiencies, etc.). Topical treatments are fine, so long as you also address the internal imbalances that are creating the symptom.

• **Fatigue.** People who experience high levels of stress for long periods of time can suddenly find that their adrenal glands can no longer produce balanced levels of stress hormones, such as DHEA, pregnenolone and cortisol. As a result, fatigue, poor memory, blood-sugar problems, decreased resistance to illness and hormonal imbalance can occur.

Some doctors immediately recommend using hormone replacement, and in some cases this is necessary. However, it is worth trying a gentler approach, using supplements such as licorice root, especially to balance out cortisol levels. A typical adult dosage would be 1,000 to 2,000 milligrams of licorice root extract taken daily for two months or longer.

Other supplements that work synergistically to treat this condition include adrenal glandular, ginseng, pantothenic acid, vitamin C, beta carotene and zinc. In more serious cases, hormones such as DHEA, pregnenolone, and even cortisol may need to be used.

•**Hormone imbalance.** Licorice is one of the better hormone-balancing herbs. It appears to have a balancing effect between estrogen and progesterone, and reduces excess testosterone levels. It is commonly included in formulas for PMS and menopause.

•**Infections.** As mentioned earlier, licorice root is very good for the immune system. The soothing and anti-inflammatory effect of licorice makes it especially good for respiratory tract infections.

•**Inflammation.** Licorice has potent anti-inflammatory properties. Glycyrrhizin is an important constituent that improves the effects of cortisol in the body (powerful anti-inflammatory and antiallergy effects), without the side effects seen with pharmaceutical anti-inflammatory agents such as prednisone. It also inhibits the formation of prostaglandins, which are substances in the body that cause inflammation.

•**Inflammatory bowel disease.** Licorice root is often included in formulas designed to heal conditions such as Crohn's disease and ulcerative colitis.

•**Mouth sores.** Mouth sores, also called *aphthous ulcers*, can be helped by licorice root. One study of 20 people found that a DGL mouthwash improved the symptoms of 15 of the participants by 50% to 75% within 1 day, and complete healing of the sores within 3 days.

•**Ulcers.** One of the most popular uses of licorice extract is for ulcers of the digestive tract. The recommended form is DGL.

It has an interesting mechanism of action: It stimulates cell growth of the stomach and intestinal linings, increases the natural mucous lining of the stomach, increases blood flow to the damaged tissues and decreases muscle spasms.

In a single-blind study of 100 people with peptic ulcers, participants took either DGL (760 milligrams three times daily) or the medication *Tagamet* (cimetidine). Both groups showed equally significant healing of ulcers after 6 and 12 weeks, demonstrating that DGL is as effective as pharmaceutical medications for this condition. Another study of 874 people also demonstrated that DGL was as effective as antacids and the antiulcer drug *cimetidine* in persons with duodenal ulcers.

More important, DGL actually works to heal ulcerated tissues instead of simply suppressing stomach acid in the way antacids and drug medications do. Remember, with insufficient stomach acid, you cannot digest proteins, minerals and other nutrients very efficiently. Stomach acid also acts as a natural barrier that keeps bacteria, parasites and other microbes from penetrating the digestive tract.

Natural Remedies for Celiac Disease

Jamison Starbuck, ND, naturopathic physician in family practice in Missoula, Montana. She is past president of the American Association of Naturopathic Physicians and a contributing editor to *The Alternative Advisor: The Complete Guide to Natural Therapies and Alternative Treatments* (Time-Life).

The next time a waiter puts a basket of fresh bread on your restaurant table, think twice before you eat it. Experts believe that at least one out of every 100 American adults has celiac disease, a condition that can make sufferers ill after eating even a single slice of bread. The culprit is gluten—a type of protein found in wheat, barley, rye and, in some cases, oats that creates an autoimmune, inflammatory reaction in the small intestine. The usual symptoms are bloating and diarrhea, but some people also experience abdominal pain and/or constipation. In some cases, celiac disease causes only a blistery, itchy skin condition (*dermatitis herpetiformis*) or fatigue.

If you think you might have celiac disease, discuss it with your doctor. A diagnosis requires specific blood tests and, in some cases, an intestinal biopsy. If you do have celiac disease, your medical doctor will tell you to completely avoid gluten. This may sound like hard work, since gluten is in all sorts of things you might not suspect, such as many kinds of soy sauce, creamed soups and salad dressings. But it is definitely doable and gets easier as you learn where gluten-free products (even bread and pasta) are available—for example, in many health-food stores and a growing number of restaurants.

Payoff: Once you start avoiding gluten, your celiac symptoms will disappear over a period of weeks and months. *Other steps to consider...**

•**Take supplements.** Inflammation in the small intestine interferes with the absorption of key nutrients. I advise my celiac patients to take a daily regimen that includes 5 mg of folic acid...800 international units (IU) each of vitamins E and D...25,000 IU of vitamin A...and 2 mg of vitamin K.

Note: Vitamin K supplements should be avoided by patients taking *warfarin* (Coumadin) or another blood thinner. I also recommend taking a botanical formula that contains one or more of these herbs (in powdered form)—deglycyrrhizinated licorice root, slippery elm and marshmallow root. Follow label instructions and take until inflammatory bowel symptoms abate.

•**Eat healthful fats daily and fish twice a week.** Olive oil, avocado, soy milk and small portions of unsalted nuts (eight to 12) are good sources of healthful fat. (However, celiac

---

*To minimize inflammation, follow the dietary advice indefinitely—and also continue to take the vitamin supplements to guard against a nutritional deficiency.

patients should avoid peanuts, which can be hard for them to digest.) Fatty fish, such as salmon or halibut, is an easily digested protein source.

Warning: In people with celiac disease, high-fat dairy products, as well as fried foods, tend to worsen diarrhea.

•**Use plant-based enzymes.** Enzyme supplementation helps break down food and reduces post-meal bloating. Plant-based enzymes (available at natural-food stores) are usually derived from pineapple or papaya, and they are safe for just about everyone unless you have ulcers or you are allergic to pineapple or papaya.

Typical dose: One or two capsules per meal.

•**Get support.** Avoiding gluten isn't easy, but you'll feel much better if you do. For more advice, consult the Celiac Sprue Association/ USA, 877-272-4272, *www.csaceliacs.org.*

Natural Ways to Improve Digestive Health

Jamison Starbuck, ND, naturopathic physician in family practice in Missoula, Montana. She is past president of the American Association of Naturopathic Physicians and a contributing editor to *The Alternative Advisor: The Complete Guide to Natural Therapies and Alternative Treatments* (Time-Life).

Though sometimes overlooked by doctors, gastrointestinal (GI) health is fundamental to overall wellness. The GI tract, also known as the "gut," allows us to draw nourishment from our food and eliminate toxins. A variety of medications claim to promote intestinal health, but I prefer my own eight-step natural approach, which is both inexpensive and easy to follow. Add one new step each day. If you're like most people, your GI tract will be healthier within two weeks. *My advice...*

1. Avoid foods that cause indigestion. Indigestion is your body's way of telling you that a certain food is not readily digestible. Instead of trying to make a food digestible by taking drugs, choose foods that you can easily digest, such as fish, brown rice and steamed vegetables.

2. Shortly after awakening in the morning, drink an eight-ounce glass of room-temperature water. This "wakes up" the GI tract, preparing you for both digestion and elimination. Repeat this step five to 10 minutes before each meal. Avoid iced beverages, including water, with meals and 15 minutes before and afterward. Some research suggests that cold beverages decrease the secretion of digestive enzymes.

3. Squeeze fresh lemon or sprinkle vinegar on your food. For most people, one-half teaspoon of lemon or vinegar per meal fights indigestion by increasing stomach acidity and improving the digestion of fats.

4. Take a 15-minute walk after meals. Doing so will improve your digestion and elimination. If you can't do this after every meal, do so following the largest meal of the day.

5. Practice simple home hydrotherapy. This practice increases blood flow to your intestines, which helps them function properly.

What to do: Finish your daily shower or bath with a 30-second spray of cool or cold water to your entire abdomen. Towel dry with brisk strokes immediately after the cool water spray.

Caution: If you have a history of stroke, check with your doctor before trying hydrotherapy.

6. Drink chamomile or peppermint tea after dinner. These herbs soothe the lining of the stomach and intestines. Add one tea bag or two teaspoons of loose herb to eight ounces of water.

7. Use foot reflexology to relieve intestinal pain. Massaging reflexology points on the feet is thought to help increase blood flow to and improve the function of corresponding organs or body parts.

What to do: Whenever you have GI discomfort, firmly massage (for five to seven minutes) with your thumb and forefinger the outside portion of the middle one-third of the soles of the feet. According to reflexologists, this area

corresponds to the colon. Your strokes should move toward the heel.

8. Never eat when you are stressed. Our bodies are not designed to simultaneously manage both stress and digestion. Studies show that just a few moments of relaxation, such as deep breathing or prayer, before a meal will improve the digestive process.

Nature's Detox Program

Jamison Starbuck, ND, naturopathic physician in family practice and a lecturer at the University of Montana, both in Missoula. She is past president of the American Association of Naturopathic Physicians and a contributing editor to The Alternative Advisor: The Complete Guide to Natural Therapies and Alternative Treatments *(Time Life).*

Cleansing the liver with so-called "detox" products is becoming more and more popular these days. Such products are theoretically designed to help the liver more efficiently perform its many functions that are crucial to your daily health. For example, the liver makes bile, a substance stored in the gallbladder and used in digestion and elimination. But the liver also synthesizes nutrients, including hormones and proteins, and plays an important role in the metabolism of fats and carbohydrates. In addition, the liver breaks down potentially dangerous compounds, including most medications, turning them into particles that the body can excrete via urine or stool.

But anyone who considers using one of these detox products should remember "buyer beware" and proceed only with the advice of a doctor. I see many patients each year who experience ill effects from over-the-counter "liver detox" pills. They typically suffer liver or gallbladder pain, diarrhea, constipation and/or gastrointestinal cramping. Instead of liver detox pills, I recommend trying the time-tested foods and liver "tonic" described below to promote optimal functioning of this vital organ...

Root vegetables—especially carrots and beets—have a long tradition as liver "medicine." They are rich in antioxidant vitamins and minerals that help the liver remove toxins from the body.

My advice: Eat two raw carrots daily...or add one-quarter cup each of shredded carrots and beets to a salad. As an alternative, eat a baked beet salad (bake fresh beets 25 to 45 minutes at 400°, slice and add olive oil, vinegar and any seasoning you like) and include steamed carrots in your diet several times a week.

"Bitter" leafy greens, such as dandelion, mustard, kale and beet tops, also promote good liver health. Leafy greens assist with fat metabolism and bile production and are high in folate, a nutrient that is essential for healthy cell development.

My advice: Include at least one portion (one-half cup cooked or one cup raw) of these bitter greens (steamed or added to soup or stew or finely chopped raw in a salad) in your daily diet.

Caution: People who take a blood thinner, such as *warfarin* (Coumadin), should not add more greens to their diet—the vitamin K in greens can interfere with the drug.

Milk thistle. Research has shown that this herb can help reduce elevated liver enzymes in people recovering from such conditions as viral hepatitis, alcoholism and medication-induced liver damage.

For a short-term liver tonic: Add one teaspoon of ground or powdered milk thistle seeds to your food each day for one month. You can buy the whole seeds in natural-food grocery stores and grind or powder them at home in a coffee mill. If you find it to be more convenient, you also can buy ground or powdered milk thistle at most natural-food stores. Ground and powdered milk thistle are equally effective. Use this tonic daily for two weeks—it will do its job by then—and repeat once every six months.

14

Anxiety and Depression Cures

Soothe Anxiety with Probiotics

You already know that chocolate can do wonders for a dark mood …but yogurt? If you buy the kind that contains active probiotics, it may indeed brighten your spirits. A new study from Canada demonstrated that probiotics can help modulate anxiety.

The study involved 35 patients with *chronic fatigue syndrome* (CFS) who experienced a host of gastrointestinal problems, including *irritable bowel syndrome* (IBS) and constipation. Participants were divided randomly into two groups, one taking a probiotic drink containing *Lactobacillus casei strain Shirota* (LaS), and the other taking a placebo that was identical in taste and appearance but had no probiotics.

Results: After two months, the probiotic group had a significant decrease in anxiety symptoms, while the placebo group did not. The probiotic group also showed a significant increase in *Bifidobacteria*, which are beneficial for gastrointestinal health, compared with the placebo group.

INTESTINAL FLORA AND YOUR BRAIN

A. Venketeshwer Rao, MSc, PhD, the study author and professor emeritus of nutritional science at University of Toronto, says that there has been skepticism in the medical world about the role intestinal flora plays in the system of gut-brain communication (the enteric nervous system, often called "the second brain"). This study provides evidence that through their metabolism in the gut, probiotic bacteria can boost levels of the mood-elevating chemicals *tryptophan* (an amino acid) and *serotonin* (a neurotransmitter). Dr. Rao adds that the regions of the brain affected by CFS also house anxiety and depression. "These parts of the brain seem to respond to changes in the microflora, and most of our behavior patterns are controlled by these areas," he says.

A. Venketeshwer Rao, BSc MSc, PhD, professor emeritus of nutritional science, University of Toronto.

Dr. Rao says there still is much to learn about the role of gut flora. But many, if not most people, could improve their health by taking probiotics. The study used a probiotic drink, but Dr. Rao says that probiotic supplements may be even more effective, depending on what types and how many of the live microbes they contain. He advises looking for a product that contains *Lactobacillus Shirota* and *Bifidobacteria*, with 100 to 120 billion live probiotic bacteria.

Six Self-Help Ways to Ease Anxiety

Michael McKee, PhD, cognitive-behavioral therapist in private practice in Scarsdale, New York, and research scientist at the Anxiety Disorders Clinic, New York State Psychiatric Institute, New York City.

Here are six simple ways to ease anxiety on your own—without help from a therapist…

• **Exercise.** Research shows that all kinds of exercise will make you feel more confident and at ease. Aerobic exercise stimulates release of endorphins, neurotransmitters that are the body's natural "feel good" drug. Yoga can calm nerves.

• **Deep breathing.** Slow breathing from deep in the diaphragm (belly breathing) slows racing thoughts and restores a sense of control.

• **Progressive muscle relaxation.** To remove tension from your muscles, clench them tightly for a full five seconds, then slowly release. Do this for individual body parts starting with your toes and working all the way up to your face.

• **Cut back on coffee.** The caffeine in coffee is a stimulant, so if you are nervous, it will make you more so. Switch to green tea—it has much less caffeine. Green tea also contains amino acids that researchers believe have a calming effect on the brain.

• **Limit alcohol consumption.** It stimulates stress hormones, so have no more than one alcoholic beverage a day.

• **Keep a "joy journal."** Write down on a piece of paper a list of all the good things in your life. Take notes during the day of any funny, entertaining or rewarding things that occur. By consciously thinking about them, they will become more meaningful than stressful parts of your life.

Bananas Fight Depression, Heartburn And More

Ara DerMarderosian, PhD, professor, department of biological sciences and research professor of pharmacognosy (the study of natural products used in medicine) at the University of the Sciences in Philadelphia. He also is the scientific director of the University's Complementary and Alternative Medicines Institute. Dr. DerMarderosian has published more than 100 scientific papers and chapters in books as well as two books.

Most people know that bananas are an excellent source of potassium (one ripe banana supplies more than 10% of an adult's daily requirement of the mineral). That's important because people with a low dietary intake of potassium are 28% more likely to suffer a stroke than those who consume higher levels, according to a study conducted at Tulane University.

Lesser-known medicinal uses of bananas…

• **Depression.** Bananas are a good source of tryptophan (a precursor to serotonin, a brain chemical that helps regulate mood).

• **Diarrhea.** Unripe bananas and plantains (high-starch, green bananas that are typically cooked) are a rich source of tannins, astringent plant compounds that help stop water accumulation in the intestines, thus diminishing diarrhea.

• **Heartburn and ulcers.** Bananas neutralize acidity and soothe and coat esophageal tissue with pectin (a substance used as a thickener and stabilizer in jellies).

Important: In rare cases, bananas may cause an allergic reaction. Bananas with blackened skin can increase blood sugar levels. Because bananas have high levels of potassium, people with kidney problems should check with their doctors before eating this fruit.

Unique Help for Weight Loss, Insomnia, Depression, Pain And More

Jeffrey C. Zimmerman, OMD, LAc, once a classical musician, is a Doctor of Oriental Medicine, licensed acupuncturist, martial artist and Qigong master in Westport, Connecticut.

At a family picnic a few months ago, my cousin raved about a form of acupuncture that brought her almost immediate relief from the depression, anxiety and insomnia she'd wrestled with for months. Called *auricular* (ear) *therapy*, this sub-type of acupuncture involves insertion of very small needles or taping tiny metal "seeds" onto various places in the ear. Auricular therapy can be useful in beating back demons like smoking, alcohol or drug addiction…helpful for people seeking to lose weight…soothing for chronic pain, as with arthritis…useful for treating nausea and high blood pressure…and for numerous other problems, including those related to mood. My cousin told me that the night after her first treatment, she slept soundly and woke up feeling free from the sense of doom that had long engulfed her.

HOW DOES IT WORK?

Acupuncture of the ear has been popular in China for centuries, but what's been known as auricular therapy was developed in the 1950s when a French doctor named Paul Nogier, MD, mapped specific sites, called points, on the ear based on the shape of a fetus (or *homunculus*). Take a careful look at a human ear, probably someone else's, and see if you can detect the outline of an inverted fetus. This may challenge your imagination, but the concept is important—it is the key to understanding how auricular therapy works. This "ear map" is how the acupuncturist finds the particular points that correspond to the problem area of the patient's body.

Though the exact mechanism that makes auricular therapy effective isn't clear, a possible explanation is that stimulating certain nerves sends signals to the brain, generating a reflex response that sends soothing sensations to the targeted body part.

EXPERT INSIGHTS INTO AURICULAR THERAPY

To find out more about this unusual therapy, we spoke with Jeff Zimmerman, OMD, LAc, a doctor of Oriental medicine and licensed acupuncturist in Westport, Connecticut. He told me he likes to use auricular therapy in conjunction with other types of acupuncture, though many practitioners treat certain types of problems with ear therapy alone. Most practitioners begin a session with a discussion of your motivation for wanting to, say, cut back on or stop drinking alcohol. You may be asked what obstacles have presented challenges in previous efforts, since treatment is tailored not just to your problem but also to how it interacts with your life. Depending on the specific way you experience the problem (e.g., drink until you pass out versus become a loud and angry drunk), different points will be used.

How many seeds or needles a practitioner uses varies—Dr. Zimmerman says he secures about five to seven seeds per ear under a small adhesive dressing (like tape), which should stay in place until the next treatment. Patients learn how to massage the points where the seeds are, thereby activating their effect at least three times a day and/or when they need relief from pain or anxiety or have an urge for the forbidden substance. This massaging may even help them when the seeds are removed.

Dr. Zimmerman says some of his patients have triumphed over a bad smoking habit after just one session, but that the general routine for an addiction treatment is six weekly sessions and then perhaps continuing another month or two after those. Some patients need "tune-up" therapy from time to time, and he noted that patients who seek auricular therapy for chronic pain or depression may want to return for a treatment every few months or so to keep their energy flowing freely.

PRACTICAL POINTERS

Auricular therapy is not covered by all health insurance plans, but may be paid for as part of acupuncture. However, even insurers who won't cover the primary cost of treatments may allow you to deduct them from a flexible spending account—check your policy. Prices vary considerably, depending on where you live and the kind of training your practitioner has had, with $50 or $60 per half-hour session a good ballpark estimate.

When looking for a practitioner, Zimmerman says to check for certification by the NC-CAOM (National Certification Commission for Acupuncture and Oriental Medicine, *www. nccaom.org*) and licensing by your state specifically for acupuncture. Before you book, inquire about his/her experience in treating your particular problem. He adds that it is important to be an educated consumer—ask around for information about the person you are considering and trust your instincts when you meet.

Best Diet to Prevent Depression

In a study of more than 10,000 men and women without depression, those who most closely adhered to the Mediterranean diet (rich in fruits, vegetables, legumes, nuts, olive oil, fish and whole grains) over an average 4.4-year period were about half as likely to develop depression.

Theory: The diet enhances function of the *endothelium* (the blood vessels' inner lining), which is needed to support the brain-cell development that helps prevent depression.

If you are at risk for depression (due to family history or recent stressful life events): Try the Mediterranean diet. Learn more at *www. oldwayspt.org/mediterranean-diet-pyramid*.

Miguel A. Martínez-Gonzalez, MD, PhD, professor and chair, department of preventive medicine, University of Navarra, Pamplona, Spain.

Dr. Joy Browne on Getting the Help You Need

Joy Browne, PhD, licensed clinical psychologist in New York City and host of a daily syndicated radio show. She is author of several books, including *Getting Unstuck: 8 Simple Steps to Solving Any Problem* and *Dating Disasters and How to Avoid Them* (both from Hay House). *www.drjoy.com*

As a psychologist, I am struck by the way people tend to isolate themselves during painful times. Whether dealing with losing a job, the end of a relationship or any major disappointment, it seems that when we most need other people, we find it most difficult to ask for help.

One reason is that people believe—erroneously—that they should be able to handle problems themselves. They don't want to impose or be a burden.

The truth is that most people like being asked for help. Think about how you feel when a friend needs your help. It's flattering. It means that your friend is taking the relationship seriously. Giving and receiving make friendships stronger.

BE SPECIFIC

Some people feel it's up to friends and loved ones to recognize distress and offer help without being asked, but it's unrealistic to expect others to read your mind or catch your hints. *Here are ways to ask for the help you need...*

•**Problem solving.** "I can't figure out what to do. Would you mind brainstorming options with me?"

•**A sympathetic ear.** "It's been a tough week. Can I tell you about it?"

•**Reassurance.** "I'm discouraged. I'd love it if you could remind me of the things I'm doing right in my life."

•**Perspective.** "I'm not sure if the problem is me or him. Can I get your take on the situation?"

189

- **Sympathy.** "My boss is on a rampage. I don't need to hear about how I should handle him—I just want someone to take my side for a few minutes."

- **Affection.** "I could use a hug."

- **Company.** "Would it be OK if I came over for a few hours? I don't want to be alone this afternoon."

- **Suggestions.** "My computer crashed. Can you recommend a good repair service?"

- **Physical assistance.** "I'm too sick to go out. Could you stop by the deli and pick up some soup for me?"

- **Practice.** Don't wait until you're in a crisis to ask for help. Practice in situations that aren't so traumatic.

Example: When your car is in the shop, call a friend and say, "Would you be able to give me a ride to work?"

SHOW APPRECIATION

Helping isn't something you contract for. Treating your request as a quid pro quo ("If you do X for me, I'll do Y for you") is likely to offend. Instead, be generous with your thanks.

Examples: Send a thank-you note…flowers…or a small gift.

Depressed? Give New Eyeglasses a Try

Eyeglasses can ease depression among the elderly.

Recent finding: After two months, seniors who received properly prescribed eyeglasses had higher scores for activities, hobbies and social interaction—and fewer signs of depression—than seniors with similar visual acuity who were not given new eyeglasses.

Cynthia Owsley, PhD, professor, department of ophthalmology, University of Alabama at Birmingham, and leader of a study of 78 nursing home residents, published in *Archives of Ophthalmology*.

How You Can Calm Down

Joy Browne, PhD, licensed clinical psychologist in New York City and host of a daily syndicated radio show. She is author of several books, including *Getting Unstuck: 8 Simple Steps to Solving Any Problem* and *Dating Disasters and How to Avoid Them* (both from Hay House). *www.drjoy.com*

In prehistoric times, if you failed to feel enough anxiety to trigger a fight-or-flight response, you got eaten by a saber-toothed tiger.

Even today, the body's instant reaction to danger includes a surge of the stress hormone adrenaline—causing rapid breathing, pounding heart, tingling hands and nausea. This floods large muscles with energy-giving oxygen by increasing breathing and heart rate and by diverting blood from the extremities and digestive tract.

Problem is, this also occurs in situations that aren't physically dangerous—such as being caught in traffic on your way to an appointment.

It's tough to focus on the task at hand during an anxiety attack. Worse, repeated adrenaline surges and other anxiety responses can contribute to hypertension, digestive disorders, weakened immunity and depression.

HOW I DO IT

To ease anxiety: A technique called *square breathing* helps me regain control over my body and mind by reestablishing the proper ratio of oxygen to carbon dioxide in my system.

I inhale deeply for a count of four…hold for four…exhale slowly for four…hold for four… and repeat until anxiety subsides. It's like giving my body a mini-vacation.

You can use it any time—when preparing to make a toast, waiting for test results—because it is inconspicuous.

Drug-Free Depression Treatments

David Mischoulon, MD, PhD, assistant professor of psychiatry at Harvard Medical School and director of Research and Alternative Remedy Studies at the Depression Clinical and Research Program, Massachusetts General Hospital, Boston.

Depression remains stubbornly intractable for many of the estimated 20-plus million Americans who suffer from it. Many of these people have difficulties with the pharmaceutical drugs so often prescribed for depression, finding them either ineffective or to cause disagreeable side effects including lowered libido and weight gain. Also several of these drugs have been associated with an increased risk for suicide, though this remains a controversial issue. All this has opened the door to a growing interest in natural solutions for depression. Research into CAM (complementary and alternative medicine) treatments for depression is active in some very mainstream academic medical centers, and several natural substances have earned a respected position on the list of depression treatment alternatives.

A chief researcher in this area is David Mischoulon, MD, PhD, assistant professor of psychiatry, Harvard Medical School, and director of Alternative Remedy Studies at the Depression Clinical and Research Program, Massachusetts General Hospital. We spoke with Dr. Mischoulon recently to get an update on alternative treatments for depression.

THE "BIG THREE"

Depression researchers refer to the "big three" in natural substances for treating depression. One well-studied natural treatment is SAM-e (*S-adenosyl methionine*), a synthetic form of a chemical produced naturally in the body with numerous functions including influencing moods and emotions. Research on SAM-e and depression has been encouraging, showing that it works better than placebo and that it is as effective as *tricyclics*, a class of older antidepressants that dates back to the 1950s

and is still very popular today. Dr. Mischoulon's research group is now studying SAM-e against the newer antidepressant drugs, SSRIs (*selective serotonin reuptake inhibitors*) such as *fluoxetine* (Prozac) and *sertraline* (Zoloft). The typical prescribed dosage of SAM-e is 800 to 1,600 mg a day, and SAM-e seems to be well-tolerated, with few if any immediate side effects.

Next, perhaps surprisingly, comes omega-3 fatty acids. We have known for some time that omega-3 fatty acids help treat many physical conditions, including cardiovascular disease. But Dr. Mischoulon says there have been numerous studies on omega-3 fatty acids and their impact on mental health, including bipolar disorder as well as depression, with many suggesting that these fatty acids are indeed effective. The types of omega-3 fatty acids that help with depression are EPA and DHA, found in cold-water fish and fish oil supplements. Psychiatric benefits are commonly obtained with about 1,000 mg a day of combined EPA/DHA.

And then there is our old friend, St. John's wort (*hypericum perforatum*). Dr. Mischoulon says that it has tested well in a number of studies, including against older antidepressant drugs. Studies have shown that this substance is calming while at the same time it seems to work in part like SSRIs. Recommended doses are on the order of 900 to 1,200 mg per day, but because of subtleties regarding dosage and the fact that St. John's wort is known to interact with many other medications, it's imperative to take this supplement under the supervision of a medical professional experienced in its use.

OTHER NATURAL TREATMENTS

Yet another substance that Dr. Mischoulon says may be helpful is Valerian (*valeriana officinalis*). It has primarily been studied as a sleep aid, but Dr. Mischoulon says it may also be useful for anxiety. It's important to keep in mind that Valerian requires several weeks to work, whether for sleep purposes or for anxiety relief, although many report feeling positive effects fairly quickly. The usual dose administered is 400 mg to 600 mg of extract in capsule form, but there is considerable variety

191

among brands as to purity and active ingredients. Different brands may achieve different results in different people, so Dr. Mischoulon says not to give up if a particular one doesn't work for you.

A number of physical treatment modalities are being incorporated in depression treatment, though research remains limited. Acupuncture is one that studies have found promising, says Dr. Mischoulon. Curiously, acupuncture studies have an unusually high placebo-effect rate (subjects on placebo showing improvement), so how much acupuncture actually helps is unclear. On the other hand, most people find acupuncture to be neither painful nor harmful, so it may be worth a try.

Exercise has also been studied with regard to potential benefits for depressed people, with new studies suggesting beneficial mood-elevating effects. However, because depression tends to cause a decrease in energy and motivation, it can be difficult to get depressed people to engage in exercise programs, Dr. Mischoulon acknowledged. But if they can push past the lethargy, they may be pleasantly surprised by how good exercise makes them feel—including the sense of accomplishment.

DEPRESSION IS MANAGEABLE

Anyone who experiences depression for more than a few weeks should seek professional treatment, says Dr. Mischoulon. Though it may take a while to find the treatment that works for you, it is important to remember that depression is usually manageable. Left untreated, it can become chronic and difficult to treat.

When choosing to treat depression with natural substances, always work under the supervision of a naturopathic physician or other health care professional who can help identify the best solution for you. To find such a doctor, seek referrals from your primary care physician and consult the database of the AANP (American Association of Naturopathic Physicians) at *www.naturopathic.org*. Click on "Find a Doctor." Then speak with the doctors to find one that seems to be a good fit for you.

Patience is in order—just as with pharmaceutical drugs for depression, natural treatments often require time to take effect, from three to six weeks, says Dr. Mischoulon. Finally, some of these therapies have been found effective in treating mild to moderate depression. While some may be of help for severe depression, the evidence to date relates only to the milder forms—treatment of more serious cases may require a different strategy.

Lies and Half-Truths About Herbal Supplements

Mark A. Stengler, NMD, licensed naturopathic medical doctor in private practice, Stengler Center for Integrative Medicine, Encinitas, California...adjunct associate clinical professor at the National College of Natural Medicine, Portland, Oregon...author of many books, including *The Natural Physician's Healing Therapies* and coauthor of *Prescription for Natural Cures* (both from Bottom Line Books)...and author of the *Bottom Line/Natural Healing* newsletter. *www.drstengler.com*

I have exposed some of the lies and half-truths about nutritional supplements, including vitamins. Herbal supplements also have gotten an undeserved bashing in recent years. Yet millions of people benefit from these safe natural remedies. Also, many prescription drugs are based on plant molecules. Herbs often work as well as, or better than, medications—and they are much gentler on the body.

Lie: St. John's wort doesn't help severe depression.

Truth: A study published in the *Journal of the American Medical Association* (JAMA) claimed that St. John's wort did not help severe depression, which is difficult to treat even with pharmaceutical drugs. As a result, many headlines stated that St. John's wort was ineffective for all types of depression. At that time, the herb was most often used to treat mild-to-moderate depression—it worked well, caused few side effects and was less expensive than antidepressants. In a later study, an analysis of 29 studies in which St. John's wort was used to treat major depression was published in the

Cochrane Database of Systematic Reviews. The article concluded that the herb worked just as well as drugs, although the dose to treat severe depression was higher than that needed to treat milder forms. Yet the impression left by the earlier study remained.

Note: St. John's wort should not be taken with an antidepressant or by women who are pregnant, breast-feeding or taking birth control pills.

Lie: Garlic does not reduce blood pressure.

Truth: There's evidence that garlic supplements can reduce blood pressure in people who have high blood pressure. Analyses of studies in *Annals of Pharmacotherapy* and *BMC Cardiovascular Disorders* confirmed that garlic lowered systolic blood pressure (the top number in a blood pressure reading) or both systolic and diastolic blood pressure (bottom number). Despite this evidence, conventional medical doctors typically don't prescribe garlic to lower blood pressure.

Brand to try: Kyolic Healthy Heart Formula 106, which provides 300 milligrams (mg) of aged garlic extract (to find a retailer call 800-421-2998, or go to *www.kyolic.com*).

Lie: Echinacea does not help fight the common cold.

Truth: An analysis of 14 studies published in *The Lancet Infectious Diseases* found that echinacea supplements reduced the risk of catching a cold by 58% and reduced the length of colds by 1.4 days, on average. This herb's effectiveness may be in question because not all echinacea products are of the same quality or strength, which means dosages vary.

Brand to try: Nature's Way Echinacea (800-962-8873, *www.naturesway.com* for a store locator).

Lie: Black cohosh makes breast cancer spread.

Truth: Many women use this herb to reduce hot flashes. An old theory is that black cohosh contains weak estrogen-like plant compounds that attach to estrogen receptors on the surface of the cell that could raise the risk for breast cancer. Concern increased when research published in *Cancer Research* found that mice bred

to develop aggressive breast cancer were more likely to have the cancer spread to their lungs when given this herb. Other studies published in *Maturitas* and *BMC Pharmacology* demonstrated that black cohosh reduces estrogen levels and does not contain phytoestrogens (estrogen-like plant compounds). Also, a National Institutes of Health sponsored study published in *International Journal of Cancer* that compared the supplement use of women with and without breast cancer found that women who took black cohosh had a 61% lower risk for breast cancer. I believe that black cohosh is safe for all women, even those who have a history of breast cancer.

Lie: Saw palmetto is not effective for benign prostate enlargement.

Truth: Enlargement of the prostate gland, known as *benign prostatic hypertrophy* (BPH), commonly affects men age 50 and older. The main symptom is reduced or erratic urinary flow. One study found that saw palmetto did not help men who had severe BPH. But many other studies reviewed in the *Cochrane Database of Systematic Reviews* have found that it does help men with mild-to-moderate BPH, which is the more common condition. For men with this condition, saw palmetto works just as well as prescription drugs, with fewer side effects—and it is less expensive.

Half-truth: Licorice root raises blood pressure.

Truth: In very large amounts, licorice root can increase blood pressure and deplete potassium, so if you have heart disease, diabetes or high blood pressure, you should not have licorice root tea or black licorice candies frequently. But these warnings about licorice don't apply to people who don't have these conditions or to multi-ingredient formulas that contain very small amounts of the herb. Most licorice supplements, which help to improve digestion, heartburn and ulcers, are *deglycyrrhized*, which means that the sweet-tasting ingredient that raises blood pressure has been removed.

Lie: Ginseng increases blood pressure.

Truth: Conventional medical physicians and organizations often advise patients who have high blood pressure against taking certain types of ginseng. Studies published in

Hypertension found that different types of ginseng, including Asian ginseng (Panax ginseng), did not increase blood pressure—and a study published in *Annals of Pharmacotherapy* found that Panax ginseng actually reduced it. I believe that ginseng can safely be used by those with high blood pressure.

Natural Remedies a Pharmacist Has in Her Own Medicine Cabinet

Suzy Cohen, RPh, registered practicing pharmacist for over 20 years and author of *The 24-Hour Pharmacist* (Collins). Her syndicated newspaper column, "Dear Pharmacist," reaches more than 24 million readers. Based in Florida, she is a member of the American College for Advancement in Medicine, American Academy of Anti-Aging Medicine, and American Pharmacist's Association. *http://dearpharmacist.com*

As a pharmacist for more than two decades, Suzy Cohen knows the importance of medication—but she also has learned to "think outside the pill" and recommend natural options that often are just as good or better at promoting health without the risk of dangerous side effects.

Here are the remedies she recommends most often. All are free of significant side effects unless otherwise noted, but always talk with your doctor before using any supplements.

TEA TREE OIL FOR WOUNDS

This oil kills germs, reduces pain and helps wounds heal more quickly. You can use it in place of antibiotic ointment for minor cuts, scratches and burns...to treat toenail fungus... and, when diluted, as a gargle to kill the germs that cause sore throat.

How it works: It's a strong antiseptic that kills bacteria as well as fungi.

How to use: Moisten a cotton ball or swab with one or two drops of the oil, and apply it to the area two to three times daily until it heals.

For a gargle for sore throat: Mix a few drops in a cup of water, gargle and spit it out.

Caution: Do not swallow it.

GINGER FOR NAUSEA

Studies have shown that ginger can relieve nausea—due to pregnancy, seasickness, etc.—as well as or better than over-the-counter drugs.

How it works: Ginger increases the pH of stomach acid, reducing its acidity. In one study, published in *The Lancet*, volunteers were given either ginger or Dramamine (a nausea-preventing drug), then were seated in a chair designed to trigger motion sickness. Those given ginger were able to withstand the motion 57% longer than those given the drug.

How to use: Put one teaspoon of peeled, grated fresh gingerroot in a cup of boiling water. Let it steep for 10 minutes, then drink (you can filter out the ginger if you want). Or chew and swallow a piece of crystallized ginger, sold in health-food stores.

Caution: Ginger can increase the risk of bleeding when taken with blood-thinning drugs, such as *warfarin* (Coumadin).

RHODIOLA ROSEA FOR STRESS

This herb acts like a natural form of Valium by reducing physical and emotional stress. The supplement is made from the root of the Siberian plant.

How it works: Herbalists classify Rhodiola as an adaptogen, a class of herbs that "sense" chemicals in the body and either raise or lower them. It normalizes levels of brain chemicals that affect mood, such as monoamines and beta-endorphins, which help counter the effects of stress. Rhodiola also may increase serotonin, which enhances feelings of well-being.

How to use: During times of stress, take 100 milligrams (mg) of rhodiola rosea in capsule form, two to three times daily. It's best taken on a cyclical basis—two months on, two weeks off.

CALCIUM PLUS MAGNESIUM FOR CRAMPS

People who experience frequent and/or painful menstrual or muscle cramps often have a deficiency of calcium and magnesium.

How it works: Calcium and magnesium regulate the contraction and relaxation of muscles.

How to use: Before going to bed, take 500 mg to 600 mg of calcium, along with 150 mg to 200 mg of magnesium (using the chelate or glycinate forms—check the label). Combination formulas are easy to find and fine to use.

For menstrual problems, start 10 days before you expect your period to begin each month and continue until your period is complete.

GABA FOR INSOMNIA

Gamma-aminobutyric acid (GABA) is a neurotransmitter (mood-related brain chemical) that is naturally present in the body. It's taken in supplement form to reduce insomnia, as well as anxiety and depression.

How it works: GABA is an inhibitory neurotransmitter that slows activity in the brain and makes it easier to fall asleep.

How to use: Take 500 mg to 1,000 mg one hour before bedtime if you have trouble getting to sleep. If your problem is that you wake in the middle of the night and can't get back to sleep, take it then. Don't exceed recommended doses on the package. Do this for two weeks. If it doesn't help, talk to your doctor.

Caution: Combining GABA with prescription or over-the-counter sleep aids can cause excessive sedation.

CAPSAICIN CREAM FOR PAIN

Capsaicin is the chemical compound that puts the "hot" in chili peppers. It is effective for easing muscle aches, back and joint pain and nerve pain caused by the herpes virus (*post-herpetic neuralgia*).

How it works: When applied as a cream, it causes nerve cells to empty their reservoirs of substance P, a pain-causing chemical. This results in less pain from the underlying disorder.

How to use: Start with a 0.025% concentration. Apply it two to three times daily—the initial burning sensation diminishes with continued use. If needed, you can always buy the stronger 0.075% concentration—but it's best to work your way up to this strength.

Caution: Wear latex gloves when applying capsaicin—and wash your hands thoroughly after using to prevent residual cream from getting into the eyes, nose, etc.

PROBIOTICS FOR DIGESTIVE DISCOMFORT

A healthy digestive tract contains trillions of bacteria, many of which have beneficial effects. These so-called "good" (probiotic) organisms promote digestive health, improve immunity and aid in the synthesis of B vitamins, among many other functions.

How they work: Probiotic supplements replenish beneficial bacteria and crowd out harmful organisms that can cause gas, bloating, diarrhea and other digestive problems.

How to use: Take a daily supplement of at least 10 billion organisms that contains a variety of living organisms, such as *L. bulgaricus*, *L. bifida* and *B. longum*. Some yogurts contain these live active cultures, but avoid those that contain sugar or artificial sweeteners.

BIOTIN FOR CRACKED NAILS

The B vitamin biotin is the only nutrient that has been shown to improve nail health in generally healthy adults. People with a deficiency of biotin often have fragile nails that crack easily.

How it works: Biotin is absorbed by the nail matrix, the part under the fingernail where nail cells are generated.

How to use: Take 2,000 micrograms (mcg) to 4,000 mcg of biotin daily, as well as a B-complex supplement. Most people will notice an improvement in nail strength and thickness in one to two months.

Meditation for Women Who Hate To Sit Still

Judith Boice, ND, naturopathic physician and acupuncturist in private practice in Montrose, Colorado. She conducts wellness seminars nationwide and is author of eight books, including *Menopause with Science and Soul: A Guidebook for Navigating the Journey* (Celestial Arts). *www.drjudithboice.com.*

Meditation is good for us—it can relieve tension by shifting brain activity away from the stress-prone right frontal cortex and into the calmer left frontal cortex. But some people have trouble finding time to meditate.

Solution: Combine exercise and meditation through rhythmic, repetitive motions, such as walking, swimming or rowing, so you strengthen the body and soothe the mind.

Bonus: "Meditation in motion" makes exercise easier, because while you do it, you won't be thinking about tired muscles or tasks that await after your workout. *Begin with walking meditation...*

• **Pick a spot.** Find a secluded outdoor area where you won't feel self-conscious.

• **Begin walking.** Start slowly, focusing on the rhythm of your heels striking the ground and your toes pushing off. Keep your eyes open for safety, but don't get distracted by the sights around you.

• **Recite a mantra.** Choose or invent a rhythmic chant, such as "I am one with the world, I am filled with peace." Repeat it over and over, out loud or in your mind, melding its rhythm with the movement of your feet. I recommend not listening to music—it may distract you from your mantra.

• **Try to stay focused.** At first you may succeed for only a few minutes before thoughts of daily life intrude. Work your way up to a 30-minute session daily.

• **Meditate at the gym.** Once you've mastered walking meditation, try the technique while using a treadmill or elliptical machine or while swimming laps.

Saffron, the Happiness Spice

From *Bottom Line's Breakthroughs in Drug-Free Healing* by Bill Gottlieb. (Bottom Line Books). *www.bottomlinepublications.com.*

Think saffron, and you probably think of the world's most expensive spice, and the golden-yellow color of saffron-containing dishes, such as Spanish paella or Indian biryani. What you probably don't think of is depression. But some psychiatrists do.

BREAKTHROUGH STUDIES

Doctors at the Psychiatric Research Center at the Tehran University of Medical Sciences in Iran (the country that produces 80% of the world's saffron) studied 40 people with depression, dividing them into two groups. One group received the antidepressant *fluoxetine* (Prozac). The other group received saffron capsules.

Result: After six weeks, both groups had the same level of relief from depression.

"The results of this study indicate the effectiveness of *Crocus sativus* [saffron] in the treatment of mild to moderate depression," say the researchers, in the *Journal of Ethnopharmacology.*

In another study by the same team of researchers, saffron matched the depression-ending power of *imipramine* (Tofranil), a drug in the tricyclic class of antidepressants.

Suggested intake: The researchers used 30 mg a day.

• **EXIR Saffron Dietary Supplements** are available at *www.amazon.com.*

Natural Remedies for Depression

Tod Cooperman, MD, founder and president of ConsumerLab.com, the leading independent evaluator of nutritional and vitamin/mineral supplements, White Plains, New York. Reports can be found at *www.consumerlab.com* (subscription required). He also is editor of *ConsumerLab.com's Guide to Buying Vitamins & Supplements* (ConsumerLab.com).

Most people assume that prescription medications are stronger and more effective than supplements. But some supplements can be just as effective—without the side effects that often accompany prescription drugs.

Also, people with chronic conditions who have no insurance or are under-insured or who have been hit with higher co-pays can save hundreds or even thousands of dollars a year by using supplements in place of drugs.

Caution: Always check with your doctor before stopping a prescription drug or taking a supplement.

Here, natural alternatives to commonly prescribed medications. If there are two alternatives, try one. If that doesn't work, try the other. Dosages are those typically prescribed, but always follow directions on the supplement label or from your health practitioner.

DEPRESSION

Antidepressant medications, including *selective serotonin reuptake inhibitors* (SSRIs), such as *paroxetine* (Paxil), *escitalopram* (Lexapro) and *citalopram* (Celexa), have revolutionized the treatment of depression. Many people who take them, however, experience troublesome side effects, including heightened anxiety and reduced libido.

Alternative 1: **St. John's wort.** It appears to be as effective for mild-to-moderate depression as SSRIs but with milder side effects. It is not effective for patients with major depression and should not be taken with prescription antidepressants. It also may interact with other medications, including blood thinners, such as *warfarin* (Coumadin).

Dose: 300 mg, three times daily. Look for a product that contains 1% to 3% *hypericin*, the active ingredient.

Alternative 2: **Fish oil.** It improves a number of emotional and mental disorders, including depression and bipolar disorder. A study found that those who combined EPA with an antidepressant medication did better than those using either treatment alone.

Dose: 1 g of EPA, once daily, or eat three or more fish servings a week.

Caution: Fish oil may interact with blood-thinning drugs such as *warfarin* (Coumadin).

15

Diabetes Cures

Cures from the Kitchen— Common Foods that Help Stave Off Serious Diseases

I f we could reduce the incidence of diabetes, high blood pressure and osteoporosis, we'd slash medical expenses in this country by tens—maybe hundreds—of billions of dollars. What's especially compelling about these three illnesses is that the cost of prevention is virtually nothing, while the cost of treatment is exorbitant...but obvious as it is, people are resistant. We recently spoke with nutritionist Joy Bauer, MS, RD, the author of *Joy Bauer's Food Cures* (Rodale) and nutrition expert for the *Today* Show about how eating the right foods can significantly reduce the incidence and effects of diabetes, high blood pressure and osteoporosis, among other maladies. She shared with me her favorite food fighters to

help keep these particularly common age-related medical problems at bay.

DIABETES

It's not news. Type 2 diabetes is a serious disease and one that's skyrocketing in the US, yet it can often be controlled through closer attention to diet and exercise. This is especially true among younger people, in whom the greatest number of new cases are seen, and who can still reverse damage, which gets harder as people age. Two-thirds of Americans are now overweight, and research has shown that losing just a few of those extra pounds —say, 10 pounds over two years—can reduce your risk of diabetes by up to 30%. Even people who already need medication to manage their blood sugar and insulin levels can improve their diabetes and overall health by

Joy Bauer, MS, RD, CDN, nutritionist and author of *Joy Bauer's Food Cures* (Rodale) and *The Complete Idiot's Guide to Total Nutrition* (Alpha Books). Bauer is the nutrition expert for the *Today* show and Yahoo. com, and monthly nutrition columnist for *Woman's Day* magazine. *www.joybauer.com*

eating the right foods—ones that successfully control blood sugar and weight—to ward off common and dangerous complications such as heart disease, nerve damage and illnesses of the eye. *Your best bets...*

●**Ground flaxseed.** Flaxseed contains a high percentage of soluble fiber, a component of plant cell walls that slows the absorption of glucose from food in the stomach, reduces the glycemic index and keeps blood sugar on an even keel. Other excellent sources of soluble fiber are beans (kidney, lima, black, navy, pinto), legumes (peas, lentils), oatmeal and vegetables.

Tip: A good way to eat flaxseed is to sprinkle a handful, ground, along with a few berries over a bowl of whole-grain cereal.

●**Broccoli, peppers as well as cauliflower.** These, along with a host of other high-quality, low-glycemic index foods contain many vitamins, minerals and fiber. This attribute is particularly important for diabetics, because it means these foods raise blood sugar slowly. Other healthful carbs include not just fiber-rich veggies but also unsweetened oatmeal, chickpeas, lentils, blueberries, strawberries, apples, etc., all of which are better than high-glycemic snacks like soft drinks, candy, cakes and "white" carbs such as white bread, pretzels, donuts, etc. Empty carbohydrates will not only make you fat, they also raise blood sugar quickly, leading to spikes and crashes in energy that aggravate diabetes.

●**Meat, seafood as well as fish.** For optimal blood sugar control, eat high-quality protein with those high-quality carbs as it slows their absorption, Bauer explains. Good choices include organically raised poultry and wild salmon, herring or mackerel—but not king mackerel, which like other large ocean fish is prone to mercury contamination.

HIGH BLOOD PRESSURE

High blood pressure, or hypertension, is often called "the silent killer," since many have it without experiencing obvious symptoms. But don't make the mistake of thinking the lack of symptoms means all's well inside your body—high blood pressure damages healthy blood vessels and causes inflammation. Ac-cording to Bauer, you can help control high blood pressure by making sure you get enough calcium, vitamin D, magnesium and potassium in your diet. (Look for good sources of calcium and vitamin D below under osteoporosis.) *Your best bets...*

●**Unsalted pumpkin seeds, sunflower seeds, almonds and cashews.** Research shows that these magnesium-rich foods bring a variety of cardiovascular benefits. They can reduce high blood pressure, lower blood fats known as triglycerides and lower "bad" LDL cholesterol.

Tip: Instead of reaching for chips or candy, snack on a daily handful of healthful seeds or nuts.

●**Bananas, avocados and sweet potatoes.** Potassium-packed foods help your body maintain a normal balance between sodium and potassium, which in turn helps regulate blood pressure. There are plenty of foods rich in potassium including beans, lentils, split peas, kale, Swiss chard, radicchio, arugula, papaya, pistachio nuts, butternut squash, mushrooms, cantaloupe and carrots.

Tip: Make a batch of lentil, split pea, mushroom or other tasty homemade soup each week, and refrigerate or freeze individual portions for quick and healthful snacks and meals.

OSTEOPOROSIS

When it comes to fighting osteoporosis, the key nutrients to focus on are calcium and vitamin D in order to help maintain bone strength and density. *Your best bets...*

●**Kale, broccoli and white beans.** Everyone knows that milk and other dairy products such as yogurt and cheese are good sources of calcium, but these three non-dairy sources can also help you meet your daily requirements.

Tip: For bone support, enjoy a vegetable salad tossed with raw broccoli, white beans and salmon or sardines with bones, drizzled with a teaspoon of olive oil and a squeeze of fresh lemon.

●**Shiitake mushrooms.** Calcium is ineffective without vitamin D, notes Bauer, which it requires for efficient absorption. While the sun is the primary source of vitamin D, there are food sources as well. Shiitake mushrooms are one rich source, and others include canned sardines and wild salmon (no bones are needed for vitamin D...but include the bones and you'll get a two-in-one bonus for both calcium and vitamin D), shrimp, egg yolks and vitamin D-fortified whole grain cereals or soy milk.

Bauer notes that it is important to remember that eating healthful foods will go a long way toward supporting optimal health—but if you have or suspect you have a medical problem, be sure to see your physician. As the old saying goes, "You are what you eat," so therefore, the healthier you eat, the healthier you'll be.

Whole Grains to The Rescue

Joanne L. Slavin, RD, PhD, food science and nutrition professor at the University of Minnesota in St. Paul. She is author of dozens of medical articles on dietary fiber.

Everyone knows that if you eat ample amounts of fruits and vegetables you can lower cholesterol, promote weight control and help prevent heart attack, stroke, diabetes and some types of cancer. But few people realize that whole grains are just as good as fruits and vegetables—and sometimes even better—at fighting many of these serious illnesses.

Fiber gets most of the credit for the healthful properties of whole grains, but studies have found that the phytochemicals, antioxidants, vitamins and minerals found in whole grains, which contain all parts of the grain, are just as important. The whole grains described below can be found at most health-food stores and many grocery stores...*

AMARANTH

What it's good for: This tiny grain with an earthy, faintly grassy taste may protect against

*For recipes using whole grains, read *Whole Grains Every Day Every Way* (Clarkson Potter) by Lorna Sass or visit the Web site of the Whole Grains Council, *www.wholegrainscouncil.org.*

heart disease and cancer. It is also an excellent source of complete protein—that is, one that contains all eight essential amino acids.

Major effective ingredients: Vitamins E and B. Amaranth is also rich in calcium, phosphorus and iron.

How to add it to your diet: As it cooks, amaranth releases a glutinous starch that adds body to soups and stews.

BROWN RICE

What it's good for: Helps fight eye disease (macular degeneration) and certain cancers, including lung cancer.

Major effective ingredients: Vitamin E and other antioxidants.

How to add it to your diet: Season brown rice as you would white rice, or it can be added to soups, casseroles, stir-fry dishes as well as salads.

CORN

What it's good for: Helps fight heart disease and cancer...and may guard against cataracts.

Major effective ingredients: Of all the grains, whole-grain corn is the richest source of antioxidants.

It's also a good source of insoluble fiber, which cannot be digested but adds bulk to the stool.

How to add it to your diet: Choose whole-grain corn-based cereals, whole-grain cornmeal breads and cornmeal tortillas.

OATS AND BARLEY

What they are good for: Lowering your cholesterol.

Major effective ingredient: Soluble fiber. When soluble fiber is digested, it changes to a gummy consistency that lowers blood cholesterol.

The exact mechanism of this effect is not yet known.

How to add oats to your diet: Choose an oat cereal or oatmeal or you can make oatmeal cookies.

How to add barley to your diet: Use it to thicken soups and make creamy risottos, or cook it with carrots.

RYE

What it's good for: Protects against heart disease and hormone-dependent cancers, such as breast and prostate malignancies.

Major effective ingredient: Rye is a rich source of lignans, a class of phytoestrogens (plant compounds that help protect against the harmful effects of excess estrogen).

How to add it to your diet: Use whole-grain rye bread or whole-grain rye crackers.

WHEAT

What it's good for: It has a laxative effect that aids digestion and also is high in vitamins, minerals and antioxidants.

Major effective ingredient: Insoluble fiber.

How to add it to your diet: Replace white bread with whole-wheat bread...and highly processed cereals with whole-grain cereals.

Helpful: To ensure that a bread product contains whole grain, the label must include the word "whole."

Example: For whole wheat, look for whole-wheat flour or whole-wheat grain. Breads that contain seven, 12 or even 15 grains are not necessarily whole-grain breads.

Get More Legumes

Eating legumes may lower diabetes risk. In a recent finding, women who consumed the most peanuts, soybeans and other legumes had significantly lower risk for type 2 diabetes. Legumes are good sources of magnesium, isoflavones and fiber, and they have a low glycemic index, which may explain why they help lower diabetes risk. Of all legumes, soybeans (though not most processed soy products) appear to be the most beneficial. Women who consumed the most soybeans were 47% less likely to develop diabetes than women who consumed the least.

Raquel Villegas, PhD, assistant professor of medicine, School of Medicine, Vanderbilt University, Nashville, and lead author of a study of 64,227 women, published in *The American Journal of Clinical Nutrition.*

Chamomile Tea May Fight Diabetes

An animal study suggests that chamomile tea can help prevent diabetic complications, such as blindness, nerve damage and kidney failure, by lowering blood glucose levels and reducing levels of enzymes linked to nerve, eye and kidney damage.

Atsushi Kato, MD, department of hospital pharmacy, University of Toyama, Japan, and coauthor of a study published in *Journal of Agricultural and Food Chemistry.*

Black Tea Helps Treat Diabetes

When researchers compared concentrations of *polysaccharides* (a type of carbohydrate) in black, green and oolong teas, the polysaccharides in black tea were the best blood sugar (glucose) inhibitors.

Theory: Polysaccharides in black tea block an enzyme that converts starch into glucose.

If you have diabetes or prediabetes: Consider drinking three cups of black tea daily to better control blood sugar.

Haixia Chen, PhD, associate professor, School of Pharmaceutical Science and Technology, Tianjin University, Tianjin, China.

Coffee and Green Tea Cut Diabetes Risk

In a study of 17,413 adults, those who reported drinking six or more cups of green tea or at least three cups of caffeinated coffee daily were one-third less likely to develop type 2 diabetes than those who drank less than one cup of green tea or coffee a week.

Theory: Caffeine stimulates oxidation (burning) of fat.

Caution: High caffeine intake—more than 500 mg daily—has been linked to arrhythmia (irregular heartbeat). One eight-ounce cup of coffee contains about 100 mg of caffeine… green tea, about 35 mg. Ask your doctor how much caffeine is appropriate for you.

Hiroyasu Iso, MD, PhD, MPH, professor of public health, Osaka University Graduate School of Medicine, Osaka, Japan.

Milk Thistle Improves Diabetes

Mark A. Stengler, NMD, licensed naturopathic medical doctor in private practice, Stengler Center for Integrative Medicine, Encinitas, California…adjunct associate clinical professor at the National College of Natural Medicine, Portland, Oregon…author of many books, including *The Natural Physician's Healing Therapies* and coauthor of *Prescription for Natural Cures* (both from Bottom Line Books)…and author of the *Bottom Line/Natural Healing* newsletter. *www.drstengler.com*

A recent study reported that milk thistle, an herbal supplement, reduced blood sugar levels in people with type 2 diabetes. Along with their regular diabetes medication, 51 men and women (ages 40 to 65) took either 200 mg of *silymarin* (the active ingredient in milk thistle) three times daily before meals or a placebo. After four months, the average fasting blood glucose level (the amount of sugar in the blood eight hours after a person's last meal) fell by 15% in the silymarin group, while rising 13% in the placebo group.

My view: Milk thistle has long been used to treat liver conditions, such as hepatitis. Now it appears to be useful in treating type 2 diabetes, too—perhaps because its antioxidant properties help to control the metabolic abnormalities of diabetes. It is safe for everyone.

Moderate Drinking May Cut Diabetes Risk

In a recent finding, people who consume one or two standard alcoholic drinks per day are about 30% less likely to develop type 2 diabetes than people who don't drink at all. The risk reduction is the same whether a person has one or two drinks.

Caution: Drinking more than three alcoholic beverages a day raises diabetes risk. Ask your doctor if daily alcohol is right for you.

Lando L.J. Koppes, PhD, researcher at VU University Medical Center, EMGO Institute, Amsterdam, the Netherlands, and leader of a meta-study analyzing data from 15 studies involving alcohol use and diabetes risk in nearly 370,000 people, published in *Diabetes Care*.

Indian Herb Fights Diabetes

Mark A. Stengler, NMD, licensed naturopathic medical doctor in private practice, Stengler Center for Integrative Medicine, Encinitas, California…adjunct associate clinical professor at the National College of Natural Medicine, Portland, Oregon…author of many books, including *The Natural Physician's Healing Therapies* and coauthor of *Prescription for Natural Cures* (both from Bottom Line Books)…and author of the *Bottom Line/Natural Healing* newsletter. *www.drstengler.com*

Salacia oblonga is an herb commonly used in traditional Ayurvedic medicine to treat diabetes and obesity. Researchers fed 66 people with type 2 diabetes test meals on three separate occasions. Study participants were given a high-carbohydrate liquid meal or the liquid meal plus *Salacia oblonga* (S. oblonga) at a dosage of either 240 milligrams (mg) or 480 mg.

Result: Compared with the control meal alone, the 240-mg dose of S. oblonga lowered blood sugar by 14%…and the 480-mg dose lowered it by 22%. The amount of insulin, a hormone that regulates blood sugar, produced in response to the meal was reduced by 14% and 19%, respectively (high insulin contributes to inflammation in the body). These reductions were especially impressive given the high-carb meal (carbs raise blood sugar and insulin).

This herb prevents carbohydrates from being broken down in the digestive tract, allowing less glucose into the bloodstream—and resulting in lower blood glucose and insulin levels. Studies have shown it to be safe, and side effects are uncommon. People with mild-to-moderate elevation in glucose levels, as well as those with diabetes, should talk to their doctors about S. oblonga.

Note: Three of the study authors are employed by Abbott Laboratories, which funded the research. However, two other studies with humans also have shown the benefits of S. oblonga.

How to Help Your Diabetic Heart Naturally

Seth J. Baum, MD, medical director of Integrative Heart Care in Boca Raton, Florida, author of *The Total Guide to a Healthy Heart* (Kensington), and fouder of VitalRemedyMD, a scientifically-based nutritional supplement company. *www.vitalremedy.com*

Kenneth Madden, MD, assistant professor of geriatric medicine at the University of British Columbia.

Robb Wolf, co-owner of NorCal Strength and Conditioning, Chico, California and author of *The Paleo Solution: The Original Human Diet* (Victory Belt Publishing).

I f you have type 2 diabetes, you've already had a heart attack—whether you've had one or not!

"The guidelines for physicians from the American Heart Association are to treat a person with diabetes as if that individual has already had a heart attack," says cardiologist Seth J. Baum, MD, medical director of Integrative Heart Care in Boca Raton, Florida, and author of *The Total Guide to a Healthy Heart* (Kensington).

HOW DOES DIABETES HURT YOUR HEART?

As excess sugar careens through the bloodstream, it roughs up the linings of the arteries.

Insulin resistance (the sub-par performance of the hormone that moves glucose out of the bloodstream and into muscle and fat cells) raises blood pressure, damaging arteries.

Diabetes also injures tiny blood vessels called capillaries, which hurts your kidneys and nerves—damage that in turn stresses the heart.

The end result—an up to seven-fold increase in the risk of heart disease and stroke, the *cardiovascular diseases* (CVD) that kill four out of five people with diabetes.

But recent studies show there are several natural ways for people with diabetes to reverse the risk factors that cause heart disease…

RECENT RESEARCH

It's never too late to exercise—and a little goes a long way. Researchers at the University of British Columbia in Vancouver, Canada, studied 36 older people (average age 71) with type 2 diabetes, high blood pressure, and high cholesterol, dividing them into two groups.

One group walked on a treadmill or cycled on a stationary bicycle for 40 minutes, three days a week. The other group didn't.

To find out if the exercise was helping with CVD, the researchers measured the elasticity of the arteries—a fundamental indicator of arterial youth and health, with arterial stiffness increasing the risk of dying from CVD.

Results: After three months, the exercisers had a decrease in arterial stiffness of 15 to 20%.

"Aerobic exercise should be the first-line treatment to reduce arterial stiffness in older adults with type 2 diabetes, even if the patient has advanced cardiovascular risk factors" such as high blood pressure and high cholesterol, conclude the researchers, in *Diabetes Care*.

WHAT TO DO

Kenneth Madden, MD, the study leader, and assistant professor of geriatric medicine at the University of British Columbia, says "You can improve every risk factor for diabetes and heart disease—and you can do it in a very short period of time."

Dr. Madden recommends that older people with diabetes and cardiovascular disease see a doctor for a checkup before starting an exercise program.

Once you get the okay from your physician, he says to purchase and use a heart monitor during exercise, so you're sure that you're exercising at the level used by the participants in his study—60% to 75% of maximum heart rate.

Example: An estimate of your maximum heart rate is 220, minus your age. If you're 60, that would be 220 – 60 = 160. Exercising at between 60% to 75% of your maximum heart rate means maintaining a heart rate of between 96 and 120 beats per minute.

Finally, Dr. Madden advises you exercise the amount proven to improve arterial elasticity—a minimum of three sessions of aerobic exercise a week, of 40 minutes each.

• **Maximize magnesium.** Researchers in Mexico studied 79 people with diabetes and high blood pressure, dividing them into two groups. One group received a daily 450 milligrams (mg) magnesium supplement; one didn't.

Results: After four months, those on magnesium had an average drop of 20 points systolic (the higher number in the blood pressure reading) and 9 points diastolic (the lower number). Those on the placebo had corresponding drops of 5 points and 1 point.

"Magnesium supplementation should be considered as an additional or alternative treatment for high blood pressure in people with diabetes," says Fernando Guerrero-Romero, MD, the study leader.

What to do: "Magnesium acts as a natural vasodilator, relaxing arteries and lowering blood pressure," says Dr. Baum. "People with diabetes should incorporate a magnesium supplement into their regimen."

He suggests a daily supplement of 400 mg, about the level used in the study.

"People with diabetes and high blood pressure should also be encouraged to increase their dietary intake of magnesium, through eating more whole grains, leafy green vegetables, legumes, nuts and fish", says Dr. Guerrero-Romero.

• **Eat like a Neanderthal.** Researchers in Sweden tested two diets in 13 people with type 2 diabetes—the diet recommended by the American Diabetes Association (ADA), a generally healthful diet limiting calories, fat and refined carbohydrates; and a "Paleolithic" diet, consisting of lean meat, fish, fruits, vegetables, root vegetables, eggs and nuts—and no dairy products, refined carbohydrates or highly processed foods, whatsoever.

In terms of lowering risk factors for heart disease, the Paleolithic diet clubbed the ADA diet.

Results: After three months, it had done a better job of decreasing…

• **High LDL "bad" cholesterol,**

• **High blood pressure,**

• **high triglycerides (a blood fat linked to heart disease) and**

• **Too-big waist size** (excess stomach fat is linked to heart disease).

The diet was also more effective at increasing HDL "good" cholesterol.

And it was superior in decreasing *glycated hemoglobin* (A1C), a measure of long-term blood sugar control.

"Foods that were regularly eaten during the Paleolithic, or 'Old Stone Age', may be optimal for prevention and treatment of type 2 diabetes, cardiovascular disease and insulin resistance," concludes Tommy Jönsson, MD, in *Cardiovascular Diabetology.*

What to do: "Eating a Paleolithic Diet is far easier than most people think," says Robb Wolf, co-owner of NorCal Strength and Conditioning in Chico, California and author of *The Paleo Solution: The Original Human Diet* (Victory Belt Publishing).

THE BASIC DIET

Eat more—lean meat, fish, shellfish, fruits, vegetables, eggs and nuts.

Eat less (or eliminate)—grains, dairy products, salt, refined fats and refined sugar.

Resource: You can order pre-packaged Paleolithic snacks and meals at *www.paleo brands.com*.

•**Have a cup of hibiscus tea.** Researchers in Iran studied 53 people with type 2 diabetes, dividing them into two groups. One group drank a cup of hibiscus tea twice a day; the other drank two cups a day of black tea. (The hibiscus tea was made from Hibiscus sabdariffa, which is also known as red sorrel, Jamaican sorrel, Indian sorrel, roselle and Florida cranberry.)

Results: After one month, those drinking hibiscus had…

•**Higher HDL "good" cholesterol,**

•**Lower LDL "bad" cholesterol,**

•**Lower total cholesterol and**

•**Lower blood pressure.**

The black tea group didn't have any significant changes in blood fats or blood pressure.

The findings were in *The Journal of Alternative and Complementary Medicine* and the *Journal of Human Hypertension*.

What to do: Consider drinking a cup or two of hibiscus tea a day, says Hassan Mozaffari-Khosravi, PhD, an assistant professor of nutrition, Shahid Sadoughi University of Medical Sciences, Yazd, Iran and the study leader.

Apple Cider Vinegar

Mark A. Stengler, NMD, licensed naturopathic medical doctor in private practice, Stengler Center for Integrative Medicine, Encinitas, California…adjunct associate clinical professor at the National College of Natural Medicine, Portland, Oregon…author of many books, including *The Natural Physician's Healing Therapies* and coauthor of *Prescription for Natural Cures* (both from Bottom Line Books)…and author of the *Bottom Line/Natural Healing* newsletter. *www.drstengler.com*

Patients often tell me that apple cider vinegar has helped them with a variety of ailments. This intrigued me because, until recently, there was little research to back up these claims.

CURE-ALL?

Apple cider vinegar has been singled out as beneficial for a variety of conditions, including leg cramps, stomach upset, sore throat, sinus problems, high blood pressure, obesity, osteoporosis and arthritis. It also has been used to help rid the body of toxins, improve concentration, slow aging, reduce cholesterol and fight infection.

It is used topically to treat acne, sunburn, shingles and insect bites…as a skin toner…and to prevent dandruff. Many women add it to bathwater to treat vaginitis. Two of its most common uses are for weight loss and arthritis.

THE SCIENTIFIC EVIDENCE

Recent studies have found that consuming apple cider vinegar can improve insulin resistance, a condition in which muscle, fat and liver cells have become resistant to the uptake of the hormone insulin and the blood sugar glucose needed to provide fuel for energy.

This is common among people who have diabetes as well as in some people we consider prediabetic—that is, their blood glucose and insulin levels are approaching the numbers that define diabetes.

People with insulin resistance are more likely to be overweight and have increased cholesterol and triglyceride levels as well as high blood pressure.

A study at the University of Arizona examined the effects of apple cider vinegar on 29 participants (10 had type 2 diabetes, 11 had signs that they could become diabetic and eight were healthy but "insulin sensitive"). All participants fasted and were randomly asked to drink either a vinegar solution (two tablespoons or 20 g of apple cider vinegar, some water and a bit of saccharin for flavor) or a placebo drink. The drinks were followed by a high-carbohydrate meal of one white bagel, butter and orange juice.

Researchers found that postmeal spikes of insulin and glucose in the vinegar group were significantly lower in those who had insulin resistance and slightly lower in those who had diabetes, compared with those in the placebo group. Other research has shown that apple cider vinegar helps control insulin and glucose spikes in healthy people.

HOW IT WORKS

Researchers theorize that the acetic acid in any vinegar, including apple cider vinegar, interferes with the enzymes that digest carbohydrates, so carbs pass through the digestive tract without being absorbed.

Acetic acid also has been shown to affect enzymes that alter glucose metabolism in liver and muscle cells, reducing insulin spikes.

Because high levels of insulin promote inflammation, taking vinegar to maintain better insulin levels will control any inflammatory response in the body. This may explain why vinegar eases arthritis pain.

DOSAGE

People can try apple cider vinegar for weight loss, blood sugar balance and other traditional uses, including arthritis relief.

Dilute one to two tablespoons (some people use as little as two teaspoons to start with) in an equal amount of water, and drink it at the beginning of a meal.

Sometimes it is more convenient to take it in supplement form. A good product is Advanced Apple Cider Vinegar Plus, which is made by Indiana Botanic Gardens (800-644-8327, *www. botanicchoice.com*).

Take one capsule with each meal for a total of three capsules a day. Ninety capsules cost $29.99.

Apple cider vinegar can cause digestive upset in some people. If you have active ulcers, use caution when taking apple cider vinegar.

Banaba—Ancient Herb, Modern Success

From *Bottom Line's Breakthroughs in Drug-Free Healing* by Bill Gottlieb (Bottom Line Books). *www. bottomlinepublications.com*

It's called *banaba* in the Philippines, *banglang* in Cambodia, *bungor* in Malaya and *jalal* in India. For thousands of years, folk healers in these southeast Asian countries have used the many-named plant to lower blood sugar. Scientists are catching on.

BREAKTHROUGH STUDIES

Japanese researchers in the Department of Diabetes and Clinical Nutrition at Kyoto University gave 31 people with diabetes and other blood sugar problems either *corosolic acid* (the active ingredient of banaba) or a placebo. Then they gave them a big dose of dietary sugar, in what's called a glucose tolerance test. An hour later…90 minutes later…and 2 hours later…those taking the banaba had much lower blood sugar levels.

In a similar study* conducted in the United States, 10 people with diabetes were given banaba for 2 weeks—and their high blood sugar dropped by 30%.

Why it works: Corosolic acid stimulates cells to absorb glucose, say the researchers.

Suggested intake: 32 to 48 mg a day of a banaba extract standardized to 1% corosolic acid (CRA), the active ingredient.

*The US study used Glucosol, a soft-gel formulation found in many products, including Glucotrim from NSI, Gluco Trim from NOW Foods and Glucosol/Rx-Blood Sugar from Nature's Plus.

16

Memory Loss Cures

Natural Ways to Power Up Your Brain

You can improve your memory, your energy, your productivity and your general well-being throughout your entire life by developing everyday habits that are very good for your brain...

• **Get exercise that requires quick movements.** Exercise increases blood flow to the brain, ensuring a healthy supply of oxygen and the nutrients on which the brain depends. Insufficient blood flow can lead to poor coordination and difficulty processing complex thoughts.

Exercise also increases the supply of *brain-derived neurotrophic factor* (BDNF), a protein that helps with the creation of new cells.

A recent study of people in their 70s found that those who exercised moderately or vigorously at least once a week were 30% more likely to maintain their cognitive skills than people who exercised less often.

Any type of exercise is good, but the ideal exercise for a healthy brain combines an aerobic workout with complex movements requiring quick reactions.

Examples: Dancing, tennis, table tennis, racquetball and juggling.

• **Eat berries, beans and salmon.** Be sure that your diet includes...

• Fruits as well as vegetables. Antioxidants in fruits and vegetables fight damage from free radicals—unstable molecules that damage cells, contribute to aging and promote inflammation, which is a factor in Alzheimer's disease. Berries are particularly rich in antioxidants.

Daniel G. Amen, MD, distinguished fellow of the American Psychiatric Association and CEO and medical director of Amen Clinics, Inc., headquartered in Newport Beach, California, *www.amenclinics.com*. He is assistant clinical professor of psychiatry and human behavior at University of California, Irvine, School of Medicine, and his work has been the basis of several PBS specials. Dr. Amen is author of many books, including *Change Your Brain, Change Your Body* (Three Rivers).

•Complex carbohydrates—such as cooked dried beans and whole grains. The brain uses sugar as its main energy source. Complex carbohydrates release sugar slowly. In contrast, white bread and other refined starches and sugars cause dramatic spikes and drops in blood sugar, leading to concentration problems and fatigue.

•Cold-water fish. Any lean protein, including chicken and lean pork, helps build neurons. Salmon, cod and other cold-water fish have the added benefit of providing omega-3 fatty acids, which play an important role in maintaining nerve cell membranes. Other sources of these healthy fats are avocados, nuts and olive oil.

•**Boost vitamin D.** Vitamin D is believed to play a role in mood and memory. A recent study published in *Journal of Geriatric Psychiatry* and *Neurology* found a possible association between dementia and low levels of vitamin D.

The best source of vitamin D is sunlight—at least 15 minutes a day without sunscreen. If you spend most of the day indoors or live in a northern latitude, take a supplement with 400 international units (IU) of vitamin D daily.

•**Avoid food additives, such as mono-sodium glutamate, and artificial sweeteners, such as aspartame.** Though studies are inconclusive, anecdotal evidence suggests that these additives may have a hyperstimulating effect, causing confusion and/or mood swings.

•**Limit caffeine and alcohol.** Caffeine and alcohol reduce blood flow to the brain, depriving cells of nutrients and energy. Both can interfere with sleep, which is essential to healthy brain activity.

Both also can be dehydrating—the brain is 80% water, so anything that dehydrates has the potential to cause problems in thinking.

One or two cups of coffee or tea a day are harmless and enhance alertness, but heavy caffeine consumption—more than 500 milligrams (mg) to 600 mg a day, or about four to seven cups of coffee—should be avoided.

Alcohol has additional dangers—it blocks oxygen from reaching cells' energy centers and reduces the effectiveness of neurotransmitters involved in learning and memory. Heavy drinkers—people who consume four or more alcoholic drinks a day—have a higher risk for dementia.

Some people drink wine daily because of evidence that it may be good for the heart. However, there are other ways to help the heart—such as exercise and diet—that don't put the brain at risk. If you are accustomed to having a drink every day, consider cutting back to one or two drinks a week.

•**Avoid airborne toxins.** Fumes from paint, pesticides and other chemicals have been associated with brain damage. If you are exposed to strong fumes—for example, while painting the interior of your house or having your nails done—be sure that the area is well-ventilated.

•**Don't smoke, and avoid being in rooms where others are smoking.** Oddly, smoking can make you feel smarter by stimulating the release of neurotransmitters that improve reaction time, but nicotine constricts blood vessels, reducing blood flow and depriving the brain of nutrients.

•**Don't overdo your electronic interaction.** Computers, mobile devices and other electronic tools can interfere with optimal brain function in several ways. They have an addictive quality, stimulating release of the neurotransmitter *dopamine*, which acts on the brain's pleasure centers. Over time, greater amounts of dopamine are required to get the same pleasurable feeling.

E-mail and text-messaging can interfere with concentration, encouraging a state of mind that is alert to the next distraction, rather than focused on the task at hand. One study at London University found a temporary IQ loss of 10 points in people who constantly checked for messages during the day.

Best: Process e-mail and text messages at set times of day, not as each message comes in. Take frequent breaks that are away from the computer.

•**Protect your skull.** The brain is very soft. The hard skull that covers it has many ridges that can damage the brain during trauma. Yet people are astonishingly careless with this precious organ.

Take precautions to protect yourself from head injury. Stabilize ladders carefully. Use nonslip mats in the bathtub and shower. Keep the floor in your house and the pathways outside it clear of debris that could cause you to trip and fall. If you bicycle or ski, be sure to wear a helmet.

•**Manage stress.** Long-term exposure to high levels of the stress hormone cortisol is associated with a smaller-sized hippocampus—the brain area involved with memory—and with poor performance on memory tests.

Cope with stress by finding daily activities that calm you, such as exercise, meditation, prayer or yoga. During difficult times, focus on what you are grateful for and talk things out with someone who can help you keep an optimistic perspective.

Dr. Gary Small's Secrets For Getting Your Memory Back in Gear

Gary Small, MD, professor of psychiatry and biobehavioral sciences, and director, University of California, Los Angeles, Center on Aging. Dr. Small is one of the world's leading physician/scientists in the fields of memory and longevity. He is author of *The Memory Bible* and *The Longevity Bible* (both from Hyperion). *www.drgarysmall.com.*

Age is the biggest factor for memory loss. We all have memory problems of some sort by age 60, such as momentarily forgetting someone's name, or briefly wondering why we just walked into a room. We can't stop the effects of aging, but we can slow them down.

At the University of California, Los Angeles, Center on Aging, where I am director, we find that using very simple techniques and lifestyle changes—such as reading regularly and playing board games—can have a positive impact on memory retention. Scientific research shows that whenever we push ourselves to solve problems in a new way, we may be strengthening the connections between our brain cells.

MEMORY TECHNIQUES

Some people are so good at memorizing things that they test their talent in competitive matches involving knowledge of trivia or the recall of remarkably large numbers. Scientists have found that those people are no different from the rest of us. There is nothing out of the ordinary in their brain structure nor are there any indications of unusual intelligence. They simply often tap into a memory technique used since antiquity called the Roman Room method.

This method is simple. Visualize yourself walking a familiar route, such as the rooms of your home. Mentally place images of the items to be remembered on specific points on the route. It may be helpful to place items where they may logically be—if you want to remember to buy coffee beans, perhaps they're best mentally placed on the kitchen counter. When you want to recall them, mentally retrace your steps.

Over time, you can add more objects to the rooms. If one day you want to remember to pick up the newspaper, add it next to the coffee beans on the counter. If it's airline tickets, visualize them taped to the fridge door. You can also extend your route or even add other familiar locations for certain kinds of memory tasks.

The Roman Room method is a very useful technique. Orators back in Ancient Rome would remember lengthy speeches this way, imagining each progression of a speech by mentally walking through rooms where they had placed objects to remind themselves of lines. Yet since today we have much more clutter coming at us, I also teach my patients an additional memory technique that I call Look, Snap, Connect...

•**Look reminds us to focus our attention.** The most common explanation for memory loss is that the information never gets into our minds in the first place. Because we are distracted, we don't take in the information or don't allow ourselves to absorb it. Simply reminding ourselves to focus our attention will dramatically boost memory power.

•**Snap stands for creating a mental snapshot or visual image in your mind's eye** of the information to be remembered. For most people, visual images are much easier to remember than other forms of information.

•Connect means we need to link up the visual images from snap in meaningful ways. These associations are key to recalling memories when we want them later. When linking your mental images, create a story that has action and detail.

Example: Say that you want to remember five words on your "to do" list: Mail, gasoline, grandson, sweater, airline. Come up with a story linking them. For instance, I imagine a grandson knitting a sweater on a plane, then mailing it at the airport, when the plane lands to refuel.

Whatever the story ends up being, having detail, action and, for me, humor, all help to imprint the information.

This linking technique works very well with everyday memory tasks, such as grocery lists or errands to run.

When trying to remember faces and names, create an image either linked to the person whose name you need to remember or a distinguishing feature of his/her face. A redhead named Lucy could be remembered by noting that the red hair reminds you of Lucille Ball. You could remember the last name of a woman named Potvin by imagining that she landscaped her yard with pots full of vines.

MENTAL AEROBICS

It's never too late to improve your memory. Recent studies show that even people in the early stages of Alzheimer's can be taught significant face and name retention under the guidance of a professional. For those of us looking to overcome the common forgetfulness in daily life, we can tackle much of that ourselves by doing activities that involve lateral thinking.

Lateral thinking means that we are trying to solve a problem from many angles instead of tackling it head on. Here are some mental aerobic exercises to get you started and, hopefully, suggest further how to invoke lateral thinking in your life.

QUIZ TIME

A lot of memory loss is simply being too busy to absorb what people are saying. These exercises are meant to remind you to slow down, pay attention and consider what is at hand. *In doing so, your memory will improve...*

1. Brush your hair using your nondominant hand. You may find it awkward at first, but over a few days notice how much easier it gets. This and other exercises don't directly help your memory (after all, how often will any of us need to remember to brush with the opposite hand?). What these mental aerobics do is challenge your mind to think differently and examine tasks we often do without thinking, and which lead to our minds getting "flabby."

2. Fill in a grid so that every row, column and two-by-two box contains the numbers 1, 2, 3 and 4.

3. Say "silk" six times. Then answer the following question: What do cows drink?

This exercise will help you be more thoughtful about things, which in turn is conducive to better memory.

4. See how many words you can spell from these letters:

LIGOBATE

No letter may be used twice in any given word, and each word must contain the letter L.

5. How many months have 28 days?

6. All of the vowels have been removed from the following saying. The remaining consonants are in the correct sequence, broken into groups of two to five letters. What is the saying?

STRK WHLTH RNS HT

How well did you do? Regardless, this is just a start to remembering more and living better.

ANSWERS TO QUIZ

Q2: Across row 1: 1, 2, 3, 4 or 1, 2, 4, 3. Row 2: 4, 3, 1, 2. Row 3: 2, 1, 4, 3 or 2, 1, 3, 4. Row 4: 3, 4, 2, 1.

Q3: Cows drink water. If you said "milk," you need to focus your attention.

Q4: agile, ail, aale, bagel, bail, bale, blog, boil, el, Gail, gale, gel, glib, glob, globe, goal, goalie, lab, lag, lea, leg, lib, lie, lob, lobe, log, loge, oblige.

Q5: All of them. (If you say only one month has 28 days, it's an example of not paying attention to the matter at hand—all months have 28 days, after all.)

Q6: Strike while the iron is hot.

Antioxidant Improves Memory

In a study of 6,000 men, half took pills containing 50 mg daily of the antioxidant beta-carotene (roughly the amount in four carrots), and the others took a placebo.

Result: Those who took beta-carotene for at least 15 years scored higher on memory tests than those who took a placebo.

Theory: Beta-carotene protects against oxidative stress, which can lead to brain aging.

If you're concerned about memory loss: Ask your doctor about taking 50 mg daily of a beta-carotene supplement.

Francine Grodstein, ScD, associate professor of medicine, department of epidemiology, Brigham and Women's Hospital, Boston.

Vitamin B-12 May Prevent Brain Shrinkage Among Seniors

Recent study: Individuals ages 61 to 87 who initially had no cognitive problems were followed for five years.

Finding: Participants among the one-third who had the lowest blood levels of vitamin B-12 were six times more likely to lose brain volume, as measured by MRI scans, than were those among the one-third with the highest

B-12 levels. Loss of brain volume is associated with memory loss and other cognitive problems.

What to do: After age 55, it may be a good idea to take B-12 supplements to avoid risk of deficiency of the vitamin.

A. David Smith, MD, founding director, Oxford Project to Investigate Memory and Ageing, University of Oxford, Britain.

Green Tea Boosts Brain Power

In a recent Japanese study of cognitive function in people age 70 or older, participants who drank two or more cups of green tea daily had a 54% lower prevalence of cognitive decline—measured via memory, attention and language-use tests—than those who drank three cups or less weekly. Theory: Antioxidants in green tea may reduce the buildup of a type of plaque in the brain that is responsible for memory loss in Alzheimer's disease. Self-defense: Drink two or more cups of green tea daily to help promote brain health.

Shinichi Kuriyama, MD, PhD, associate professor of epidemiology, Tohoku University Graduate School of Medicine, Sendai, Japan.

Green, Leafy Vegetables Protect Memory

Recent finding: People who eat about three servings of vegetables a day have a 40% slower rate of cognitive decline than people who eat less than one serving a day. All vegetables provide protection, but green, leafy ones, including spinach, provide the most protection.

Surprising: Fruits don't help slow memory loss, but researchers are not yet sure why.

Theory: Vitamin E is believed to prevent cognitive decline. Vegetables contain high amounts of it and are typically eaten with added fats, such as salad dressing, which increase vitamin E absorption.

Bottom line: Eat at least three servings of green, leafy vegetables every day.

Martha Clare Morris, ScD, associate professor, department of internal medicine, Rush University Medical Center, Chicago, and leader of a study of 3,718 people, age 65 and older, published in *Neurology*.

Memory Busters

Mark A. Stengler, NMD, licensed naturopathic medical doctor in private practice, Stengler Center for Integrative Medicine, Encinitas, California...adjunct associate clinical professor at the National College of Natural Medicine, Portland, Oregon...author of many books, including *The Natural Physician's Healing Therapies* and coauthor of *Prescription for Natural Cures* (both from Bottom Line Books)...and author of the *Bottom Line/Natural Healing* newsletter. *www.drstengler.com*

A number of environmental and health factors can contribute to short- and long-term memory loss. *Among the most common...*

•**Prescription drugs can adversely affect memory.** If you are taking any medications, ask your doctor whether memory loss is a known side effect.

•**Low thyroid function also can cause poor memory and concentration.** With a simple blood test, your doctor can check thyroid levels. If they are low (hypothyroidism), he/she can prescribe medication.

•**Toxic metals, such as lead, mercury and aluminum, can lead to brain degeneration.** A holistic doctor can test your urine levels of these metals and recommend treatment, such as chelation therapy, if necessary.

Strengthen Your Brain, Naturally—What You Can Do to Stay Sharp and Healthy

Dharma Singh Khalsa, MD, one of the world's leading experts in integrative or complementary medicine, Alzheimer's disease and memory loss. Dr. Khalsa is an associate fellow of the University of Pennsylvania Medical School, and has formulated a holistic medicine program for the prevention and treatment of Alzheimer's disease and memory loss (The Brain Longevity Program). He is author of numerous books including *The Better Memory Kit* (Hay House) and *Brain Longevity* (Grand Central) and is president and medical director of the Alzheimer's Research and Prevention Foundation (*www.alzheimersprevention.org*). Visit his Web site at *www.drdharma.com*.

Recent headlines have trumpeted the exponential growth in the number of people with Alzheimer's disease—according to one report we read, someone in this country develops the disease every 72 seconds. It is estimated that within a few decades, that rate will more than double, with Alzheimer's striking a new victim every 33 seconds. Researchers are working to isolate the causes and develop effective treatments... but more important is finding ways to prevent the disease—and certainly those who already have it would benefit from avoiding or minimizing side effects caused by treatments.

Keeping memory sharp with brain teasers and other mental activities won't stave off Alzheimer's disease altogether (if only it were so simple) but, we recently learned, it actually can help decrease the intensity and persistence of symptoms and help maintain functionality.

Wondering whether there were particular foods we should eat, supplements we could take or exercises to do to fortify memory, we called Dharma Singh Khalsa, MD, a leading expert in integrative medicine, Alzheimer's disease and memory loss. An Associate Fellow of the University of Pennsylvania Medical School and the medical director of the Alzheimer's Research and Prevention Foundation, Dr. Khalsa has created a program for avoidance and treatment of Alzheimer's disease and memory loss, called the Brain Longevity Program. Understanding that age-related memory loss (normal forgetfulness that occurs with advancing years) and full-out Alzheimer's exist on a continuum, it's important for all people to work to keep their memory skills sharp and strong. "Just like your muscles, the brain gets weak as we age—but it doesn't have to be that way," he said.

INVESTING IN THE MEMORY BANK

As opposed to dementia, Dr. Khalsa believes that mild cognitive impairment is something of a "disease of lifestyle." He said that some intriguing new research is focused on a concept called cognitive reserve, which he likened to a savings account for your brain in that its capacity can be built up over time. "By building up your cognitive reserve through healthy diet and mental and physical exercise, you will not only have better brainpower now, you'll have better ability to resist challenges to the brain later in life," he said.

The three basic strategies Dr. Khalsa recommends to accomplish this aren't exactly new—but they bear repeating…

• **Eat well and take supplements.** Research shows that people eating plenty of vegetables each day (around three or four servings or more) seem to have a slower rate of cognitive decline. Interestingly studies suggest that fruits are not as protective as vegetables in this regard—Dr. Khalsa speculates that since vegetables are so loaded with natural anti-inflammatories, they reduce inflammation, which is known to figure in cognitive impairment and Alzheimer's. Basic supplements, including a multivitamin, and B vitamins (including folic acid), vitamin C and vitamin E, are also helpful.

• **Manage stress.** Stress causes the release of cortisol into the bloodstream, which in chronic and excessive amounts can cause cell death in the brain's memory center, Dr. Khalsa told me. He said that meditation and other relaxation techniques are excellent ways to reduce damagingly high levels of stress hormones.

• **Exercise.** Can you walk and talk at the same time? According to Dr. Khalsa, "for optimal impact on the brain, both physical and mental exercise need to happen—preferably at the same time." For instance, he suggests taking a walk—but instead of daydreaming, sing a song or talk aloud, mindfully. "Say, 'I'm walking up a hill, the tree over there is green with a brown trunk, and there goes Dave driving his new Ford,'" he suggests. "This kind of mental involvement literally lights up the brain." You could also just walk with a friend, discussing current events or anything else you find interesting.

Though we hear an awful lot about mental exercise nowadays, Dr. Khalsa explained that it does not have to be sophisticated or difficult to be effective. "You don't need to do Sudoku puzzles or crosswords to benefit. Going to a museum with friends and talking about what you've just seen is great. Many recent studies have shown that merely being mentally engaged, no matter what the topic, actually increases blood flow, leading to the building of new brain cells along with enhanced cognitive function. You're literally increasing your cognitive reserve!"

FORTIFY YOUR MEMORY WITH SUPPLEMENTS

Finally, Dr. Khalsa closely follows research on dietary supplements and cognitive function, and told me he believes that certain ones are quite helpful. *He likes…*

• **Phosphatidylserine.** This naturally occurring molecule, known as a *phospholipid*, is important for the integrity and maintenance of the brain cell membranes. Because it is depleted by stress hormones like cortisol, it is often deficient in people with chronic stress.

• **Fish oil.** The anti-inflammatory properties of fish oil are very helpful in reducing inflammation in the brain which many scientists believe increases vulnerability to Alzheimer's. Interestingly, the National Institutes of Health has begun to study omega-3 oils and their effect on cognitive function, though no conclusive findings are yet available.

• **Ginkgo biloba.** "A recent study showed that patients taking gingko performed no differently on standard memory tests than a matched group of patients taking *donepezil* (Aricept), a common medication for Alzheimer's," said Dr. Khalsa.

• **Turmeric/curcumin.** This spice is a significant anti-inflammatory and therefore thought to be helpful to all brain function. Take in supplement form or simply use the spice when cooking as much as possible.

• **L-Alpha Glycerylphosphorylcholine (Alpha-GPC).** Naturally present in all cells, this molecule can also be taken as a supplement. It is a pro-phospholipid, used by the body to build cell membranes. Numerous studies have shown that, used as a supplement, it benefits attention, mental focus, recall and other higher mental functions.

While there is no proven way to prevent Alzheimer's, employing some or all of these strategies may help you stay sharper and more functional longer. Who among us wouldn't benefit from doing that?

The Truth About Brain Food...and Supplements that Keep Your Memory Intact

Mark A. Stengler, NMD, licensed naturopathic medical doctor in private practice, Stengler Center for Integrative Medicine, Encinitas, California...adjunct associate clinical professor at the National College of Natural Medicine, Portland, Oregon...author of many books, including *The Natural Physician's Healing Therapies* and coauthor of *Prescription for Natural Cures* (both from Bottom Line Books)...and author of the *Bottom Line/Natural Healing* newsletter. *www.drstengler.com*

Everyone forgets something from time to time. Some people have trouble remembering names. Others can't keep track of their car keys. Whether we suffer everyday absentmindedness or moments of real memory loss, all of us are concerned about keeping our brain power intact.

In recent years, a great deal of research has focused on the most severe kinds of memory loss—senile dementia and Alzheimer's disease. In the US, these closely related conditions affect up to 10% of people over age 65 and nearly half of those over age 85.

Many studies have identified ways to lower risk of these age-related problems. Popular methods include stress-reduction strategies, such as daily exercise, positive mental imagery, biofeedback and close personal relationships, to prevent spikes in the memory-draining stress hormone cortisol..."brain workouts," including crossword puzzles, word games and challenging card games...and eight to nine hours of sleep each night. Good nutrition—and the right kind of supplementation—also can help protect our brains and safeguard our memories at any age. The sooner you get started with a brain-protecting regimen, the more you'll benefit.

For optimal brain function, your diet should be well-balanced with carbohydrates (40%), protein (30%) and fats (30%). You can accomplish this by eating meals that include whole grains, fruits and vegetables (for complex carbohydrates)...fish, poultry, lean meats, legumes, nuts and seeds (for protein)...and fish oil, olive oil, avocados, almonds, walnuts and ground flaxseed (for fats). Steer clear of dairy products and packaged and processed foods, such as cookies, white bread and pasta, which are packed with simple carbohydrates that wreak havoc on glucose levels, contributing to diabetes, stroke/vascular disease and dementia.

THE VALUE OF FISH

Fish provides *docosahexaenoic acid* (DHA) and *eicosapentaenoic acid* (EPA), the most plentiful fatty acids in the brain. DHA, an omega-3 fatty acid, is found in abundance in cold-water fish such as mackerel, sardines, salmon and herring. You also can get it from fish-oil supplements, egg yolks, DHA-enriched eggs and some algae supplements, such as Neuromins, a product that is available at most health-food stores. Foods such as walnuts... leafy, green vegetables...and supplements including flaxseed and hemp oil contain *alpha-linolenic acid*, an omega-3 fatty acid that can be converted by the body into DHA and EPA.

How essential is DHA to memory? It has been known for some years that people have a higher risk of Alzheimer's if they have low blood levels of DHA. A study in *Archives of*

Neurology revealed that people who ate fish one to three times a month had a 40% lower risk of Alzheimer's than those who never ate fish. Those who consumed fish once a week or more had a 60% lower risk. Fish may be baked, broiled or grilled.

It also makes sense to take a fish-oil supplement daily. I suggest 1,000 mg of combined DHA and EPA. Good brands are Nordic Naturals (800-662-2544, *www.nordicnaturals.com*) and Carlson Laboratories (888-234-5656, *www. carlsonlabs.com*), both available at health-food stores.

Caution: Fish oil can thin blood, so check with your doctor before using it if you take blood-thinning medications such as *warfarin* (Coumadin).

GLA IS ESSENTIAL

Omega-6s make up another class of essential fatty acids that are necessary for good brain function. Omega-6 is found in vegetable oils, including safflower, sunflower and corn oils. Most American diets contain too much of these oils due to consumption of packaged and fried foods. However, the most important omega-6 fatty acid is linoleic acid, which is converted in the body to *gamma-linolenic acid* (GLA). This essential fatty acid plays a big role in the formation of healthy brain-cell membranes, the part of the cell that stores information. Taking borage oil or evening primrose oil are healthful ways to increase GLA intake—hempseed and hempseed oil also are good sources. Another way to get GLA in the diet is by consuming flaxseed (with water to prevent constipation) or flaxseed oil.

COUNT ON CHOLINE

Just as a car needs spark plugs, an active brain needs quick-firing neurotransmitters. As the name implies, a neurotransmitter sends a signal that jumps from one brain cell to another. Substances that act as neurotransmitters—the most important of which is a brain chemical called *acetylcholine*—are vital components of the brain's communication system.

There's one hitch. In order for your body to manufacture enough acetylcholine, you need to get a closely related nutrient called *choline*. The best source of choline is *phosphatidylcholine* (PC), which occurs naturally in fish, egg

yolks, legumes, nuts, meat and vegetables. It also is found in breast milk. To help prevent memory problems, you can boost your PC intake by taking a 1,500-mg to 2,000-mg PC supplement daily. (Doses of more than 3,000 mg can cause digestive upset, including diarrhea, nausea and stomachache.)

PC is only part of the neurotransmitter equation. To turn PC into brain-friendly choline, you also need to get healthy doses of vitamin C and certain B vitamins. You can get plenty of these vitamins in your diet by eating red, yellow and green peppers, citrus fruits and cantaloupe for vitamin C and sweet potatoes, tuna and avocados for B vitamins. Also, I recommend taking a balanced daily multivitamin/mineral supplement.

Deficiencies of folic acid and other key B vitamins have been associated with an increased risk of Alzheimer's disease. These nutrients help to lower levels of homocysteine, a harmful by-product of protein metabolism that is increased in people who are genetically susceptible. That's why it is important to have your blood levels of homocysteine, folic acid and B-12 tested by your doctor to see if you need additional supplementation of folic acid and/or B-12.

THE EUROPEAN CURE

For years, European doctors have recommended a supplement called *L-alpha-glycerylphosphorylcholine* (GPC) to promote mental acuity (the ability to respond quickly and appropriately to mental challenges). GPC actually is used by the brain more effectively than PC to form acetylcholine—but it costs twice as much and is less widely available in the US. A good GPC supplement by Source Naturals is sold in some health-food stores under the brand name Alpha GPC (to find a retailer, go to *www.sourcenaturals.com*). Take two 300-mg capsules twice daily for the first four weeks, then two 300-mg capsules once daily as a maintenance dosage. Side effects are rare, but take GPC with a meal if it seems to interfere with your digestion.

PS: BE SURE TO GET MORE

Phosphatidylserine (PS) is a fat that the brain needs to preserve the key brain chemicals serotonin and dopamine. It also has been shown to reduce levels of the stress hormone cortisol. PS is found in fish, soy and leafy, green vegetables. As we age, PS levels in the body start to decline, so most people need to take a supplement once they're past age 50.

A normal daily diet has about 70 mg of PS. You need about four times that much if you have memory problems. Nearly anyone can benefit from a 300-mg daily supplement of PS. You're likely to notice improvements in mental alertness after four to eight weeks. A small percentage of people have digestive upset, such as bloating and diarrhea, but you can reduce the dosage if this is a problem. PS is available at health-food stores and pharmacies. Make sure you buy a product that lists "*phosphatidylserine*" on the label. (Some supplements contain "phosphorylated serine," a nutrient complex that doesn't provide the same benefits as PS.) A high-quality PS supplement is made by Jarrow Formulas called PS 100 (to find a retailer, call 800-726-0886 or go to *www.jarrow.com*).

HELP FROM ALC

When taken as a supplement, a nutrient known as *acetyl-L-carnitine* (ALC) has been shown to improve cognitive function and memory in older adults. Researchers also have found that ALC slows the progression of early-stage Alzheimer's disease. By improving communication between the two main hemispheres of the brain, ALC helps enhance the interplay of creative and cognitive brain activity.

For people with mild memory problems, I recommend taking 500 mg of ALC daily on an empty stomach. For those with more severe problems such as dementia, I suggest the same dose three times daily. Cut back if you have digestive upset. Most health-food stores carry a reliable Acetyl-L-Carnitine formula produced by Now Foods (888-669-3663, *www. nowcatalog.com*).

ADD ANTIOXIDANTS

In all likelihood, Alzheimer's disease and other types of dementia are related to excessive damage by free radicals (normal by-products of metabolism that can destroy cells, organs and tissues). Free radicals irreversibly injure our cells and contribute to accelerated aging, but studies have shown that this damage can be warded off by getting enough antioxidant nutrients to help guard our brain-cell membranes.

There's ample evidence that a daily dose of 2,000 international units (IU) of the powerful antioxidant vitamin E can slow the decline of cognitive function in people who have moderate to severe Alzheimer's disease. There have been controversial vitamin E studies that seemed to show a link to worsening chronic disease. However, I don't have much confidence in those studies because they were performed on unhealthy people. When it comes to Alzheimer's, results of vitamin E studies have been quite good.

All fresh fruits, vegetables and other plant foods provide multiple naturally occurring antioxidants. Juices are an especially concentrated source of antioxidants. In fact, a study of nearly 2,000 Japanese Americans found that those who reported drinking fruit and vegetable juices at least three times a week had a 75% lower risk of developing dementia than those who drank juices less than once a week. The most nutritious fruit juices include cranberry, pomegranate, apple and blueberry. I also like mixed vegetable juices containing any combination of spinach, celery, lettuce, parsley, watercress, carrot and tomato.

If there is a strong family history of dementia or you have beginning signs of it, take up to 2,000 IU of vitamin E daily. Green tea also is an excellent source of antioxidants. I recommend drinking two to four cups of green tea daily and eight ounces of fresh juice.

GINKGO—THE BRAIN PLEASER

Ginkgo biloba is an herbal remedy that has been shown to improve memory and cognitive processing by promoting blood flow to the brain. I recommend a 24% *flavoglycoside* extract. Start with a dose of 120 mg to 240 mg daily, and increase to 360 mg daily over a four-week period. Some people begin to see results in four to eight weeks. If you're already taking a blood-thinning medication such as aspirin or warfarin, consult your doctor before taking ginkgo.

Exercise Rejuvenates Your Brain

John J. Ratey, MD, associate clinical professor of psychiatry at Harvard University, Boston, *www.johnratey. com*. He is author of *Spark: The Revolutionary New Science of Exercise and the Brain* (Little, Brown).

Staying active is a key to a vigorous, healthy body as we grow older. But exercise is just as important for mental health. Walking, biking or swimming helps keep your memory and reasoning ability sharp and your mood bright while it strengthens your heart, arteries—and muscles.

Like every organ, the brain requires a steady supply of oxygen and nutrients to maintain vigor. A sound mind needs a healthy body, and a healthy body needs exercise. Heart disease, diabetes and other illnesses can have a devastating effect on the brain, and exercise cuts the risk that you'll get them.

In recent years, scientists have learned a lot about what happens inside the brain when we think, form memories and learn new things... and what determines whether our moods are up or down. They've found solid evidence that exercise—even a modest amount—can have a positive effect on biological events within the brain cells themselves.

YOUR GROWING BRAIN

Not that long ago, everyone believed that after maturity, no new brain cells were born—your supply of several hundred billion declined gradually but inexorably with advancing years. Now we know that like other parts of the body, the brain constantly renews itself, generating blank cells that, under the right circumstances, can turn into thinking, functioning tissue.

At work are naturally occurring chemicals called growth factors. They are produced by the brain itself and by blood vessels and muscles. They act like fertilizer on a flowerbed, stimulating new brain cells to grow and new blood vessels to support them.

Brain cells are constantly dying, succumbing to a mix of toxins and overstimulation called molecular stress. With age, the balance shifts—growth factors decline, along with the cells' ability to withstand stress. After age 40, we lose 5% of our brain cells per decade, on average. The network of capillaries feeding the brain withers.

Nothing can stop the effects aging has on the brain, but exercise can dramatically slow it down. Animal experiments have shown that exercise boosts growth factors and the number of new brain cells produced. Other studies found that when animals were active, their brains worked better—exercise increased their ability to learn new things.

KEEP YOUR MENTAL EDGE

There's evidence that just a modest amount of exercise can have a powerful anti-aging effect on the human brain.

A study at the University of Illinois divided 59 sedentary people aged 60 to 79 into groups that did one hour of stretching three times a week, or had sessions of aerobic exercise (activity that gets your heart rate up and keeps it up) for the same amount of time. After six months, magnetic resonance imaging scans found that brain volume had increased in the aerobic exercisers—the frontal and temporal lobes, which are involved in thinking, decision-making and learning, had actually grown bigger.

These results "suggest a strong biological basis for the role of aerobic fitness in maintaining and enhancing central nervous system health and cognitive functioning in older adults," the researchers concluded.

Looking at actual performance on tests of mental ability, scientists have found that a regular aerobic program can apparently push back age-linked decline in brain function by seven to 10 years.

Exercise also protects against the worst brain-killers of all—diseases such as Alzheimer's and Parkinson's. Besides generally strengthening brain circuits, it helps keep arteries healthy and blood sugar under control, cutting the risk for dementia.

IMPROVE YOUR MOOD

Low moods can strike no matter how old you are, but the stresses and losses that frequently

217

come with age—illness, ending a career, retiring to an unfamiliar place—make depression a special danger. Biology also plays a role. The neurotransmitters that carry messages between brain cells dwindle as the years pass. Low levels of these chemicals—*serotonin, dopamine* and *norepinephrine*—are associated with depression, and antidepressants appear to work by raising them.

Exercise stimulates neurotransmitter production and can battle depression as effectively as medication. In a Duke University study, an aerobic program proved as potent as the antidepressant Zoloft in relieving depressive symptoms.

You needn't be clinically depressed to benefit. The neurotransmitter boost of exercise raises mood, increases motivation and can charge up anyone's zest for life.

AEROBICS AND BEYOND

Your goal should be to get some physical activity nearly every day. But, especially if you've been sedentary, get there slowly. The good news is that noticeable benefits start at a much lower level—with as little as an hour a week of exercise.

Important: Check with your doctor before starting any exercise program.

Aerobic exercise appears to be the most beneficial to the brain. Swimming, biking and jogging are good, but for most, brisk walking is perfect.

How hard you should work out: To calculate your "maximum heart rate," subtract your age from 220. Your goal is walking (or doing another activity) strenuously enough to get your pulse up to 60% to 65% of maximum. Vary your workouts from 30 minutes to an hour, four days a week.

After you've become used to exercising, pick up the pace—go for 70% to 75% of maximum for 20 to 30 minutes, then back down to 60% to 65%—during two of the four workouts.

Keep it interesting. Many find that walking is more stimulating out of doors. Team up with a friend so that you can motivate each other and add the pleasures and benefits of social interaction. Variety spices up routine. If you

have access to a health club or gym, try the treadmill, exercise bike or elliptical trainer.

Strength training: The brain benefits of strength training (with weights or resistance machines) haven't been researched as thoroughly as those of aerobics, but it's well worth the effort anyway—to counter the muscle deterioration that otherwise comes with age. Try to include strength training in your workouts twice a week. If you're new to it, have a personal trainer design a program for you.

FEED YOUR BRAIN

The same diet recommended for general good health maintains the strong circulation and metabolic balance that protect your brain—lots of fruits, vegetables and whole grains, abundant fiber and limited fats. *Particularly beneficial…*

• **Berries, broccoli, spinach, beets, garlic and onions, green tea and red wine.** These contain antioxidants and other nutrients that activate cellular repair.

• **Omega-3 fatty acids**—the kind found in fish—have been linked to a host of health benefits and seem especially vital for brain vigor. The Framingham Heart Study found that a diet with the omega-3s found in three servings of fish weekly cut dementia risk in half. If you don't like fish, take a daily supplement that includes EPA and DHA, the key fatty acids.

Brain-Boosting Nutrients Women Need

JoAnn E. Manson, MD, DrPH, professor of medicine and women's health at Harvard Medical School and chair of the division of preventive medicine at Brigham and Women's Hospital, both in Boston. She is one of the lead investigators for two highly influential studies on women's health—the Harvard Nurses' Health Study and the Women's Health Initiative. Dr. Manson is author, with Shari Bassuk, ScD, of *Hot Flashes, Hormones & Your Health* (McGraw-Hill).

Certain foods may help ward off subtle age-related cognitive decline or even full-blown dementia, recent research suggests. *Nutrients linked to a clear mind and sharp memory…*

• **Folate.** In studies of people age 70 and older, those with low blood levels of folate had about twice the risk for Alzheimer's disease as those with normal levels.

Folate reduces homocysteine, a dietary by-product linked to inflammation, blood clots and small blood vessel damage.

Best: Each day, eat two or more servings of folate-rich dark green leafy or cruciferous vegetables, such as spinach, romaine lettuce, broccoli and brussels sprouts.

As insurance, consider taking a daily multi-vitamin that provides 400 micrograms of folic acid (synthetic folate). Many doctors recommend up to 1,000 mcg.

• **Marine omega-3 fatty acids.** Fish provide the omega-3s *eicosapentaenoic acid* (EPA) and *docosahexaenoic acid* (DHA). Studies show that people who eat fish five or more times weekly are 30% less likely to suffer a stroke than those who rarely eat fish.

Frequent fish consumption also is associated with fewer "silent" (symptomless) brain lesions, as seen on imaging tests…and may reduce Alzheimer's risk.

Fish oil also improves function of nerve cell membranes and boosts the production of brain chemicals that allow nerve cells to communicate.

Wise: Eat salmon, tuna, herring, sardines or mackerel at least twice weekly…or take daily fish oil supplements with 400 mg to 1,000 mg of combined EPA and DHA.

Important: Watch consumption of large fish such as tuna and salmon. These may have higher levels of mercury and PCBs.

• **Flavonoids.** Oxidation, a chemical reaction that can damage blood vessels, may be a key contributor to brain aging.

Antioxidant plant pigments called flavonoids may counteract this—particularly the *anthocyanins* in deep-colored fruits such as berries, cherries and Concord grapes. In animal studies, berry extracts reversed age-related declines in spatial learning and memory as measured by how quickly the animals learned to navigate a maze.

Goal: Eat berries or deep-colored fruit at least two to three times per week.

• **Coffee.** In a study of 7,017 people age 65 and older, women who drank at least three cups of caffeinated coffee or six cups of caffeinated tea per day experienced less decline in memory over four years than those who drank one cup or less.

However, caffeine can trigger digestive upset, insomnia and migraine.

Advised: Have no more than four eight-ounce cups of coffee daily.

The alcohol question: Moderate alcohol intake is linked with less cognitive decline—though this may simply reflect that people who already have cognitive problems are less likely to imbibe.

Recommended: Do not start drinking alcohol specifically to prevent cognitive decline. If you already drink, limit consumption to no more than one alcoholic beverage daily.

Cinnamon Can Help You Stay Focused

It speeds the rate at which the brain processes visual cues. Try chewing cinnamon-flavored gum before doing something that will require quick responses, such as playing tennis.

To make cinnamon a regular part of your diet, sprinkle one teaspoon of it on oatmeal or cereal at breakfast.

Daniel G. Amen, MD, Amen Clinics, Newport Beach, California, writing in *AARP*, 601 E St. NW, Washington, DC 20049.

The Most Powerful Brain-Building Nutrients And Herbs

Mao Shing Ni ("Dr. Mao"), PhD, DOM (doctor of oriental medicine), LAc (licensed acupuncturist), chancellor and cofounder of Yo San University in Los Angeles, and codirector of Tao of Wellness, a clinic in Santa Monica, California. He is author of numerous books, including *Second Spring: Dr. Mao's Hundreds of Natural Secrets for Women to Revitalize and Regenerate at Any Age* (Free Press). *www.taoofwellness.com*

You open your cupboard but then can't recall what you wanted…you're introducing two friends and suddenly draw a blank on one's name.

Such instances of "brain fog" are common, but they are not an inevitable part of aging. Many people remain remarkably sharp all their lives—and the right nutritional strategies can help you be one of them.

Cognitive declines can result from hormonal changes and reductions in neurotransmitters, chemicals that help brain cells communicate with each other. Increasing your intake of certain nutrients helps balance hormones and protect neurotransmitters. *You can get these nutrients from…*

•**Foods.** Eating brain-boosting foods is an ideal way to get needed nutrients.

Reasons: The body is designed to absorb nutrients from foods rather than from isolated or manufactured chemicals (such as in supplements)…and foods contain complementary components that enhance nutrient absorption.

•**Herbs.** The healthful aromatic oils are most active when herbs are fresh, but dried herbs also will do.

•**Supplements.** These are an option if you cannot find the foods that provide certain nutrients, or if you need specific nutrients in quantities beyond what you typically get from food. Unless otherwise noted, the following supplements generally are safe, have few side effects and may be used indefinitely. All are sold at health-food stores.

Important: Ask your doctor before supplementing, especially if you have a health con-

dition…use medication…or are pregnant or breast-feeding. To reduce the risk for interactions, do not take supplements within 30 minutes of medication…and limit your use of these supplements to any four of the following.

NUTRIENTS YOUR MIND NEEDS

For the foods recommended below, one serving equals four ounces of meat, poultry, fish, or soy products…eight ounces of milk… two ounces of nuts…two eggs (with yolks)… one-half cup of vegetables or fruit…and one cup of leafy greens.

•**Choline.** The neurotransmitter *acetylcholine* plays a key role in learning and memory. Choline is a precursor to acetylcholine that is produced in the liver. Production of choline declines with age, as does the body's ability to efficiently use the choline that remains.

Brain boost: Eat one or more servings daily of choline-rich broccoli, cauliflower, eggs, kidney beans, navy beans, liver, milk or even peanuts.

Supplement option: 1,200 milligrams (mg) daily.

•**DMAE (2-dimethylaminoethanol).** The body uses fatty acids to create brain cells and neurotransmitters. DMAE, a chemical in fatty acids, helps produce acetylcholine.

Brain boost: Have two servings weekly of DMAE-rich anchovies or sardines. If fresh fish is not available, have canned water-packed sardines or anchovies and rinse before eating to reduce salt.

Supplement option: 500 mg twice daily after meals.

•**L-carnitine.** Mitochondria are the engines of cells. The amino acid L-carnitine transports fatty acids to mitochondria for use as fuel and provides nutrients to brain cells.

Brain boost: Have two weekly servings of lamb or poultry, which are rich in L-carnitine.

Supplement option: 500 mg to 1,000 mg before breakfast and again in the afternoon.

•**Vitamin B-12.** This is key to red blood cell formation and nerve cell health. The body's ability to absorb vitamin B-12 diminishes with age—about 10% to 15% of people over age 60 are deficient in it.

Brain boost: Have two servings weekly of beef or lamb…halibut, salmon, sardines or sea bass…eggs…or vitamin B-12–enriched soybean products (miso, tempeh).

Supplement option: 500 micrograms (mcg) to 1,000 mcg daily.

THE MOST HELPFUL HERBS

An easy way to get the benefits of mind-sharpening herbs is to brew them into a tisane, or herbal infusion—more commonly called herbal tea.

To brew: Pour eight ounces of very hot water over one heaping tablespoon of fresh herbs or one teaspoon of dried herbs. Steep for five minutes, strain and drink.

Convenient: To reduce the number of cups needed to meet the daily recommendations below, brew two or more herbs together.

• **Chinese club moss.** This herb contains the chemical *huperzine A*, which helps conserve acetylcholine.

Brain boost: Drink one to two cups of Chinese club moss tea each day.

Supplement option: 50 mcg of huperzine A twice daily (discontinue if supplements cause gastric upset or hyperactivity).

• **Ginkgo biloba.** This herb increases blood flow to the brain's tiny capillaries and combats DNA damage caused by free radicals.

Caution: Do not use ginkgo if you take blood-thinning medication, such as *warfarin* (Coumadin).

Brain boost: Drink three cups of ginkgo tea daily.

Supplement option: 120 mg daily.

• **Kitchen herbs.** Oregano, peppermint, rosemary and sage have oils that may increase blood flow in the brain and/or support neurotransmitters, promoting alertness.

Brain boost: Use any or all of these herbs to brew a cup of tea for a pick-me-up in the morning and again in the afternoon.

Also: Use herbs liberally when cooking.

Supplement option: About 150 mg each of any or all of these herbs daily, alone or in combination.

• **Mugwort (wormwood).** This herb improves circulation, aiding delivery of nutrients to brain cells.

Brain boost: Twice a week, drink one cup of mugwort tea…add a half-dozen leaves of fresh mugwort to salad…or sauté leaves with garlic or onions.

Supplement option: 300 mg daily.

Caution: Avoid mugwort during pregnancy —it may stimulate uterine contractions.

Don't forget: Green Tea

Strictly speaking, an herb is a flowering plant whose stem above ground does not become woody. In that sense, the leaf of the Camellia sinensis shrub—otherwise known as tea—is not an herb. Yet green tea (which is less oxidized than black) is so helpful that it must be listed among the top brain boosters.

Along with antioxidant polyphenols, green tea provides the amino acid *theanine*, which stimulates calming alpha brain waves and improves concentration. Green tea also has been linked to a reduced risk for Alzheimer's disease.

To brew: Pour eight ounces of very hot water over one teaspoon of loose, fresh green tea leaves (or a tea bag if fresh is not available) and steep for three to five minutes. You needn't strain the tea. As you empty your cup, you can add more warm water to the remaining leaves—as long as the water turns green, the tea still contains polyphenols.

Brain boost: Drink three cups of green tea (caffeinated or decaffeinated) daily.

Supplement option: 350 mg of green tea extract daily.

221

Breakthrough Jellyfish Treatment Makes You Smarter Within Days

Mark A. Stengler, NMD, licensed naturopathic medical doctor in private practice, Stengler Center for Integrative Medicine, Encinitas, California...adjunct associate clinical professor at the National College of Natural Medicine, Portland, Oregon...author of many books, including *The Natural Physician's Healing Therapies* and coauthor of *Prescription for Natural Cures* (both from Bottom Line Books)...and author of the *Bottom Line/Natural Healing* newsletter. *www.drstengler.com*

Scientists have found that a naturally occurring protein in one of the planet's oldest sea creatures—the jellyfish—might hold the key to improved memory and comprehension. The substance, *apoaequorin* (a-poh-ee-kwawr-in), found in the Aequorea victoria jellyfish species, has a unique way of working in the brain that is different from other natural memory enhancers. Many of my patients already are benefiting from it. Apoaequorin not only seems to reverse some of the effects of aging on the brain but also might help alleviate the effects of serious neurodegenerative diseases such as Alzheimer's disease, Parkinson's disease and ALS (Lou Gehrig's disease).

THE JELLYFISH CONNECTION

Scientists first discovered apoaequorin and its companion molecule, green fluorescent protein (GFP), in the Aequorea jellyfish, found off the west coast of North America, in the 1960s. The natural glow of GFP enables researchers to observe microscopic processes within cells that were previously invisible, such as how proteins are transported or how viruses enter cell membranes. Apoaequorin, which binds to calcium and becomes luminescent once it does, has been used since the 1990s in a similar way to track the activity of calcium in the body's cells. In 2008, three researchers who played key roles in developing these chemical markers were awarded the Nobel Prize in Chemistry. Apoaequorin's value as a memory-boosting supplement also depends on its calcium-binding properties but in a different way.

In the brain, calcium plays an important role in the chemical process that allows nerve cells to recharge before firing. It has to be present in just the right amounts. If too much calcium builds up inside a nerve cell, it interferes with the nerve-firing process and causes the cell to die. One of the key roles of calcium-binding proteins is to prevent the toxic buildup of calcium by removing excess calcium from the nerve cells. In the normal course of aging, beginning at around age 40, the number of calcium-binding proteins in our brain cells starts to decline, resulting in the gradual buildup of toxic calcium inside these cells. This leads to impaired cellular function and eventually brain damage as the toxic calcium kills off brain cells. The symptoms of this age-related deterioration start slowly but then accelerate as we get older. Because apoaequorin is similar to the naturally occurring calcium-binding proteins in the brain, the theory is that by taking daily supplements, you can replace the calcium-binding proteins that are lost through the aging process—allowing your brain cells to function optimally again while also preserving them from the long-term toxic effects of excess calcium.

A "EUREKA" MOMENT

The jellyfish protein went from "scientific" discovery to "supplement for the brain" because of the efforts of Mark Underwood, cofounder of the biotech firm Quincy Bioscience, the company that makes Prevagen (888-814-0814, *www.prevagen.com*), the only commercially available form of apoaequorin. Underwood's "eureka" moment came when he was reading about an Australian swimmer who developed multiple sclerosis–like symptoms after being stung by a jellyfish. Underwood wondered what protected the jellyfish from its own venom...and whether apoaequorin's calcium-binding abilities could have neuroprotective properties.

His company conducted a number of studies in conjunction with the University of Wisconsin–Milwaukee that found that apoaequorin did seem to have a powerful protective effect on brain cells. In one study, 56 people ranging in age from 20 to 78 showed significant improvements in memory after taking 10 mg of

Prevagen daily for 30 days. More than half the group reported gains in general memory and information retention...two-thirds did better at word recall...and 84% showed improvement in their ability to remember driving directions. Most of my patients and others report that taking Prevagen helps them feel mentally sharper, improves their memory and gives them more mental energy. Some even say that their mood is enhanced and that they sleep more soundly.

HOW TO USE IT

Prevagen is best taken in the morning (because cognitive function is more important during the day than at night), with or without food. I recommend it for anyone over age 40 who wants to improve memory and focus. While 10 mg daily is the recommended starting dose, apoaequorin also is safe at higher doses. I recommend that my own patients who have suffered a noticeable decline in cognitive function start out with 10 mg daily for four weeks. If they don't notice an improvement in memory and focus, they can increase to 20 mg daily. Most of my patients benefit from taking 10 mg or 20 mg daily. Research has shown that Prevagen is safe to take with other memory-enhancing supplements, such as omega-3 fish oils, or medications, such as *donepezil* (Aricept). People with allergies to fish or shellfish can use it because jellyfish is neither. The manufacturer of Prevagen is exploring apoaequorin's potential as a medical treatment for conditions such as Alzheimer's disease and Parkinson's disease. It's a good choice for those who need safe, natural memory support.

Rejuvenate Your Mind With Acupressure

Applying pressure to certain areas of the body opens energy pathways by increasing blood circulation.

How to do it: Gently place your thumb and middle finger of one hand on your forehead above each eyebrow, making a bridge. Meanwhile, with your other hand, reach around to the back of your head and apply firm pressure just below the base of the skull on either side of the spine. Use light pressure in front and firm pressure in back for three minutes to refresh your mind.

More information: *www.acupressure.com.*

Michael Reed Gach, PhD, founder, Acupressure Institute, Berkeley, California.

Exercise Your Brain by Using the Internet

Brain scans show that searching the Internet for information may take more brain power than reading and can be a great mental exercise. Activities that keep the mind engaged may help preserve brain health and cognitive ability with advancing age. Traditionally, these activities include reading, games and puzzles, but now Internet use may be among the best.

Gary Small, MD, professor of psychiatry and biobehavioral sciences, Jane and Terry Semel Institute for Neuroscience and Human Behavior, University of California, Los Angeles, and coauthor of *iBrain: Surviving the Technological Alteration of the Modern Mind* (Harper).

17

Fatigue Cures

Feeling Tired All the Time? How to Get Your Energy Back

All too often, conventional medical practitioners mistakenly assume that fatigue is a red flag for depression—especially if the patient complains only of a vague yet constant tiredness. But fatigue typically results from a complex constellation of physical and emotional issues. That's why treatment should be based on an assessment of the patient's physical health and lifestyle. *Before you see your doctor with a complaint of fatigue, spend two weeks completing this checklist...*

•**Monitor your breathing.** Shallow breathing, which is commonly caused by anxiety, fear and poor posture, reduces your oxygen supply and, as a result, often leads to fatigue. To monitor your breathing, pay attention to your breathing patterns throughout the day.

In addition, practice deep breathing for five minutes several times a day.

What to do: As you inhale deeply, allow your lungs to fully expand (your belly should rise if you're doing this correctly), then exhale to a count of five. If you have trouble taking a deep breath, or if you cough or wheeze during deep breathing, discuss this with your physician. These reactions could be signs of disease or injury.

•**Note your caffeine intake.** If you need more than 20 ounces of a caffeinated beverage to get through the day, ask your doctor to order blood tests to check your levels of blood sugar (glucose) and the adrenal hormones *dehydroepiandrosterone* (DHEA) and cortisol as well as your thyroid function (TSH, T3 and T4). Each may be linked to fatigue.

Jamison Starbuck, ND, naturopathic physician in family practice, Missoula, Montana. She is past president of the American Association of Naturopathic Physicians and a contributing editor to *The Alternative Advisor: The Complete Guide to Natural Therapies and Alternative Treatments* (Time-Life).

224

•**Do a media and computer "fast" for the weekend.** Keeping up with media reports is enough of a job. When you add in the deluge of information most of us receive via the computer, it can be a tremendous energy drain. A time-out will tell you if you need to cut back on these activities.

•**Keep a diet diary for one week.** Each day, write down what you eat and drink and a description of your energy levels in the morning, afternoon and evening. Look for patterns. Skipping meals and consuming foods that can trigger allergic reactions, such as wheat, dairy, eggs or soy, are common causes of fatigue. Not drinking enough plain water, which is important to overall physiological function, also may be a culprit.

My advice: Drink one-half ounce of plain water for every pound of body weight—for example, if you weigh 150 pounds, drink 75 ounces of water daily.

•**Assess your emotional state.** Fatigue can result from painful emotions, such as grief or anger, but some doctors are too quick to prescribe an antidepressant. It's often better to first try keeping a journal, talking to a close friend and/or meeting with a counselor.

Of course, fatigue can be caused by medical conditions, such as diabetes, anemia and even cancer. That's why you should see a doctor if your fatigue does not improve after trying these steps. If you experience extreme fatigue accompanied by pain, fever or disorientation, see your doctor immediately.

Energy Drinks

Energy drinks can raise blood pressure, cause faster heartbeat and lead to irritability, nervousness and nausea. Many contain as much caffeine as one or two cups of coffee and as much sugar as one can of soda. Some also include herbal stimulants. An occasional energy drink may be a useful stimulant—but regularly drinking several energy drinks a day can damage health.

Also: It is dangerous to consume energy drinks with alcohol or when you are dehydrated. The caffeine and other ingredients can increase risk for fainting and even a heart attack.

Mayo Clinic Health Letter, 200 First St. SW, Rochester, Minnesota 55905. *https://healthletter.mayoclinic.com*

10 Quick Energy Boosters

Jon Gordon, best-selling author of *Energy Addict: 101 Physical, Mental and Spiritual Ways to Energize Your Life* (Perigee) and *The 10-Minute Energy Solution* (Putnam). His performance-energy consulting firm The Jon Gordon Companies, is based in Ponte Vedra Beach, Florida. Clients include the PGA Tour, the Jacksonville Jaguars football team, General Electric, State Farm Insurance and Wachovia Bank. *www.jongordon.com.*

Three-quarters of the people I meet complain of tiredness during the day. This epidemic of exhaustion is brought about by mental and physical stress, including too much caffeine and sugar as well as too little sleep and exercise.

Here are easy ways to feel more alert and energetic...

•**Stop hitting the snooze button on your alarm clock in the morning.** Your brain goes through periods of light and heavy sleep. Falling back to sleep for just five more minutes can cut short a new sleep cycle, leaving you groggier when you do arise.

Better: Set your clock for when you really have to get up. Open your shades right away, and get as much light as possible—bright light wakes you up and invigorates you. Raise your heartbeat for at least five minutes in the morning by running in place or doing sit-ups, push-ups or jumping jacks.

•**Eat a power breakfast.** It will energize you as you start the day.

My favorite power breakfast: Mix low-fat plain yogurt and one-half cup of old-fashioned raw oatmeal when you first get up. The yogurt will soften the oats while you shower and dress. Add a few chopped walnuts, one-half cup of pineapple or one-quarter cup of blueberries.

• **Sit up straight.** Bad posture can decrease your oxygen intake, and slouching exhausts your neck, shoulders and upper-back muscles.

Correct posture for sitting: Your back should be aligned against the back of the chair, so that you can work without leaning forward. Your knees should be a bit higher than your hips. Keep both feet flat on the floor and your arms flexed at a 75- to 90-degree angle.

• **Replace coffee with green tea.** The rich taste of coffee and the mental alertness it imparts make coffee drinking a tough habit to break. But coffee raises stress hormones, and just a few cups a day creates an energy roller coaster that increases overall fatigue. I have found that people who have the most success giving up coffee switch to green tea. It contains one-third the amount of caffeine (20 mg to 25 mg per six-ounce cup), so you get an energy boost without feeling irritable or experiencing a slump later on.

Bonus: Green tea is loaded with disease-fighting antioxidants.

If you have no intention of giving up your daily coffee, at least try cutting back to half regular/half decaffeinated.

• **Consume protein with meals.** It helps your body absorb sugar at a slower rate, so your energy levels don't fluctuate so much during the day.

Examples: Fish, eggs, hummus, skinless poultry breast, lean red meat.

• **Go for a 10-minute walk after lunch.** It raises your metabolism and prevents you from falling into the familiar, post-meal "coma."

If it's inconvenient to go outside, try chair squats.

How to do that: With a chair behind you, stand with your feet positioned shoulder-width apart. Keep your back straight and your chin up. Squat down, and push out your rear as if you were going to sit in the chair behind you. Just as your rear touches the chair, return to your starting position. Repeat five to 30 times—or until you feel your muscles have had enough.

• **Take a short nap, no more than 25 minutes.** Longer than that and you move into a deeper phase of sleep, which, if interrupted, can leave you groggier than before your nap. The optimal time to take a nap is eight hours after you wake up.

• **Eat an energy snack, such as a banana or a handful of walnuts or almonds.** Avoid commercial energy drinks and energy bars— they often work by introducing caffeine and/ or sugar into your system.

Helpful: I do recommend a caffeine-free, multivitamin energy powder that I use myself each day—Fatigued to Fantastic! from Enzymatic Therapy, available at health-food stores.

Cost: About $30 or more for a month's supply.

• **Try peppermint.** It boosts mood and motivation. Have a cup of peppermint tea, or dab peppermint oil (available at health-food stores) on your wrists.

• **Breathe.** We tend to hold our breath when we work intensely or are under stress—and this contributes to fatigue.

To practice energy-boosting breathing: Stand up straight with your arms at your sides. Inhale for two seconds as you raise your arms slowly over your head with your palms open. Continue lifting your arms until they are directly over your head with fingertips touching. Exhale for three seconds as you bring your arms down. Repeat 10 times.

12 Powerful Ways to Boost Your Energy

Kenneth H. Cooper, MD, MPH, pioneer in the fields of preventive medicine and physical fitness. He is founder and chairman of Cooper Aerobics Center, Dallas, and author of 19 books, including *Regaining the Power of Youth at Any Age* (Nelson). His books have sold more than 30 million copies worldwide. *www.cooperaerobics.com*

As we get older, we often complain that we're "running on empty." I call this age-related loss of energy youth drain—but we don't have to be victims of it. At 74 years of age, I work 60 hours a week, travel widely and still feel energetic.

Youth drain can be caused by a variety of factors, including obesity...chronic medical problems, such as anemia, diabetes, emphysema or an under-active thyroid gland...depression...cancer...use of sedatives and sleeping pills...menopause...poor diet...inadequate sleep...and stress. These factors batter us over the years and drain our vitality—unless we learn how to respond to them and counter their effects.

Here, 12 revitalizing strategies for us all...

1. Eat less but more frequently. Consuming large meals (more than 1,000 calories per sitting) makes you feel sluggish, as your body's resources are directed toward digesting all that food.

Instead, graze on small meals and snacks that contain a mix of carbohydrates and protein (but little fat) to provide a steady stream of fuel.

Examples: Yogurt smoothie (one cup light nonfat yogurt, one-half cup fat-free milk, one-half peach, blended)...peanut butter and banana sandwich (one slice wholewheat bread, one-half tablespoon peanut butter, one-half banana, sliced)...fruity cottage cheese (one-half cup 1% low-fat cottage cheese, one-half cup pineapple chunks in juice, drained).

2. Exercise. The health benefits of exercise are well-known, but many people tell me they continue to exercise year after year because it makes them feel good and gives them more energy. I recommend at least 30 minutes of sustained activity five times a week. The best activities for most people tend to be brisk walking, jogging, swimming, cycling and aerobic dance.

3. Take a multivitamin. In a clinical trial, people who took multivitamins daily not only had improved immunity against infectious diseases but also had more energy. In general, it is best to get vitamins from food, but many people don't get the necessary amounts, so I suggest taking a multivitamin/mineral supplement daily.

4. Prevent dehydration. Consuming an inadequate amount of fluids, particularly if it's hot outside or you're exercising, can deplete energy and lead to weakness, dizziness and headaches. Drink at least six to eight eight-ounce glasses of water daily. On days that you exert yourself to the point of perspiring, increase that to up to 13 glasses.

5. Watch what you drink. Drink no more than one caffeinated beverage a day. Coffee, tea, cola and other caffeinated beverages provide a temporary energy boost, but energy levels plunge when the stimulant's effects wear off.

Caffeinated drinks also have a diuretic effect, which may cause you to lose fluids because you urinate more frequently.

Also, limit alcohol consumption to no more than one drink a day—any more can lead to fatigue.

6. Practice the "relaxation response." This technique, developed by Herbert Benson, MD, of Harvard University, has been shown to reduce blood pressure and heart rate. For me, doing this for just five minutes in the middle of the day is rejuvenating.

How to do it: Sit in a chair in a quiet room. Close your eyes. Starting with your feet, begin to relax your muscles, progressively moving up the body to the top of the head. While you do this, breathe in slowly and naturally through your nose and out through your mouth. As you exhale, silently repeat a focus word or phrase that has meaning for you, such as "peace." Push away distracting thoughts by focusing on your breathing and the word you have chosen to repeat.

For more information, read *The Relaxation Response* by Herbert Benson, MD (Harper-Torch).

7. Take naps. Surveys show that most Americans don't get as much sleep as they need (most of us require seven to eight hours a night). Daily naps of 15 to 20 minutes are energizing—and longer naps can help you catch up if you are sleep-deprived. I sleep only five to six hours a night, so I often take a two-hour nap on Saturdays.

8. Don't immerse yourself in bad news. The glut of negative information coming our way from TV, radio, newspapers, the Internet, etc. can hurt the psyche, causing stress and fatigue. Reduce the amount of time you spend watching, listening to or reading the news, and focus on things that bring you joy.

9. Be social. Studies show that isolation can lead to depression and early death. We gain energy by being with others (both humans and animals). Make time for family, friends and pets.

10. Explore your creativity. Boredom leads to a lack of motivation and energy. Finding a creative outlet that absorbs you is invigorating. Developing your creativity also teaches you new skills...challenges your brain...and leads to the release of endorphins, feel-good brain chemicals. Take up a new hobby...learn a musical instrument...take on an unusual project at work.

Added benefit: Mentally stimulating activities such as the ones mentioned above, can lower your risk of Alzheimer's disease.

11. Laugh. Laughter appears to release endorphins just as creative pursuits do. By improving your outlook, you'll feel more energetic and ready to tackle life.

Helpful: Watch funny movies...read cartoons...share humorous stories and jokes with friends.

12. Think young. To a large extent, your mindset dictates how much energy you have as you age. If you expect the worst, you're likely to feel tired and unwell. If you expect to stay vital, you'll fight off disease that can sap energy and well-being—and you'll add years to your life.

Boost Your Energy In Eight Minutes Or Less

Evangeline R. Lausier, MD, director of clinical services at Duke Integrative Medicine and assistant clinical professor of medicine at Duke University School of Medicine, both in Durham, North Carolina.

When you feel drowsy or droop with fatigue, every task you undertake seems monumental—and even fun activities you normally enjoy feel like work.

Helpful: Take a double-pronged approach to invigoration—including on-the-spot techniques for an immediate energy burst...plus simple strategies that take just minutes to do, yet give you long-lasting stamina day after day.

For An Instant Energy Surge...

•**Wake up your nose—and the rest of you will follow.** Aromatherapy stimulates the brain's olfactory center and heightens awareness of your surroundings. Dab a drop of therapeutic-grade rosemary essential oil (sold at health-food stores) on the pulse points behind both ears, as you would perfume...or dampen a cloth with cool water, sprinkle it with four drops of therapeutic-grade lemon essential oil, then place it on your forehead or the back of your neck for five minutes. Do not dab full-strength essential oil directly under your nose—it could be too strong.

To Refuel Energy Reserves...

•**Eat a stamina-boosting breakfast—one cup of fortified, whole-grain cereal.** Whole grains are complex carbohydrates that enter the bloodstream slowly, providing sustained energy by keeping blood sugar levels stable. Avoid starting your day with simple carbohydrates, such as white toast or a doughnut, which cause blood sugar and energy levels to spike and then plummet by mid-morning.

Also: With your cereal, have one-half cup of low-fat milk or fortified soy milk. Its calcium and vitamin D nourish your bones...its protein is used to build and repair muscle and other tissues.

● **For snacks, go nuts.** A handful of almonds, cashews, walnuts or other type of nut provides a sustained energy boost, thanks to blood sugar–stabilizing complex carbohydrates and tissue-building protein.

More benefits: Though relatively high in calories at about 160 per ounce, nuts tend not to cause energy-depleting weight gain because they promote long-lasting satiety and stave off hunger. Nuts also are rich in unsaturated fats that promote cardiovascular health.

18

Insomnia Cures

New and Natural Sleep Aids

Oh for a sweet sleep—and, goodness, how Americans are clamoring to get one. Naturopathic physician Chris D. Meletis, ND says that if this is a new situation, first consider what may be causing it. Is there something in your life that has increased stress—perhaps conflicts at work or a problem with your child—anything, in fact, causing anxiety that might interfere with sleep? Maybe the problem is something less apparent, for instance, your sleep environment. A mattress that has become uncomfortable or a pillow that is too hard or soft can be just enough of an irritant to intrude on good sleep. Is the bedroom dark enough and the temperature just right for you? Also consider—have you started any new medications (or changed dosages) that might impact the quality of your sleep?

Dr. Meletis also reminds people that food and drink can impact sleep. Caffeine, of course, is often a culprit. Some people must avoid having caffeine after 2:00 pm, but supersensitive types should stay away from caffeine completely. Only by eliminating or vastly reducing it for a few weeks will you know if you are in that group. Remember, too, that caffeine lurks in chocolate, colas and tea as well as coffee. As to food, Dr. Meletis recommends having the last meal of the day provide a balance of protein and complex carbs—vegetables (except tomatoes and peppers)...whole grains and the like. This will fill you enough that hunger won't wake you up. Avoid spicy, fried and fatty foods and mint, all of which may increase acid reflux, and don't eat or drink liquids for two or three hours before bed to avoid middle-of-the-night treks to the bathroom. The ban includes alcohol, which also interferes with the quality of sleep.

Chris D. Meletis, ND, executive director and officer of Academic Affairs for the Institute of Healthy Aging, Beaverton, Oregon.

Anyone who is taking sleeping pills may need to be careful when weaning off of them, he says.

The reason: You can become dependent on the drug and need time to recover. Under supervision of the prescriber, gradually decrease dosage until you are off the medication completely. This process often takes several weeks. Dr. Meletis says that drinking green tea (during the day since it also has caffeine) will help in this process because it has *L-theanine*, an amino acid that potentially helps induce relaxation. He adds that B-complex vitamins also combat stress and, as a bonus, often make dreams more vivid. (Although necessary to take at least twice daily, unduly high B vitamin supplementations can contribute to sleeplessness because they can be energizing.) Certain herbs are also calming and can help produce a more restful sleep, including valerian, Passion Flower and chamomile tea.

Dr. Meletis says there are also herbal formulas that some people find helpful for occasional sleeplessness.

He likes Herbal Sleep by Vitamin Research Products (*www.vrp.com*) that contains the following…

- **L-theanine (150 mg)**
- **Hops (133 mg)**—Humulus lupulus extract, (strobiles)
- **Lemon Balm (133 mg)**—(Melissa officinalis extract, leaf)
- **Valerian (100 mg)**—(Valeriana officinalis extract, root with 0.8% valerianic acid)
- **Passion Flower (133 mg)**—(Passiflora incarnata, arial)

Consult a knowledgeable physician before you take any of the herbs or supplements above, as all botanicals can have side effects or interact with other pharmaceuticals or other supplements.

OTHER IDEAS

Some nights, though, you may need other ways to quiet a mind that continues to churn. Dr. Meletis suggests keeping a note pad and pen next to your bed so that you can jot down a few words that capture the worry or great idea so that you can relax knowing you have a reminder for the morning. He also suggests the following self-healing techniques, based in part on existing sleep-inducing methods. Studies show a stressful experience during the day can inhibit sleep at night and so it is important to combat one with relaxation techniques right away.

Try this for a brief mid-day meditation: Sitting up, close your eyes and observe your breathing without changing the way you breathe in any way. How much time do you spend breathing in and how much time breathing out? Pay attention to where the breath goes inside of you and what parts of you don't participate in the breath process. Again, don't change the way you breathe, merely observe it until you feel completely relaxed.

For soothing yourself into sleep, try these techniques, both of which you should do slowly, gently and in bed…

- **On your back, rest your palms on either side of your belly.** As you breathe in, notice how your fingers go along for the ride as your belly gently swells on breathing in and recedes as you exhale. After many breaths, begin to gently, minimally lift one set of fingers, such as your thumbs, then switch to index fingers, just slightly so that ultimately the tips are barely off your skin as you finish breathing in. Allow them to return to the belly as you exhale and your belly recedes. The idea is not to breathe bigger or differently in any way, which is enough to induce stress. Instead simply observe what you do and repeat as necessary.

- **On your back, rest your arms at your sides and bend your elbows so that one forearm is now perpendicular to the bed with your hands in a soft-fist position.** Keeping your forearm upright, gently bend your wrist so that the palm faces the bed. Do this slowly enough that you can feel that pull of gravity on your hand. (Your forearm position does not change.) You will see that your fist gradually and naturally unfolds as you do this. Gently, slowly, return your hand to its original position where it will return to a soft fist, again, naturally. Repeat as necessary.

Better Insomnia Relief

In a study of 46 people with chronic insomnia, one group was trained in *cognitive-behavioral therapy* (CBT) techniques, including relaxation practices and stimulus (noise, light) control. Two other groups took either the sleeping pill *zopiclone* (Imovane) or a placebo every night.

Result: After six weeks, time spent awake dropped 52% in the CBT group compared with 4% in the zopiclone group and 16% in those taking a placebo.

Theory: CBT helps patients identify and change negative thoughts, which can be an underlying cause of insomnia.

Børge Sivertsen, PhD, researcher and psychologist, department of clinical psychology, University of Bergen, Norway.

Healing Herb for Insomnia

Kathy Abascal, RH, registered herbalist who practices in Vashon, Washington. A member of the American Herbalists Guild, she is coauthor of *Clinical Botanical Medicine* (Mary Ann Liebert).

Until recently, if you peeked inside the medicine cabinet of a typical American household, you were likely to find such items as aspirin for headaches...an anti-inflammatory ointment for sore muscles and joints...an antihistamine for colds—and perhaps even a prescription sedative for sleep problems and/or an antidepressant.

Latest development: With the recent economic downturn and rising drug costs, many Americans are turning to medicinal alternatives. Recently, nationwide sales of herbal supplements totaled $4.8 billion, up more than 4% from the previous year. Perhaps due to the recession, Americans now appear to be trying many of the same herb-based products that

have been used for generations in other parts of the world as the front-line treatments for many common conditions.

How herbs can help you: Compared with many medications widely used in the US, herbal therapies tend to have fewer side effects, are generally just as effective—if not more so—and are often less expensive.*

An herb to have on hand in your home...

VALERIAN FOR INSOMNIA

Compounds in valerian act on brain receptors to induce drowsiness and relaxation.

How to use: Take one-half teaspoon of valerian tincture, diluted in water according to the instructions on the label, one hour before bedtime and one-half teaspoon at bedtime, as needed. In small doses—about one-quarter to one-half of the insomnia dose—valerian also can help reduce mild anxiety. Most people avoid valerian tea due to its unpleasant odor.

*If you have a chronic condition and/or take prescription medication, consult your doctor before taking herbs.

Insomnia Remedy

Certain aromas have a calming effect that can help bring on sleep.

Helpful: Make a sachet to place under your pillow. You'll find most of the items you need at natural-food stores.

In a bowl, toss together two tablespoons of corncob chips (sold as bedding at pet shops) and four drops each of lavender essential oil and lemon essential oil...cover and let stand overnight. Uncover and stir in one-half cup of dried hops...and one-quarter cup each of dried lavender buds and lemon verbena leaves. Place mixture inside a small fabric drawstring sack (about six inches square). Refill the sack with a fresh batch of herbal stuffing every two to three weeks or when the aromas start to fade.

Dorie Byers, RN, master gardener and herbalist, Bargersville, Indiana, and author of *Natural Beauty Basics: Create Your Own Cosmetics and Body Care Products* (Vital Health).

The Hidden Risks of Sleep Problems

Lawrence J. Epstein, MD, instructor in medicine at Harvard Medical School in Boston, medical director of Sleep HealthCenters, based in Brighton, Massachusetts and author of *The Harvard Medical School Guide to a Good Night's Sleep* (McGraw-Hill).

Most people assume that lack of sleep is more of an annoyance than a legitimate threat to their health. But that's a mistake. Lack of sleep—even if it's only occasional—is directly linked to poor health. If ignored, sleep problems can increase your risk for diabetes and heart disease.

About two out of every three Americans ages 55 to 84 have insomnia, but it is one of the most underdiagnosed health problems in the US. Even when insomnia is diagnosed, many doctors recommend a one-size-fits-all treatment approach (often including long-term use of sleep medication) that does not correct the underlying problem.

Everyone should have a comfortable mattress...keep the bedroom cool (about 68°F to 72°F)...and dim or turn out the lights (production of the sleep hormone melatonin can be inhibited in the presence of light). Keep TVs and computers out of the bedroom—both can be stimulating, rather than relaxing. But these basic steps may not be enough.

To treat specific sleep problems...

IF YOU WAKE UP TOO EARLY IN THE MORNING

Early risers often have *advanced sleep phase syndrome* (ASPS), which is seen most commonly in older adults. With this condition, a person's internal body clock that regulates the sleep-wake cycle (circadian rhythm) is not functioning properly. ASPS sufferers sleep best from 8 pm to 4 am.

My solutions: To be able to reset your circadian rhythm, try a light box (a device that uses lightbulbs to simulate natural light). Light boxes don't require a doctor's prescription and are available for $100 to $500 online or from retailers, such as Costco. Most people use a light box for 30 minutes to an hour daily at sundown. (Those with ASPS may need long-term light therapy.) If you have cataracts or glaucoma or a mood disorder (such as bipolar disorder), consult your doctor before trying light therapy. Patients with retinopathy (a disorder of the retina) should avoid light therapy.

Also helpful: To help regulate your internal clock so that you can go to bed (and get up) later, take a 3-mg to 5-mg melatonin supplement each day. A sleep specialist can advise you on when to use light therapy and melatonin for ASPS.*

IF YOU CAN'T STAY ASLEEP

Everyone wakes up several times a night, but most people fall back to sleep within seconds, so they don't remember waking up.

Trouble staying asleep is often related to sleep apnea, a breathing disorder that causes the sufferer to awaken repeatedly during the night and gasp for air. Another common problem among those who can't stay asleep is *periodic limb movement disorder* (PLMD), a neurological condition that causes frequent involuntary kicking or jerking movements during sleep. (Restless legs syndrome, which is similar to PLMD, causes an uncontrollable urge to move the legs and also can occur at night.)

My solutions: If you are unable to improve your sleep throughout the night by following the strategies already described, consult a sleep specialist to determine whether you have sleep apnea or PLMD.

Sleep apnea patients usually get relief by losing weight, if necessary...elevating the head of the bed to reduce snoring...using an oral device that positions the jaw so that the tongue cannot block the throat during sleep...or wearing a face mask that delivers oxygen to keep their airways open. PLMD is usually treated with medication.

IF YOU CAN'T GET TO SLEEP

Most people take about 20 minutes to fall asleep, but this varies with the individual. If your mind is racing due to stress (from marital strife or financial worries, for example) or if you've adopted bad habits (such as drinking

*To find a sleep center near you, consult the American Academy of Sleep Medicine (630-737-9700), *www.sleepcenters.org.*

caffeine late in the day), you may end up tossing and turning.

My solutions: Limit yourself to one cup of caffeinated coffee or tea daily, and do not consume any caffeine-containing beverage or food (such as chocolate) after 2 pm. If you take a caffeine-containing drug, such as Excedrin or some cold remedies, ask your doctor if it can be taken earlier in the day.

Helpful: If something is bothering you, write it down and tell yourself that you will deal with it tomorrow—this way, you can stop worrying so you can get to sleep.

Also helpful: When you go to bed, turn the clock face away from you so you don't watch the minutes pass. If you can't sleep after 20 to 30 minutes, get up and do something relaxing, such as meditating, until you begin to feel drowsy.

IF YOU CAN'T GET UP
IN THE MORNING

If you can't drag your head off the pillow, sleep apnea or a *delayed sleep phase* (DSP) disorder might be to blame. DSP disorder makes it hard to fall asleep early, so you stay up late at night and then struggle to get out of bed in the morning.

My solutions: To treat DSP disorder, progressively stay up for three hours later nightly for one week until you reach your desired bedtime. By staying up even later than is usual for you, you'll eventually shift your circadian rhythm. Once you find your ideal bedtime, stick to it. Also consider trying light-box therapy each morning upon arising. Light helps advance your body clock so that your bedtime should come earlier. Taking 3 mg to 5 mg of melatonin one hour before bedtime should also make you sleepy at an earlier hour.

IF YOU CAN'T STAY AWAKE
DURING THE DAY

If you're getting ample rest—most people need seven and one-half to eight hours a night—and still are tired, you may have narcolepsy. This neurological disorder occurs when the brain sends out sleep-inducing signals at inappropriate times, causing you to fall asleep and even temporarily lose muscle function.

Sleep apnea or periodic limb movements also can leave people feeling exhausted.

My solutions: Figure out how much sleep you need by sleeping as long as you can nightly (perhaps while on vacation) for one to two weeks. At the end of that period, you should be sleeping the number of hours you need. Give yourself that much sleep time nightly. If you remain sluggish, ask your doctor about tests for sleep apnea, PLMD or narcolepsy, which is treated with stimulants, such as *modafinil* (Provigil), that promote wakefulness.

Can't Sleep? Surprising Causes of Insomnia

Andrew L. Rubman, ND, medical director, Southbury Clinic for Traditional Medicines, Southbury, Connecticut. *www.southburyclinic.com*

Every night, millions of Americans have trouble falling asleep or staying asleep. Quite often this is caused by stress, anxiety, caffeine or overstimulation before bed. But there is another common cause that few people even know to consider—a nutritional deficiency of one kind or another. If you have such a deficiency, once it is identified you can easily correct it—and start enjoying peaceful slumber once again.

This is a far superior approach to prescription sleeping pills, which not only fail to address the underlying reason for sleeplessness but often are also addictive and have side effects such as disorientation and next-day fatigue and sluggishness.

One example: My usually bubbly and energetic colleague Kathryn suddenly started dragging at work, even nodding off during meetings. At night she would awake with unpleasant and uncontrollable urges to move her legs. The surprising cause turned out to be related to Kathryn's new vegetarian diet, which she had started several months before—without meat, her diet no longer included the iron she needed. As a result, she had developed restless legs syndrome, which makes sleeping a real challenge.

The simple solution: Her doctor prescribed iron supplements and began monitoring her levels. Now Kathryn sleeps like a baby and is once again bursting with energy at the office.

NUTRITIONAL DEFICIENCIES INTERFERE WITH SLEEP

Iron and restless legs syndrome is just one of the hidden dietary deficiencies affecting sleep. For more insight on potentially sleep-disturbing dietary deficiencies and how to address them, we turned to our nutrition guru, contributing medical editor Andrew L. Rubman, ND. If you suffer from insomnia, he recommends consulting a doctor who is knowledgeable about nutritional biochemistry to assess your nutrient levels and offer diet advice and/or supplements to support your body's natural sleep processes.

Dr. Rubman told me that the following nutrients are strongly related to sleep...

CALCIUM: NATURE'S SEDATIVE

When you run short on calcium, you are apt to toss and turn and experience frequent awakenings in the night. This mineral has a natural calming effect on the nervous system. It works by helping your body convert *tryptophan*—an essential amino acid found in foods such as turkey and eggs—into the neurotransmitter *serotonin*, which modulates mood and sleep. Serotonin, in turn, is converted into *melatonin*, a hormone that helps regulate the sleep cycle.

Dr. Rubman suggests: It's always better to get the nutrients you need from food rather than supplements. Milk and dairy products are the most common dietary sources of calcium, but Dr. Rubman notes that many people have trouble digesting cow's milk, especially as they grow older. Excellent nondairy sources of calcium are leafy green vegetables such as kale and collard greens, canned sardines, sesame seeds and almonds. The Recommended Dietary Allowance (RDA) for adults over age 18 is 1,000 to 1,200 mg/day. For those not getting enough from dietary sources, Dr. Rubman often prescribes the calcium-magnesium sup-

plement *Butyrex* from T.E. Neesby. Take it half an hour before going to bed.

RELIEVE LEG CRAMPS WITH MAGNESIUM

Nighttime leg cramps, often due to a magnesium deficiency, are a common cause of sleeplessness. Magnesium helps your body's cells absorb and use calcium, so this mineral pair works hand in hand to relax muscles, relieve painful cramps or spasms and bring on restful slumber.

Dr. Rubman suggests: Leafy green vegetables are the best source of dietary magnesium, followed by artichokes, nuts, legumes, seeds, whole grains (especially buckwheat, cornmeal and whole wheat) and soy products. The Butyrex Dr. Rubman prescribes for calcium deficiency contains magnesium, so it helps solve this problem too. (The RDA for magnesium for adults is 400 mg/day for men and 310 mg/day for women.)

VITAMIN B-12 FOR SEROTONIN PRODUCTION

Vitamin B-12 supports the production of neurotransmitters that affect brain function and sleep, helping to metabolize calcium and magnesium and working with them to convert tryptophan into the neurotransmitter serotonin. Insufficient B-12 may be a factor if you have trouble falling or staying asleep.

Dr. Rubman suggests: Foods rich in vitamin B-12 include liver and other organ meats, eggs, fish and, to a lesser degree, leafy green vegetables. For B-12 deficiency, Dr. Rubman sometimes prescribes B-12 tablets taken sublingually (dissolved under the tongue) one hour before bedtime—but notes that it's important to take a multivitamin that contains B vitamins twice daily as well, since it helps your body use the B-12 efficiently. Note: Most B multivitamins contain B-12 but only a minimal dose, Dr. Rubman said, so further supplementation is usually necessary.

VITAMIN D MODULATES CIRCADIAN RHYTHMS

Again with the vitamin D! We can't hear enough about the importance of this vital nutrient, it seems—and indeed, vitamin D turns out to be essential to support your body's uptake and usage of calcium and magnesium. Its role in sleep involves modulating your circadian rhythm (the sleep/wake cycle that regulates your 24-hour biological clock).

Dr. Rubman suggests: Pointing out that most Americans have less than optimal levels of vitamin D, Dr. Rubman said he commonly prescribes daily supplements of D-3, the form most efficiently used by the body. He noted that 10 to 20 minutes of sunshine daily helps your body manufacture vitamin D, and foods such as fish and fortified milk are rich in this nutrient.

HERBS: SOME HELP, SOME INTERFERE WITH SLEEP

Although they do not specifically address nutritional deficiencies, Dr. Rubman also recommends relaxing herbal supplements such as chamomile, hops or valerian to gently nudge you toward sleep. Try them in teas, capsules or tinctures from reputable manufacturers such as Eclectic Institute (*www.eclecticherb.com*), taken half an hour before retiring.

Though many people swear by melatonin, Dr. Rubman said that there is not enough scientific evidence yet to demonstrate that this popular sleep supplement works efficiently and without long-term ill effects. He does not prescribe it.

It's also important to be aware that a number of supplements are stimulating and may cause sleep irregularities in some individuals.

The biggest stimulators: Ginseng, ginkgo, St. John's wort, alpha lipoic acid and Sam-e. If you take any of these, do so early in the day, take the lowest dose that seems effective for you or discuss alternatives with your physician. These are all best used under professional guidance.

A SOOTHING BEDTIME SNACK

Dr. Rubman said that his favorite sleep inducer is to head upstairs each evening with a soothing bedtime beverage—either a cup of herbal tea with honey or a glass of warm milk (though not everyone's digestive system easily tolerates milk). He generally advises against late-night snacking, which can disturb sleep, but if you must have something keep it light. A high-protein, low-glycemic snack, such as a banana with peanut butter or half a turkey sandwich on whole-grain bread, can help encourage serotonin production...and sweet dreams.

19

Cold and Flu Cures

Fighting Winter Bugs

The holidays bring together families and friends…and unfortunately, all those hugs, kisses and handshakes can spread cold and flu germs. That's one major reason why the incidence of wintertime infections usually peaks in January.

And it turns out that the flu shot is not as protective as doctors have believed. Researchers recently reported that while flu shots can prevent people from contracting specific strains of influenza, they do not decrease flu-related deaths, according to the *American Journal of Respiratory* and *Critical Care Medicine*. Why not? Those who survive the flu tend to be healthier to begin with, so the shot may not be the lifesaving factor.

Luckily, you can bolster your defenses and, if necessary, ease your symptoms with the help of natural remedies. In my experience, it's easy to reduce a cold to about two and a half days with comparatively mild symptoms. The same regimen also can minimize flu symptoms and keep them from lingering.

THREE TIPS FOR PREVENTION

Of course, it is always best to avoid getting sick in the first place. *These suggestions—challenging as they may be during the holiday season—can so effectively prevent a bug from catching hold that they are worth trying…*

• **Don't indulge in a lot of sweets.** Sugary foods reduce the ability of white blood cells to fight germs. Allow yourself a small treat or two on any given day—no more.

• **Watch your stress.** People often overcommit during the holidays. Don't overdo…get lots of rest.

Mark A. Stengler, NMD, licensed naturopathic medical doctor in private practice, Stengler Center for Integrative Medicine, Encinitas, California…adjunct associate clinical professor at the National College of Natural Medicine, Portland, Oregon…author of many books, including *The Natural Physician's Healing Therapies* and coauthor of *Prescription for Natural Cures* (both from Bottom Line Books)…and author of the *Bottom Line/Natural Healing* newsletter. *www.drstengler.com*

•**Wash your hands often.** It's easy to pick up germs from handshakes and doorknobs, utensils and other objects. Wash with soap for at least 20 seconds, or use a hand sanitizer if you can't get to a lavatory.

BE PREPARED TO ACT QUICKLY

If you do start to feel sick but act quickly—as soon as you notice a slight runny nose and before sniffles turn into sneezes—you may prevent cold and flu germs from taking hold. You'll need to have a "nutritional first-aid kit" handy. Stock it with these supplements, available at drugstores and health-food stores. *You can take them all at the same time...*

•**N-acetylcysteine (NAC).** In one of the many studies on this potent antioxidant and immune-system booster, Italian researchers found that people taking 600 mg twice daily developed few if any flu symptoms, even though blood tests confirmed infection. I recommend taking 500 mg to 600 mg of NAC daily throughout the year—and doubling this dose during the cold and flu season. At the first sign of symptoms, increase your intake to 2,000 mg to 3,000 mg daily for two to three days. If you are fighting a full-fledged cold or flu, maintain this higher dose for a week.

•**Vitamin C.** Take at least 1,000 mg daily throughout the year. Consider doubling this amount during the winter. I recommend 3,000 mg to 5,000 mg during the first few days of symptoms. Warning: If you develop loose stools, you're taking too much.

•**Vitamin D.** Vitamin D boosts levels of *cathelicidin*, a powerful germ-killing agent produced by your body's immune cells. Some researchers propose that colds and flu are related to low seasonal levels of vitamin D. Take 1,000 IU of vitamin D3 daily, and increase it to 5,000 IU daily for the first five days of a cold or flu.

•**Zinc.** Studies show that zinc lozenges can reduce the duration of colds in adults (zinc must be dissolved in the mouth in order to exert its antiviral properties). Take a zinc lozenge every two hours for three days, after which you can reduce the frequency—and stop when you are symptom-free. Be sure the lozenges are made with *zinc gluconate, zinc gluconate-glycine* or *zinc acetate*—which allow the best delivery into cells for fighting colds. I recommend the Cold-Eeze brand, which contains 13.3 mg of zinc gluconate-glycine.

EXTRA AMMUNITION

I also recommend that you begin taking one or more of the following supplements on the first day you feel cold or flu symptoms. (You can take them all if you wish.)

•***Oscillococcinum* (pronounced os-sil-uh-cox-see-num).** One study found that this homeopathic remedy reduced the duration of cold symptoms by about one-fourth. A review published by the *Cochrane Collaboration* described the treatment as "promising." Follow label directions.

•**Elderberry.** Extract of elderberry (*Sambucus nigra)* rapidly reduces the aches, fatigue, coughing and fever commonly associated with flu. In one study, Israeli researchers found that 14 out of 15 people taking elderberry extract had a significant reduction in symptoms after just two days...and 13 of the patients were symptom-free after three days. I recommend the brand Sambucol, a syrup—take according to label directions.

•**Andrographis.** This Chinese herb (*Andrographis paniculata*) can reduce symptoms of upper respiratory infections, such as flu. For extra benefits, take Siberian ginseng (*Eleutherococcus senticosus*) at the same time. Stop when symptoms go away. Because herbal products vary, follow label directions.

Good brand: Nature's Way (800-962-8873, *www.naturesway.com*).

•**North American ginseng.** In a study of 323 adults with a history of catching colds, supplements of North American ginseng (also known as *Panax quinquefolium*) cut the duration of colds by one-third. I recommend the COLD-fX brand, available at many pharmacies. Take one or two capsules a day if symptoms are just beginning...increase to six to nine capsules if you already have a pronounced cold or flu symptoms.

Caution: In rare cases, Panax ginseng may increase blood pressure.

•**Echinacea.** This herb enhances the body's ability to fight infections. It is readily available in tablets, capsules and alcohol-based tinctures. In an analysis of 14 studies, University of Connecticut researchers found that echinacea supplements reduced the length of a typical seven-day cold by about a day and a half. I recommend Nature's Way Echinacea capsules and Natural Factors Echinamide. Take according to label directions.

Extra defense: If you fly on commercial aircraft between November and February, assume that you will be exposed to cold and flu germs. As a safeguard, double your dose of NAC and vitamin C starting two days before and ending two days after your flight...and take vitamin D and zinc lozenges with you. As added protection, carry antibacterial wipes to keep your hands clean, and twice daily use Xlear nasal rinse, which has antimicrobial properties and helps moisturize nasal passages. All of these products are available at drugstores and health-food stores.

• **What about Airborne?** People frequently ask me what I think of this popular product, which claims to prevent winter bugs if you start taking it at the first sign of symptoms but has not been shown in studies to do so. My view: Take my list of supplements instead—they are proven cold and flu fighters.

I do not recommend that healthy children and adults get an annual flu vaccination. There is no guarantee that it will prevent the bug from striking...and the vaccines may contain traces of the toxin mercury. However, if you are at a higher-than-average risk of contracting the flu or you live with someone who is at high risk, a vaccination is worth considering. Your risk is higher than average if you are pregnant... have suppressed immunity...live with or care for others at high risk of contracting the flu (including health-care workers)...and/or have a lung condition, such as asthma or emphysema. If you do get vaccinated, I strongly recommend thimerosal-free (mercury-free) products, such as the FluMist nasal spray (for ages two to 49) or the Fluzone single-dose, prefilled syringe. Talk to your doctor about which is best for you.

Eat Just One a Day...And Fight Colds, Flu and More

Carol S. Johnston, PhD, RD, professor and director, department of nutrition, Arizona State University in Mesa, Arizona. She has published more than 80 research papers and book chapters on nutrition subjects and received the 2004 Grace A. Goldsmith Award from the American College of Nutrition in recognition of her research.

Wouldn't it be nice if you could add one simple item to your diet each day to help your body fight colds, flu, fatigue and other ailments related to a weakened immune system?

You can, according to recent research conducted at the University of California at Los Angeles. The six-year study of 17,688 men and women, published in the *Journal of the American Dietetic Association*, found that people who eat at least a one-cup portion of salad, including raw vegetables and salad dressing, every day have high blood levels of vitamins C and E as well as folic acid, all of which help promote a healthy immune system.

But some salads provide more disease-fighting nutrients than others. *Here's how to make sure your salad is as healthful as possible...*

1. Use salad dressing. In an effort to reduce fat and calories, many people sprinkle salad greens with just lemon juice or vinegar. That's a mistake.

A small amount of fat actually helps promote the absorption of fat-soluble vitamins, such as vitamins A, E, D and K. In addition to the health benefits these vitamins themselves provide, they also aid in the absorption of certain other nutrients—for example, vitamin D helps facilitate the absorption of calcium. Aim to include about two tablespoons daily of olive oil or another healthy oil, such as canola, in your salad dressing.

Smart idea: To ensure that your salad dressing is healthful, make your own. An easy recipe: Combine one-half cup of balsamic vinegar, one-quarter cup of olive oil, two tablespoons each of finely grated Parmesan cheese and sugar, one teaspoon of oregano and one-half teaspoon of garlic salt.

Calories: About 80 per two-tablespoon serving.

Sodium: 60 mg.

Fat: 7.5 g.

If you want the convenience of a bottled salad dressing, shop carefully. Many brands contain as much as 700 mg of sodium per serving (the recommended daily allowance is 1,500 mg for people age 50 and older) as well as partially hydrogenated or hydrogenated oils—code words for trans fat, which has been shown to raise blood cholesterol and heart disease risk—and 100 calories per tablespoon. If your salad contains healthful fat from avocado or nuts, consider using a low-fat dressing.

2. Don't overdo the fat content. Even though a certain amount of healthful fat is good for you, people who try to make a meal of their salad often end up adding too much fat by piling on processed meats, fried chicken, creamy salad mixtures, such as egg salad, tuna salad or macaroni salad, and high-fat cheeses.

Smart idea: Use low- or nonfat cheeses, cubed tofu, poultry (except fried or breaded versions) or fish (salmon and tuna are good choices because of their omega-3 fats).

3. Choose lettuce that is dark green or reddish. The majority of Americans make their salads with iceberg lettuce. However, this is the least nutritious type of lettuce because it contains mostly water.

Smart idea: Select romaine lettuce for your salad, then for variety, add any combination of dandelion greens, arugula, endive, chicory, butterhead lettuce or spinach, all of which are rich in folic acid, a vitamin that is important to cardiovascular health.

In general, the darker the color of the lettuce leaf, the more vitamins and minerals the lettuce contains.

4. Choose a variety of richly colored vegetables. Americans tend to pile their salads with celery and cucumbers. Even though these vegetables make good snacks—they are very low in calories—they are also relatively low in nutrients, compared with some other vegetables.

Smart idea: Add tomatoes, broccoli, snow peas and bell peppers to your salad. They are excellent sources of vitamin C and other key nutrients.

Rule of thumb: The brighter the vegetable's color, the more vitamins and minerals it contains.

5. Get your phytochemicals. These chemicals are antioxidants or enzyme inhibitors that protect our bodies from disease-causing free radicals and help to slow down the aging process.

Smart idea: Add white, yellow or red onions, garlic (crushed or chopped) and mushrooms (such as shiitake or maitake)—all are loaded with healthful phytochemicals.

6. Add nuts. Many people like to top their salads with croutons or bacon bits to add flavor, but croutons often are high in calories and most bacon-bit products contain nitrates—which have been linked to cancers of the digestive tract and the pancreas—as well as harmful fats and sodium.

Smart idea: Add a tablespoon or two of unsalted nuts, such as almonds, pistachios, cashews, walnuts, hazelnuts or peanuts. All of them contain healthful fats and are excellent sources of vitamin E. As an alternative, add unsalted sunflower seeds, which are high in fiber, potassium, phosphorus and other nutrients.

Echinacea—The Best-Selling Immune Booster

Mark A. Stengler, NMD, licensed naturopathic medical doctor in private practice, Stengler Center for Integrative Medicine, Encinitas, California…adjunct associate clinical professor at the National College of Natural Medicine, Portland, Oregon…author of many books, including *The Natural Physician's Healing Therapies* and coauthor of *Prescription for Natural Cures* (both from Bottom Line Books)…and author of the *Bottom Line/Natural Healing* newsletter. *www.drstengler.com*

It's not unusual to get calls at my office from patients wondering what to do about the cold or flu that just hit them.

My first thought is: What natural supplements can they get quickly, right off the shelf?

Well, just about anyone can find *echinacea* (pronounced eck-in-ay'-sha) at a nearby store. It's one of the five top-selling herbs in North America. In fact, it's a worldwide best-seller, as herbalists and doctors in Europe have been prescribing echinacea for decades. Carrying the popular name of purple coneflower (so-called because of its beautiful, purple, daisy-like petals), echinacea is renowned as an herb that enhances the immune system. It's commonly used to treat a number of conditions from flu and the common cold to a range of other infectious diseases.

THE SNAKEBITE CONNECTION

Native Americans of the Plains are believed to be the first to use echinacea. As today, it was a remedy for colds, coughs and sore throats, but also toothaches, battle wounds and even rattlesnake bites.

During the latter part of the 1800s, Plains settlers adopted the purple coneflower as a common remedy; and by the 1920s, echinacea was being sold as a commercial product and prescribed by the many physicians who were comfortable with herbal medicines.

Dr. H.C.F. Meyer of Pawnee, Nebraska, was a keen commercial promoter. Adding his own recommendations to what he had learned from Native Americans, Dr. Meyer sold echinacea as a "cure all" for various ailments. His reputation was considerably enhanced by the claim that he had successfully treated 613 cases of rattlesnake poisoning. One doctor gave the following candid account of Dr. Meyer's own, personal echinacea experiment…

"With the courage of his convictions upon him, he injected the venom of the *crotalus* (rattlesnake) into the first finger of his left hand; the swelling was rapid and in six hours up to the elbow. At this time he took a dose of the remedy, bathed the part thoroughly, and laid down to pleasant dreams. On awakening in four hours, the pain and swelling were gone."

INFECTION FIGHTER TO THE RESCUE

I can't say I have had any patients come to me for the natural treatment of rattlesnake bites. (If I did, I would quickly hurry them off to a hospital emergency room for a dose of up-to-date antivenin.) But it's interesting to note that echinacea does have the special property of preventing the spread of infectious substances to tissues.

Echinacea as a healing remedy was introduced to Europe during the 1930s. Since then the preponderance of scientific research on echinacea has been done in Western Europe, especially Germany, where the government plays an active role in funding natural-medicine research. But Canadian and American researchers have recently made similar strides in echinacea research, with clinical studies and biochemical analysis of the healing herb.

Over 400 studies to date have looked at the pharmacology and clinical uses of echinacea. Not all studies have shown efficacy of the herb, but most of the research indicates that echinacea helps reinforce the immune system.

Echinacea is consistently one of the best-selling herbs in North America and Europe. Over 10 million units are sold annually in Germany alone.

Though there are nine species of echinacea, *Echinacea purpurea* and *Echinacea angustifolia* are the two most often used commercially. Most clinical studies are done with these species, especially purpurea.

TONGUE-TINGLING CHEMICALS

Scientists have not reached a consensus about the active ingredients in echinacea. Though researchers acknowledge the herb has many immune-boosting properties as well as anti-inflammatory and antimicrobial effects, they're not sure what chemicals or combination of chemicals are responsible.

It's known, however, that echinacea contains caffeic acid derivatives such as *cichoric acid* and *polysaccharides*. The plant also has compounds known as *alkylamides* that are thought to be important. (Alkylamides are the substances that make your tongue tingle and go numb if you take a hefty dose of straight echinacea.)

Some of these compounds are water-soluble and some are alcohol-soluble. When tinctures, pills, or tablets are being created from echinacea, the manufacturer must go through an elaborate process to extract the compounds.

Recent research done at the University of British Columbia in conjunction with the University of Alberta has shown that the ratio of the actives in echinacea is important for optimal immune response. So in other words, not only is it important to have active constituents in echinacea products, but to also have them in a specific ratio or blend.

AROUSING IMMUNE CELLS

Echinacea doesn't work like the pharmaceutical antibiotics that "kill" microbes like bacteria. Instead, echinacea arouses the immune cells that patrol and defend the body against these invaders. It increases the number and activity of disease-fighting white blood cells, and it activates antiviral chemicals such as interferon. Echinacea can even activate the immune cells that fight tumors. In addition, research has shown that the chemicals in echinacea have the power to inhibit an enzyme released by bacteria, called *hyaluronidase*. Bacteria normally produce this enzyme to penetrate into human tissue. Echinacea prevents this from happening.

Researchers in a German study found clear evidence that echinacea helps to promote good immune cells, called *phagocytes*. One group of people were given 30 drops of echinacea three times daily for five days, while people in the control group were given a placebo. The level of phagocytes was measured at the beginning and throughout the study. At day three, the phagocyte activity of those taking echinacea increased by 40 percent. By the fifth day, phagocyte activity had increased 120 percent. When people stopped taking echinacea, immune-cell activity dropped off sharply. After three days, there was no difference in immune-cell activity between the group taking echinacea and the control group.

Leading researchers now feel that echinacea may actually be more of an immune-modulating herb, meaning it has a balancing effect on the immune system. As research continues, this may mean that echinacea may be more valuable than just boosting immune function.

VIRUS SLAYERS

While there are a host of modern antibiotics for killing bacteria, modern medicine has a limited arsenal of weapons to defeat viral infections. This presents a problem for the many doctors who rely on conventional pharmaceuticals in their medical practice. Over 65 million people in the U.S. each year "catch" the common cold, while another 108 million get the flu—and these are just two of the infectious diseases caused by viruses. Others include genital herpes, which affects an estimated 45 million people, as well as hepatitis C, which afflicts 170 million people in the world. Even a simple viral infection like a viral sore throat poses a challenge for any doctor who relies exclusively on antibiotics and other conventional prescription medications.

Echinacea, like some other immune-enhancing herbs, has a direct antiviral effect. Even better, it seems to summon all the resources of the immune system to help destroy the viral invaders.

It also works well in combination with other antiviral plants and herbs. I like to prescribe echinacea in a formula called the "virus cocktail," which is comprised of echinacea, lomatium, astragalus, reishi and licorice root. The synergistic blend of these herbs tends to be more effective than any one herb by itself.

BACTERIA AND FUNGUS

Since echinacea enhances the action of your immune cells, it is also effective against bacterial, fungal and yeast infections. This is especially helpful if you're fighting a bacterial infection, because many bacteria are now resistant to antibiotics (because they're overprescribed by doctors for things like viral infections). If needed, there is no problem using echinacea in combination with antibiotics. As a matter of fact, I find when people are on antibiotics for a bacterial infection and use echinacea simultaneously, they recover more quickly.

At least one study—which included 4,190 patients—confirmed this observation. Researchers divided the patients into two groups and gave about half of them an antibacterial formula that included echinacea (along with two other herbs—*thuja* and *baptisia*). Along with that formula, the patients received antibiotics that were chosen by the doctors. For comparison, the rest of the patients received only antibiotics, with no herbal formula.

The results showed the effectiveness of taking herbal antibacterial agents along with antibiotics. In the group that got an echinacea-based formula plus an antibiotic, people were cured significantly faster and there was a lower incidence of recurring infection than in the group of people who just got an antibiotic. Also, the symptoms of "sore throat" and "difficulty in swallowing" were improved much more efficiently in the first group than in the second group.

Dosage: Echinacea is generally available as a tincture, capsule, tablet or cream in the U.S. It's also possible to take it in the form of an injection, though this method is mainly used in Germany.

Glycerine (alcohol-free) tinctures are available. These are good for kids, who especially enjoy the berry-flavored varieties.

• **Tincture.** I recommend 20 to 60 drops of the tincture every two to three hours for acute infections or twice daily for long-term use.

• **Capsule.** I recommend 500 to 1,000 milligrams every two to three hours for acute infections or twice daily for long-term use.

Note: High-potency, quality echinacea products are standardized to contain active ingredients such as *alkylamides, cichoric acid* and *polysaccharides.*

Some controversy surrounds the length of time one can use echinacea. Many authors state that echinacea should not be used on a long-term basis. However, there are no studies showing that long-term use is harmful or that echinacea loses its effectiveness.

I generally recommend patients use echinacea for acute infections until they are completely over the illness. For those who are very susceptible to infections, especially during the winter, and do not want to change their lifestyle, echinacea can be used on a long-term basis (although it is not so effective as improving diet, reducing stress and exercising). Long-term use of echinacea throughout the winter season is common in European countries.

Feed a Cold, Starve A Fever and Other Nutrition Myths

Edward Saltzman, MD, chief of the division of clinical nutrition and medical director of the Obesity Consultation Center at Tufts–New England Medical Center, and a scientist at the Jean Mayer USDA Human Nutrition Research Center on Aging at Tufts University, both in Boston.

Many commonly held beliefs about the health impact of certain foods are based on hearsay, not on scientific research. *Here are the realities behind some often-cited nutrition myths...*

Myth: Feed a cold, starve a fever.

Reality: Both a cold and a fever—and you can have both at once—are associated with inflammation, which increases metabolic rate, allowing you to burn calories at rest more quickly. However, eating more or less will have no real effect on how long you remain sick. There is no evidence that food shortens a cold's duration or reduces symptoms.

It's often believed that vitamin C can help a cold, but there's no firm evidence to back that claim. Recently, researchers reviewed 55 previous studies. Most showed that taking vitamin C did not prevent colds—a few showed that colds were slightly shorter with vitamin supplementation, but usually by only one day or so.

Zinc may reduce a cold's duration, but it must be taken early on—before full-blown symptoms strike. The benefit comes from zinc gluconate lozenges (see the label for the correct dosage). Zinc acetate lozenges or zinc-rich foods, such as oysters and beef, have no impact on a cold's severity or duration.

Bottom line: The real goal is to stay hydrated and loosen mucus by increasing your intake of liquids, such as water, clear soups and tea.

Myth: Fiber prevents colon cancer.

Reality: A high-fiber diet keeps your bowel movements regular and can lower cholesterol and reduce risk of insulin resistance, a precursor to diabetes. But there is no consistent evidence that fiber protects against colon cancer.

A study in *The Journal of the American Medical Association* reviewed data on 726,000 people over 20 years and found that high-fiber diets did not reduce the risk of colon cancer. Another study determined that people eating 33 grams of fiber per day—roughly 6.5 servings of fruits and vegetables—had no fewer polyps (benign growths in the colon that may become cancerous) than those eating roughly half as much fiber. Even high-fiber cereals seem to strike out when it comes to protecting against colon cancer, although they may have benefits for cardiovascular health and prevent constipation.

Bottom line: Continue to eat fiber-rich foods, such as fruits, vegetables and whole grains, for their proven health benefits, including cardiovascular health and weight control. Also, while fiber-rich foods do not protect against colon cancer, they do protect against other types of cancer—including those of the breast, mouth, throat and esophagus—probably because of their phytochemicals, protective compounds found in some foods.

Myth: Soy relieves hot flashes.

Reality: Most scientific studies have not found that soy-rich foods or supplements offer relief from hot flashes. While soy is a good source of phytoestrogens (chemicals occurring naturally in plants that act like the hormone estrogen), it provides an extremely weak estrogenic effect. Some menopausal women may benefit from a soy-rich diet, but most do not—at least not on a consistent basis.

Bottom line: Soy-rich foods are nutritious, low in fat and may help lower cholesterol and improve prostate health (so far, studies have produced mixed results). And a recent analysis of 18 previous studies found that soy may slightly lower the risk of breast cancer. To control hot flashes, however, you're better off adjusting room temperature...wearing "breathable" fabrics, such as cotton...and drinking cool beverages when a flash starts. At this time, there are no dietary supplements known to be both safe and effective for hot flashes.

Myth: Eating after 8 pm causes weight gain.

Reality: It's not when you eat that causes weight gain—it's how much. There is no evidence that calorie "burn" is slower at night. Weight gain results from overeating and lack of activity, whether that occurs in the morning, afternoon or night.

This myth likely stems from the fact that many people eat little during the day but then overeat at night, when they're relaxing at home—but these people won't gain any more weight than those who overeat earlier in the day. Some research has suggested that people who eat breakfast are less likely to gain weight or become obese—though the reason for this is unclear.

Bottom line: Watch portion sizes more than the clock. Don't go for long periods without eating, because you are more likely to overeat when you are ravenously hungry.

Myth: Olive oil is the healthiest oil.

Reality: This foundation of the Mediterranean diet is among the healthiest cooking oils—and certainly gets the best publicity—but other oils may be just as good. For example, the FDA decreed that canola oil, like olive oil, can carry a health claim for its ability to reduce the risk of coronary heart disease due to its unsaturated fat content. The important thing is to limit saturated fats, which are most often found in animal products, such as red meat, poultry, butter and whole milk.

Bottom line: Choose oils high in mono- or polyunsaturated fat, such as olive, canola, safflower, flaxseed and walnut oils. If you choose olive oil, select extra-virgin. Extra-virgin olive oil comes from the first pressing of olives, so it's less processed and contains higher levels of antioxidants, substances that slow down the natural process that leads to cell and tissue damage.

Myth: Honey is more healthful than sugar.

Reality: Honey contains more fructose than sugar—and fructose is becoming public enemy number one among some cardiologists. Some studies suggest that high-fructose diets are linked to weight gain and metabolic syndrome, a group of health problems that includes excess abdominal fat, high blood pressure, high triglycerides (a type of fat in the blood), low "good" cholesterol and high blood sugar.

Bottom line: Go easy on sugar and honey. Both offer "empty calories"—a tablespoon of honey has 64 calories and a tablespoon of sugar has about 45 calories. Neither is a good source of any nutrient. You would need to overeat honey to an unhealthy level in order to benefit from its micronutrients or other purported health benefits.

Amazing Folk Remedies For Colds, Coughs, Flu And More

Joan Wilen and Lydia Wilen are folk-remedy experts based in New York City. The sisters are coauthors of many books, including *Bottom Line's Healing Remedies: Over 1,000 Astounding Ways to Heal Arthritis, Asthma, High Blood Pressure, Varicose Veins, Warts and More!* from which this article is adapted. *www.bottomline publications.com.*

Not every winter illness requires a trip to the doctor's office. The following time-tested folk remedies offer effective, inexpensive treatments for minor health complaints.

Important: Consult your doctor if your condition persists or grows worse.

COLDS

The average adult contracts between two and four colds each year, mostly between September and May. Medical science has no cure for these highly contagious viral infections, but the following folk remedies can help ward off colds, ease symptoms and possibly shorten a cold's duration…

• **Garlic.** Garlic contains *allicin*, which has been shown to reduce the severity of a cold. Eat four cloves of freshly crushed raw garlic three times a day until you have recovered.

• **Cinnamon, sage and bay.** Cinnamon contains compounds believed to reduce congestion. Sage can help sooth sore throats. Some

Native American cultures have used bay leaves to clear breathing passages. Steep one-half teaspoon each of cinnamon and sage with a bay leaf in six ounces of hot water. Strain and add one tablespoon of lemon juice. Lemon helps reduce mucus buildup. If you like your tea sweet, add honey.

• **Chicken soup.** The Mayo Clinic has said in its health newsletter that chicken soup can be an excellent treatment for head colds and other viral respiratory infections for which antibiotics are not helpful.

FLU

• **Influenza is a potentially serious viral infection.** People often mistake colds for the flu. Colds take hold gradually and are not usually accompanied by severe aches or a fever. The onset of the flu is sudden, and symptoms include fever, severe muscle aches and fatigue.

• **Garlic and cognac.** A shot of cognac is a popular flu remedy in Germany, where it's thought to ease symptoms and help the body cleanse itself. Garlic helps clear mucus, among other potential benefits. Peel and dice a half-pound of garlic. Add one quart of 90-proof cognac, and seal the mixture in an airtight bottle. Store in a cool, dark place for two weeks. Strain out the garlic, and reseal the liquid in the bottle. Prepare a new batch each year.

To treat the flu: Add 20 drops to eight ounces of water. Drink three glasses a day, one before each meal.

For prevention: Use 10 to 15 drops, instead of 20, per glass in flu season.

Important: This treatment is not advisable for people who have drinking problems or for children.

• **Sauerkraut.** Sauerkraut's concentration of lactic acid bacteria may weaken infections. Have two tablespoons of sauerkraut juice or about one-half cup of sauerkraut each day during flu season to reduce the chances of getting an infection.

SORE THROATS

Experiment with these remedies until you find what works best for you…

245

•**Apple cider vinegar.** Vinegar is a powerful anti-inflammatory, and its acidity might help kill the bacteria that cause some sore throats. Add two teaspoons of apple cider vinegar to six ounces of warm water. Gargle with a mouthful, spit it out, then drink a mouthful. Continue this until the mixture is gone. Rinse your mouth with water to prevent the vinegar from eroding your teeth. Repeat the vinegar gargle every hour for as long as your sore throat persists.

•**Sage.** Sage is an anti-inflammatory. Add one teaspoon of dried sage to one six-ounce cup of boiling water. Steep for three to five minutes, strain, then gargle and swallow.

•**Lemon and honey.** Honey coats the throat, while lemon can temporarily reduce the mucus buildup that often accompanies a sore throat. Squeeze one lemon, add a teaspoon of honey and drink. Repeat every two hours.

•**Tongue stretching.** Stick out your tongue for 30 seconds, relax it for a few seconds, then repeat four times. This is believed to increase blood flow to the throat, speeding the healing process.

COUGHS

Try these folk remedies to figure out which works best for you…

•**Lemon, honey and olive oil.** Honey and olive oil coat and soothe, while lemon reduces mucus. Heat one cup of honey, a half cup of olive oil and the juice of one lemon over a medium flame for five minutes. Turn off the heat, and stir for two minutes to blend the ingredients. Consume one teaspoon of the mixture every two hours.

•**Vinegar and cayenne pepper.** Cayenne pepper contains capsaicin, a proven painkiller, while vinegar serves as an anti-inflammatory. Add a half cup of apple cider vinegar and one teaspoon of cayenne pepper to one-half cup of water. Add honey if desired. Take one tablespoon when your cough acts up and another tablespoon before bed.

•**Horseradish and honey.** Horseradish can help loosen mucus, while honey coats the throat. Grate one teaspoon of fresh, peeled horseradish into two teaspoons of honey. Consume one teaspoon every two to three hours.

•**Ginger.** Ginger is an anti-inflammatory that contains gingerols, which provide pain-reducing and sedative benefits. Chew a piece of fresh, peeled gingerroot when you feel the cough acting up, usually in the evening before bed. Chew until the ginger loses its kick.

•**Licorice root tea.** Licorice relieves the pain of irritated mucous membranes. Drink licorice root tea as long as your cough persists.

Note: Don't try licorice root if you have high blood pressure or kidney problems.

Relief at Your Fingertips

Michael Reed Gach, PhD, founder of the Acupressure Institute in Berkeley, California and author of self-healing instructional DVDs and CDs and many books, including *Acupressure's Potent Points* (Bantam), *Acupressure for Lovers* (Bantam), *Arthritis Relief at Your Fingertips* (Warner). *www.acupressure.com*

Y ou've probably heard of acupuncture, but there's something similar that you can do yourself—no needles involved—called *acupressure*. Acupressure can alleviate many physical, mental and emotional problems in only a few minutes—and it is free.

Acupressure involves stimulating acupoints on the body with fingertips or knuckles and is based on the principles of acupuncture, an ancient healing technique used by practitioners of *Traditional Chinese Medicine* (TCM). The acupoints often have ancient descriptive names, such as "Joining the Valley" and "Mind Clearing." Acupressure increases blood flow to the treated area and triggers the release of *endorphins*, pain-relieving brain chemicals.

Here are the acupressure techniques for various health problems. Unless otherwise noted, daily acupressure sessions, three times a day, are the best way to relieve a temporary or chronic problem.

ARTHRITIS PAIN

Joining the Valley is a truly amazing acupoint because it can relieve arthritis pain anywhere in the body.

Location: In the webbing between the thumb and index finger, at the highest spot of the muscle when the thumb and index finger are brought close together.

What to do: Rhythmically squeeze the acupoint. As you're squeezing, place the side of your hand that is closest to the little finger on your thigh or a tabletop. Apply pressure in the webbing as you press downward. This allows you to angle more deeply into the point, increasing the benefits.

Also good for: Headache, toothache, hangover, hay fever symptoms, constipation.

Caution: This point is forbidden for pregnant women because its stimulation can cause premature contraction in the uterus.

MEMORY PROBLEMS

The *Mind Clearing* acupoints are for improving recall instantly—for example, when you have forgotten a name or gone to the supermarket without your shopping list.

Location: One finger width (about one-half inch) directly above the center of each eyebrow.

What to do: Gently place your right thumb above your right eyebrow and your middle fingertip above the eyebrow on the left side. Hold very gently. You should feel a slight dip or indentation in the bone structure—the acupoints on both sides are in the dip. Press the indentation very lightly, hold and breathe deeply. After a minute or two, you'll experience more mental clarity and sharper memory.

LOWER BACK PAIN

To help prevent and relieve lower back pain, practice this exercise for one minute three times a day. You can do it standing or sitting.

Location: Place the backs of your hands against your lower back, about one inch outside the spine.

What to do: Briskly rub your hands up and down—about three inches up and six inches down—using the friction to create heat in your lower back.

If you're doing the technique correctly, you'll need to breathe deeply to sustain the vigorous rubbing, and you'll break out in a slight sweat.

Also good for: Food cravings, especially sugar cravings, chronic fatigue, sexual problems, chills, phobias and fibromyalgia symptoms.

EMOTIONAL UPSET

The *Inner Gate* acupoint can reduce emotional upset—such as anxiety, depression and irritability—in two to three minutes.

Location: On the inner side of the forearm, three finger widths up from the center of the wrist crease, in between two thick tendons.

What to do: Place your thumb on the point and your fingers directly behind the outside of the forearm between the two bones. Squeeze in slowly and firmly, hold for two to three minutes, breathing deeply. Repeat on the other arm for the same amount of time.

Also good for: Carpal tunnel syndrome, insomnia, indigestion and nausea.

COLDS AND FLU

If you think you're about to get a cold or flu, stimulating the *Heavenly Rejuvenation* acupoint may prevent infection.

Location: On the shoulders, midway between the base of the neck and the outside of the shoulders, one-half inch below the top of the shoulders, just above the tip of the shoulder blades.

What to do: There are two ways to stimulate this point...

Curving your fingers, hook your right hand on your right shoulder and your left hand on your left shoulder. You also can use your fingers on your opposite shoulder, which may be easier. With your fingertips, firmly press the point and take three slow, deep breaths.

If you don't have the flexibility to perform the first technique...lie down on your back, on a firm mattress or carpeted floor, with your knees bent and feet on the floor as close to your buttocks as possible. Bring your hands above your head, and rest the backs of your hands on the floor beside or above your head. Inhale and lift up your pelvis, pressing your feet against the floor to assist the lift. The higher your pelvis, the more weight will be transferred onto your shoulders, stimulating the acupoint. Hold this posture for one minute, taking long, slow, deep breaths, with your eyes closed. Lower your pelvis, and rest for three minutes.

Also good for: Nervous tension, stiff neck, high fever, chills, shoulder aches as well as irritability.

INSOMNIA

The acupoints *Calm Sleep* and *Joyful Sleep*—on the outer and inner ankles—can help relieve insomnia. Use these acupressure points whenever you want to deeply relax and sleep better.

Location: *Calm Sleep* is in the first indentation below the outer anklebone. *Joyful Sleep* is directly below the inside of the anklebone, in a slight indentation.

What to do: Place your thumb on one side of your ankle and your fingers on the other, and press firmly. If you're on the right spot, it will be slightly sore. Hold for two minutes, breathing deeply. Repeat on the other ankle. Do this again if you still are having trouble sleeping or if you wake up.

HEADACHES

The acupoints *Gates of Consciousness* relieve a tension headache or migraine.

Location: Underneath the base of your skull to either side of your spine, about three to four inches apart, depending on the size of your head.

What to do: Using your fingers, thumbs or knuckles, press the points under the base of your skull.

At the same time, slowly tilt your head back so that the angle of your head relaxes your neck muscles. Press forward (toward your throat), upward (underneath the base of your skull) and slightly inward, angling the pressure toward the center of your brain. Continue to apply pressure for two minutes, breathing.

Also good for: Neck pain, insomnia, high blood pressure.

ACUPRESSURE BASICS

Unless otherwise noted, use your middle finger, with your index and ring fingers for support. Firmly and gradually, apply stationary pressure directly on the acupoint for three minutes.

•**Firmly means using an amount of pressure that causes a sensation between pleasure and pain—pressure that "hurts good."** If the pressure is applied too fast or too hard, the point will hurt. If the pressure is too soft, you won't get the full benefit.

•**Gradually means moving your finger into and out of the point in super-slow motion.** Applying and releasing finger pressure allow the tissue to respond and relax, promoting healing.

•**Stationary means you are not rubbing or massaging the area.**

•**Directly means at a 90-degree angle from the surface of the skin.** If you are pulling the skin, the angle of pressure is incorrect.

•**When you apply pressure, lean your weight toward the point.** If your hands are weak or it hurts your fingers when you apply pressure, try using your knuckles. You also can use a tool, such as a golf ball or pencil eraser.

•**Breathe slowly and deeply while you apply pressure.** This helps release pain and tension.

Illustrations courtesy of Michael Reed Gach, PhD.

Exercise Fights Colds

Researchers studied 160 overweight, sedentary women ages 18 to 85. Half walked for 45 minutes five days a week for 12 to 15 weeks, while the other half remained sedentary.

Result: The walkers who got colds had 40% to 50% fewer days of illness than nonwalkers who got colds.

Theory: Thirty to 60 minutes a day of moderate exercise, such as walking at a 15-minute-per-mile pace, spurs production of germ-killing cells called *neutrophils.*

Caution: Ninety minutes or more of high-intensity daily exercise, such as long-distance running, has the opposite effect, increasing stress hormones and immune dysfunction.

David C. Nieman, MD, DrPH, professor of health and exercise science, Appalachian State University, Boone, North Carolina.

Eat Turkey to Prevent Colds

Turkey is a good source of *glutamine,* an amino acid used by cells to protect against infection. And, like other protein sources, it boosts immunity. Eat turkey often during cold season to keep protective cells functioning at their peak.

Elizabeth M. Ward, MS, RD, nutrition consultant, Boston, and author of *The Low-Carb Bible* (Publications International).

Homeopathic Help for Colds and Flu

Richard Mann, ND, chair of the department of homeopathic medicine at Bastyr University School of Naturopathic Medicine and a faculty member in clinical practice at Bastyr Center for Natural Health, both in Seattle. He is a diplomate of the Homeopathic Academy of Natural Physicians.

You may never have tried homeopathy, a form of alternative medicine that boosts the body's own healing responses. But if you get sick this winter, chances are that homeopathy can bring relief—if you pick the appropriate homeopathic remedy for your specific symptoms. *What you need to know...*

HOW HOMEOPATHY WORKS

Like vaccination, homeopathy seeks to stimulate the immune system. A vaccine contains a tiny amount of the pathogen that causes a certain disease.

Principle of homeopathy: Substances of plant, animal or mineral origin that can cause symptoms of disease also can cure symptoms when given in the form of very highly diluted remedies.

Homeopathy is not a one-size-fits-all therapy. Rather, the remedy must be carefully matched to a particular person's specific symptoms and his/her physical and mental reactions to these symptoms. This individualization makes it difficult to devise clinical studies that accurately reflect homeopathy's effectiveness.

What is known: For more than 200 years, homeopathy has helped people heal.

People who have colds or flu often respond to self-treatment using nonprescription homeopathic remedies sold in health-food stores and online.

Key: Match the right remedy with your symptoms.

What to do: Follow directions on product labels, taking 6C, 12C or 30C potency remedies. "C" stands for centesimal and indicates that one part of the active substance was mixed with 99 parts of alcohol...the numbers reflect how many times the mixture went through a dilution process. Paradoxically, the more dilute the potency, the greater the effect.

Remedies usually are sold as tiny pellets that dissolve under the tongue. Oils or other substances on your hands can inactivate pellets, so use a spoon to remove them from the container and place them in your mouth. Do not put anything else in your mouth for 30 minutes before or after taking a remedy.

Homeopathic remedies generally work quickly. *Unless otherwise directed by your practitioner or product labels, follow these instructions...*

•**If there is no change in symptoms after several hours, repeat the dose once more.** If symptoms still do not change after several hours, try a different homeopathic remedy that corresponds to your symptoms.

•If you feel somewhat better after taking a homeopathic remedy, repeat it at four-hour intervals until you feel significantly better, for a maximum of four doses in total.

•Once you feel significantly better, do not take another dose. If symptoms return, repeat dosing according to the instructions above.

When to seek help: In some cases, patients need prescription-potency homeopathic remedies and/or conventional medical treatment. *See a homeopathic physician or your primary care practitioner if…*

•None of the remedies below seem appropriate for your specific symptoms.

•You have tried three or four of the homeopathic remedies below without result.

•You are over age 65 or have a chronic health problem.

•You are pregnant or breast-feeding.

Important: The flu can be deadly, so if your symptoms are severe—for instance, you have a very high fever, have trouble breathing and/or feel extremely weak—seek immediate medical care.

THE RIGHT REMEDY FOR YOU

The following homeopathic remedies are among those most commonly indicated for colds or flu. Choose the remedy that most closely correlates to your symptoms.

Use *Arsenicum album* if you…

•Have alternating chills and fever.

•Are thirsty and prefer warm drinks to cold ones.

•Have a runny nose or burning sensation in the nose.

•Feel extremely weak.

•Are anxious or restless.

•Feel worse from 10 pm to 3 am.

Use *Belladonna* if you…

•Spike a sudden fever.

•Cough a lot.

•Have a hot, red face (though hands and feet may be cold).

•Have glassy eyes or dilated pupils.

•Have a throbbing headache.

•Cannot tolerate light.

•Feel slightly delirious.

Use *Gelsemium* if you…

•Ache all over (particularly if this comes on gradually).

•Feel exhausted and weak.

•Have a trembling sensation running up and down the spine.

•Sneeze and/or have a runny nose.

•Develop a sore throat.

•Get dizzy.

•Feel apathetic or antisocial.

Use *Hepar sulphuricum* if you…

•Have a thick nasal discharge.

•Develop a sore throat.

•Cannot tolerate cold drafts.

•Are extremely sensitive to touch.

•Perspire heavily.

•Feel bothered by everything and everybody.

Use *Nux vomica* if you…

•Are shivering.

•Sneeze frequently or feel a tickle in the nose.

•Have a backache or headache.

•Have stomach cramps, nausea or constipation.

•Get more congested at night.

•Have trouble sleeping.

•Are sensitive to noise.

•Feel irritable or anxious.

Use *Pulsatilla* if you…

•Have had symptoms for several days.

•Have a thick green or yellow nasal discharge.

•Must blow your nose often.

•Have an upset stomach.

•Crave cool, fresh air.

•Feel worse at night.

•Feel weepy or want attention.

To find a homeopath: Contact the Homeopathic Academy of Naturopathic Physicians

(541-840-2422, *www.hanp.net*) or the National Center for Homeopathy (703-548-7790, *www. nationalcenterforhomeopathy.org*).

Nature's Virus Killers for Colds and Flu

Mark A. Stengler, NMD, licensed naturopathic medical doctor in private practice, Stengler Center for Integrative Medicine, Encinitas, California...adjunct associate clinical professor at the National College of Natural Medicine, Portland, Oregon...author of many books, including *The Natural Physician's Healing Therapies* and coauthor of *Prescription for Natural Cures* (both from Bottom Line Books)...and author of the *Bottom Line/Natural Healing* newsletter. *www.drstengler.com*

Do you have to get a cold or the flu this coming season? No! This year can be different. With the right preparation, quick intervention and a lineup of powerful, natural virus fighters, there's a good chance that you can enjoy fall and winter without getting sick. *Here's how...*

KNOW YOUR ENEMY

Colds and flu are both caused by viruses. They are spread through the air by coughs and sneezes and through contact with contaminated objects, such as a doorknob or a hand that has been used to cover a cough. A virus is little more than a clump of genetic material (DNA or RNA) inside a packet made of protein. Stray viruses constantly land on your body. The trouble starts when they attach to cell receptors and get inside your cells. Viruses use the cells' own reproductive equipment to duplicate themselves—damaging more and more cells as they churn out millions of lookalikes.

It actually is a good sign when you begin to get a stuffy head or a runny nose. Your body is fighting back. Your immune system picks up signals from the by-products of viral activity—pain, redness, swelling, heat, fever and rash are results of your immune system launching a counterattack. Mucus is produced to help expel viral intruders.

Flu viruses are a lot more powerful than typical cold viruses. Cold symptoms are mainly confined to the head, neck and chest. Flu causes more generalized symptoms, such as fever, body aches, nausea, cramping, vomiting and severe fatigue. Flu also can develop into bronchitis. In the worst cases, it can lead to pneumonia and other severe respiratory diseases that are sometimes fatal, especially in the elderly or others with weakened immune systems.

START WITH PREVENTION

I'll tell you about great ways to feel better if you get a cold or flu, but prevention should be your first line of defense...

• **Avoid spending time around people who already are sick,** particularly if they're coughing or sneezing. If you live with someone who is sick, sleep in separate rooms. Wash your hands frequently during cold-and-flu season, and don't share towels—assign one to each family member or use paper towels. Keep your hands away from your face, especially your nose, mouth and eyes.

• **Take vitamins.** A good multivitamin/mineral supplement provides a base of nutrients to support a healthy immune system. A formula that I recommend as a preventive against viral infections is Source Naturals Wellness Formula (to find a retailer near you, call 800-815-2333 or go to *www.sourcenaturals.com*). It contains vitamins A and C, which are involved in the formation of antibodies...the minerals zinc and selenium...and immune-supportive herbs, such as garlic, echinacea and astragalus, which increase the activity of virus-fighting white blood cells. The dosage used to prevent infection is two capsules daily during cold-and-flu season, taken in conjunction with your year-round multisupplement.

• **Reduce exposure to toxins.** You are more vulnerable to viral infection when your body is "distracted" by having to deal with toxins that can damage or suppress the immune system. Toxins aren't necessarily exotic—they could include sugars and alcohol consumed to excess, fast food and other unhealthy food laced with artificial preservatives and/or pesticides. Toxins also include small but significant amounts of metals—mercury, arsenic and

251

lead—that you can get from food, water and air pollution.

It is even more vital to eat healthfully during cold-and-flu season because you're indoors more and are exposed to higher concentrations of germs. Go easy on holiday sweets and other treats, and you will be less likely to get sick.

Many people cut back their exercise regimens in winter months—a big mistake, since exercise strengthens your immune system. Also consider sitting in a dry sauna once or twice a week for 20 to 30 minutes...or a wet sauna for 10 to 15 minutes. Saunas increase sweating, which excretes toxins. Be sure to check with your doctor first if you have diabetes or heart disease.

For those who get colds or the flu every year, I recommend taking a super-greens formula in the fall to remove toxins from the colon, liver and lymphatic system. It also can be taken year-round for gentle continuous detoxification. One good product is Greens (800-643-1210, *www.greensplus.com)*, which contains chlorella, wheat grass, super-green foods and detoxifying herbs such as milk thistle. The dosage is one scoop a day dissolved in water or juice.

Don't forget the impact that toxic emotions have on your immune system. Anger, anxiety, resentment, loneliness and other chronic emotional difficulties trigger the release of hormones that suppress immune function. Seek support to overcome these problems if they linger.

DO CONVENTIONAL THERAPIES HELP?

At the first sign of a runny nose or scratchy throat, some people head straight to the drugstore for cold and flu remedies. However, there are no conventional drugs—available either by prescription or over the counter—that help cure the common cold. Nasal decongestants and pain medications may make you feel better, but they don't address the actual viral infection. Natural remedies also can help you feel better—with fewer potential side effects—and they simultaneously improve immune function.

For flu, on the other hand, a number of effective prescription antiviral drugs are available that may reduce the flu's severity and duration (by one or two days) if taken within 48 hours of the first signs of illness. Such medicines include *amantadine* (Symmetrel), *rimantadine* (Flumadine), *zanamivir* (Relenza) and *oseltamivir* (Tamiflu). Possible short-term side effects range from central nervous system problems, including anxiety and light-headedness, to decreased respiratory function and digestive upset. These antiviral drugs are not approved for children under age one.

All of these antiviral drugs except zanamivir also are approved for preventing the flu during outbreaks. These may benefit individuals who are immunocompromised—for example, those who have AIDS or have had organ or bone transplants. I prefer to have my otherwise healthy patients focus on effective natural therapies since they work so well and rarely cause side effects.

RELY ON NATURE'S VIRUS KILLERS

If you start to come down with a cold or the flu, my first recommendation is to change your diet. Eat lightly so that your body can focus on healing. For the first 24 hours, consume filtered water, broths and soups with lots of garlic, onions and spices, such as turmeric and cayenne, which relieve congestion, promote circulation and have a natural anti-inflammatory effect. Herbal teas (especially ginger, cinnamon and peppermint) and steamed vegetables also are good choices. When you're feeling better, move toward a more normal diet.

I have found several supplements to be effective for treating colds and flu. Consider taking these when people around you are sick or when you first feel symptoms. You can use one or any combination until you feel better. These also are safe for children when given in dosages of one-quarter to one-half of what I recommend for adults. The bigger the child, the higher the dose you can use.

•**Lomatium dissectum** is a plant once used by Native Americans to fight Spanish flu. Preliminary research shows that *lomatium* has the ability to prevent viruses from replicating and to stimulate white blood cell activity. With colds and flu, I often see improvement within 24 hours. In my experience, the only side effect has been an allergic reaction in the form of a measles-like rash in a small percentage of users. This rash disappears a few days after lomatium is discontinued.

Eclectic Institute makes a potent product called Lomatium-Osha (800-332-4372, *www. eclecticherb.com*), which soothes the respiratory tract. This product is 50% alcohol, so take only the dosage recommended on the label. For children, add one-quarter of the adult dosage to hot water and let it sit for five minutes so that the alcohol evaporates. Women who are pregnant or nursing should not use lomatium.

●**Elderberry,** as shown by research in Israel, can stimulate the immune system, enhance white blood cell activity and inhibit viral replication. Flu patients have reported significant improvement within 48 hours of taking elderberry. It also helps with colds. The elderberry used in research studies is Sambucol Black Elderberry Extract from Nature's Way (to find a retailer, call 800-962-8873 or go to *www.naturesway.com*). Adults should take two teaspoons four times daily…children, one teaspoon four times daily.

●**Echinacea.** Contrary to recent media reports, extracts from this plant can be effective for treating colds and flu. Echinacea makes the body's own immune cells more efficient in attacking viruses. The key is using a product that has been processed to contain a high level of active constituents. Ground-up echinacea root or leaves won't do much. The use of alcohol and water by the manufacturer to extract active components is critical to the product's potency. Also, be sure to use enough (many people don't).

Two potent, well-researched products are Echinamide: Fresh Alcohol-Free Echinacea Extract, Natural Berry Flavor, and Echinamide Anti-V Formula Softgels, both by Natural Factors (to find a retailer, call 800-322-8704 or go to *www.naturalfactors.com*). This echinacea has been shown to reduce the length and severity of the common cold.

If you feel a cold or the flu coming on, take 20 drops of liquid extract or two capsules every two waking hours for 24 hours, then cut back to every three waking hours until the illness has passed.

The same company makes a liquid preparation called Echinamide Anti-V Formula, which contains Echinamide (super-extracted Echinacea purpurea), lomatium and other virus fighters. It is the most aggressive product for cold and flu from the Natural Factors line and can be used instead of the other supplements. Take 1.5 ml every two waking hours for the first 48 hours and then every three waking hours until the illness is gone.

●**Homeopathic influenzinum** is an intriguing remedy that I have used with success. Made from active flu strains, it stimulates the body's own defense system to resist infection. It works along the same lines as an oral vaccine, but since it is homeopathic, none of the flu particles are left in the preparation. It can be used for prevention or treatment of flu and has no side effects.

Take two 30C-potency pellets twice daily for two weeks at the beginning of flu season (in early November). Take two pellets four times daily when exposed to flu sufferers or if you start to have symptoms. It is available from health-food stores and The Vitamin Shoppe (866-293-3367, *www.vitaminshoppe.com*).

●**Oscillococcinum** is another great homeopathic remedy for flu, which is also available from The Vitamin Shoppe, health-food stores and pharmacies or by calling Boiron, the manufacturer, at 800-672-4556 or visiting *www.oscillo.com*. It can be taken at the first sign of flu and is the number-one-selling homeopathic flu remedy in the US.

●**N-acetylcysteine (NAC).** This nutrient helps thin the mucus that may accompany a cold or the flu. In addition to making you feel better, NAC helps to prevent sinus and more serious chest infections. A study at University of Genoa, Italy, showed that NAC, when taken as a supplement, could help prevent as well as treat flu. The nutrient increases levels of the powerful antioxidant *glutathione* in the body, which, in turn, improves immune function. NAC is available at any health-food store and many pharmacies. If you tend to get the flu every year, take 600 mg twice daily when you are around people who have the flu or if you start feeling sick yourself.

• **Vitamin C enhances the activity of white blood cells.** I have found that taking 3,000 mg to 5,000 mg daily helps fight viral infections. However, some people get diarrhea from this amount. For immediate treatment of symptoms, start with 5,000 mg in divided doses. If loose stools occur, cut back to 3,000 mg (or even less).

Chamomile Tea Is Great For Colds and Other Ailments

Drinking at least five cups a day increases *phenolics*, which help the body fight colds...and boosts levels of *glycine*, which helps soothe muscle spasms and fights stress. Chamomile tea also may help relieve menstrual and other cramps.

Caution: Chamomile can cause a severe reaction in people who are allergic to ragweed.

Andrew L. Rubman, ND, medical director, Southbury Clinic for Traditional Medicines, Southbury, Connecticut.

Are You Showering Yourself with Germs?

Norman Pace, PhD, distinguished professor, Department of Molecular, Cellular and Developmental Biology, University of Colorado, Boulder.
Laura Baumgartner, PhD, researcher, applied molecular microbiology, University of Colorado, Boulder.

You assume that when you're taking a shower, you're getting clean, not sick. Read on for startling information.

Surprising: A new study shows that your showerhead might be blasting bad-for-you bacteria into the air—bacteria that can give you a respiratory infection every bit as serious as tuberculosis.

THE BACTERIAL BIOFILM

Researchers at the University of Colorado analyzed 45 showerheads from homes, hotels and health clubs in nine cities around the US, including New York, Chicago and Denver.

They found that three out of every 10 showerheads were coated inside with slimy, hard-to-remove "biofilms" of *Mycobacterium avium*, a bacteria similar to the type that causes tuberculosis (*Mycobacterium tuberculosis*).

When the shower is turned on, those bacteria are "aerosolized" in tiny droplets that are suspended in air and inhaled into the deepest part of the lungs, explains Norman Pace, PhD, a study researcher.

"If you are getting a face full of water when you first turn your shower on, that means you are probably getting a particularly high load of Mycobacterium avium, which may not be too healthy," he says.

Warning: Scientists theorize that the recent rise in serious and even fatal lung infections caused by these *nontuberculous mycobacteria* (NTM) is because people are taking more showers and fewer baths, say the researchers, in the *Proceedings of the National Academy of Sciences*. In fact, cases of infection from NTM now outnumber cases of tuberculosis in many areas of the US.

WHAT TO DO

NTM can infect anybody, but the most likely victims are people with a compromised immune system or people with chronic lung disease. *If any item on this list describes you, infection with NTM from your showerhead is a concern...*

• **Age 65 or older, with the thin,** weak "frail" elderly at greatest risk

• **Pregnant**

• **Chronic obstructive pulmonary disease (COPD)**

• **Undergoing chemotherapy or radiation for cancer**

• **Active leukemia,** lymphoma or multiple myeloma

• **HIV/AIDS**

• **Genetic immune-deficiency disease,** such as cystic fibrosis

• **Taking an immune-suppressing drug** after a transplant

• **Taking an immune-modifying drug** for rheumatoid arthritis or another disease

• **Excessive alcohol use**

• **Using illegal drugs such as heroin,** cocaine or methylamphetamine

Symptoms of lung disease caused by NTM can include fatigue; a persistent, dry cough; shortness of breath; weakness and "generally feeling bad," says Dr. Pace.

• **See your doctor.** If you have the above symptoms, see your doctor immediately—and specifically mention NTM as a possible cause. "This type of infection is not on the radar of most doctors," says Laura Baumgartner, PhD, a study researcher.

Important: Infection from NTM is not transmissible, like a cold.

For a person with a weak immune system, any one of the following precautions may be effective in preventing infection from NTM, say both Dr. Pace and Dr. Baumgartner.

• **Take a bath.** "Shower usage possibly is contraindicated for individuals with compromised immune or pulmonary systems," write the researchers. "Taking a bath is the simplest way to avoid the problem," adds Dr. Baumgartner.

• **Change your showerhead every six months.** "We haven't seen strong biofilms on any showerhead newer than six months," says Dr. Baumgartner.

Buy a showerhead with an effective filter. The Pall Corporation manufactures filtered showerheads for the immunocompromised—the Pall-Aquasafe or Pall Kleenpak Shower Filters. They are available at most medical supply stores and online.

• **Use a metal rather than a plastic showerhead.** Since plastic showerheads appear to "load up" with more bacteria-rich biofilms, all-metal showerheads may be a good alternative, says Dr. Pace.

• **Don't clean your showerhead with bleach.** The researchers tried that on one showerhead and re-installed it. Seven months later, they checked the showerhead again—and levels of NTM had tripled, covering 75% rather than 25% of the inside of the showerhead. "Chlorine might kill everything else and encourage the one bacteria you want to eliminate," says Dr. Baumgartner.

What Is Most Effective Against the H1N1 Flu?

Chemical compounds in a plant called *ferula asafoetida* were more effective against the H1N1 (swine) flu virus than an antiviral drug in laboratory studies. Ferula asafoetida has been used in folk medicine for many years, including during the 1918 Spanish flu epidemic. Compounds in the plant could become the basis for new antiviral medicines.

Fang-Rong Chang, MD, and Yang-Chang Wu, MD, researchers, Kaohsiung Medical University, Taiwan, and correspondent authors of a study published in the *American Chemical Society's Journal of Natural Products.*

Healing Herbs for Colds And Congestion

Kathy Abascal, RH, registered herbalist who practices in Vashon, Washington. A member of the American Herbalists Guild, she is coauthor of *Clinical Botanical Medicine* (Mary Ann Liebert).

A recent study reported that echinacea is not effective for the common cold. Then, another study, found that it does help. Does it or doesn't it?

Echinacea stimulates both white blood cells (which attack viruses) and natural killer cells (which destroy virus-infected cells). Most scientific studies of echinacea involve dosing patients every four to six hours. That's not enough.

How to use: Add about one teaspoon of echinacea tincture to one-half cup of water. Drink it once every waking hour at the first signs of a cold until symptoms subside.

Helpful: Add to the mixture one-half teaspoon of elderberry tincture—which also helps boost immunity—for additional antiviral effects.

EUCALYPTUS FOR CONGESTION

Used as an essential oil, eucalyptus penetrates the mucous membranes and promotes drainage—helpful for relieving symptoms caused by the common cold and/or sinusitis (inflammation of the sinuses). The oil also has antimicrobial properties that can inhibit viruses and bacteria.

How to use: At the first signs of a cold or sinusitis, put five to 10 drops of eucalyptus essential oil in a large bowl. Add one to two cups of steaming hot water. (The dose is correct if you can smell the eucalyptus.) Put a towel over your head, and lean over the bowl (with your eyes closed) and breathe in the steam for about 10 minutes. Repeat as needed, using fresh eucalyptus oil each time.

Caution: Keep your head far enough from the steaming water to avoid burning yourself.

20

Natural Remedies for Women

All-Natural Beauty Products You Can Make at Home

Skin is porous—so when you use synthetic personal-care products on your hands, face and scalp, artificial ingredients may be absorbed into your bloodstream.

Better: Create your own beauty products using all-natural ingredients available at supermarkets and health-food stores. Unless noted, products do not require refrigeration and can be stored for up to one year in a resealable plastic or glass container (new or recycled).

• **Peppermint hand smoother.** This removes dead skin and stimulates cell regeneration.

1 cup extra virgin olive oil

1 cup coarse salt

10 drops peppermint essential oil

Place all ingredients in a clean container (such as a mason jar), and mix thoroughly.

Daily: Gently massage a grape-sized dollop onto hands for two minutes…rinse with warm water.

• **Beeswax lip balm.** This soothes and protects chapped lips. For color, add a bit of left-over lipstick from the bottom of a used-up tube.

4 teaspoons castor oil

1 teaspoon beeswax

½ teaspoon honey

¼ teaspoon lipstick (optional)

5 drops sweet orange essential oil

Place all ingredients except orange oil in a small saucepan. Stirring, warm over low heat until melted. Remove from heat. Add orange oil and mix well. Fill a casserole dish with two inches of ice water and set the saucepan in the ice-water bath. Whisk the balm rapidly for

Andrea R. Frayser, ND, award-winning cosmetics formulator and founder of All Natural Diverse Eco-Friendly (ANDE) cosmetics based in Smithsburg, Maryland.

one minute. Spoon balm into a clean, shallow container (such as a baby food jar), cap and refrigerate 30 minutes or until balm solidifies.

Several times daily: Apply to lips with fingertips or a lip brush.

• **Five-oil hair therapy.** This soothes an itchy scalp and makes dry, damaged hair silkier.

¼ cup extra virgin olive oil

¼ cup grapeseed oil

4 tablespoons jojoba oil

10 drops lavender essential oil

10 drops rosemary essential oil

In a small saucepan, combine all ingredients and warm over low heat for three minutes (do not boil). Let cool, then pour into a clean plastic container with a small-hole cap (such as an empty liquid soap bottle).

Weekly: Leaning over a sink, squeeze mixture onto dry hair, using enough to coat all strands. Cover hair with a shower cap for 30 to 60 minutes. Shampoo to remove oil.

• **Two-tea shampoo.** This gentle formula is good for all hair types.

2 cups distilled water

1 chamomile tea bag

1 green tea bag

1 organic orange peel, grated

2 teaspoons chopped fresh rosemary

1 teaspoon chopped fresh sage

½ teaspoon jojoba oil

¾ cup liquid castile soap

In a small saucepan, combine water, tea bags, orange peel and herbs. Bring to a boil, then remove from heat. Let stand, covered, for 30 minutes. Strain liquid into medium-sized bowl. Add jojoba oil and castile soap, stirring until well blended. Pour into a clean, unbreakable container with a tight-fitting lid.

Daily or as needed: Wash hair using ¼ cup to ½ cup of mixture. This also makes an excellent all-over body wash.

Note: Store in the refrigerator, and use within one month for best aroma.

For containers: Check in a drugstore or a dollar store.

Herbal Aphrodisiacs

Laurie Steelsmith, ND, author of *Natural Choices for Women's Health* (Three Rivers). Her private practice in naturopathic and Chinese medicine is in Honolulu. *www.naturalchoicesforwomen.com.*

If your libido is lagging, rekindle the spark with herbs used by practitioners of *traditional Chinese medicine* (TCM). Try them one at a time, in the order presented (*epimedium* and *rehmannia* can be taken together). If you don't see results with one herb after two months, discontinue it and try the next. Typically an herb corrects the underlying problem within six months and is then discontinued. These herbs are sold in health-food stores. Do not use while pregnant or breastfeeding. If you have any health problems, talk to your doctor before beginning herbal therapy.

Cordyceps (a mushroom) improves kidney health, according to TCM, by supporting *kidney qi* (vital energy)—and abundant qi is necessary for a strong libido. Take 500 mg in tablet form two to three times daily. Do not use if you have a fever because it could worsen symptoms.

Ginseng contains compounds called ginsenosides, which may boost enzymes that help to break down or otherwise dispatch stress hormones, such as cortisol. Stress dampens libido, so decreasing stress helps to increase desire. Ginseng "modulates" the nervous system, boosting sexual energy if you are lethargic and helping you relax if you are tense. Using an extract labeled "standardized to 4% ginsenosides," take 100 mg in pill form or 50 drops in tincture form, two or three times daily. Do not use if you have hot flashes, insomnia, dry mouth or dry skin—ginseng could exacerbate symptoms.

Epimedium (horny goat weed) stimulates the nervous system, especially nerves in the genitalia, by increasing the flow of qi to the pelvis. It usually is sold in a combination herbal formula. Choose a brand that provides 800 mg of epimedium per day. Do not use if you have a fever, hot flashes or insomnia.

Rehmannia is an herb that draws energy into the reproductive organs through the body's meridians (energy pathways). Usually it is sold in combination with other herbs. Select a brand that has 300 mg of rehmannia per tablet, and take three times per day. Do not use if you have diarrhea, because it can loosen stool.

Bonus: Rehmannia eases anxiety and hot flashes—making it even easier to get into the mood for love.

Better Bones

Recent finding: In a study of 1,500 healthy women (ages 70 to 85), hip-bone density was 2.8% higher in those who drank caffeinated or caffeine-free black tea, compared with people who did not drink tea. Tea drinkers consumed an average of three cups daily.

Theory: Flavonoid antioxidants in black tea may stimulate production of new cells that build bone.

Self-defense: Drinking black tea daily may help protect your bones as you age. If your doctor has advised you not to drink caffeine, opt for caffeine-free black tea.

Amanda Devine, PhD, senior lecturer, nutrition program, Edith Cowan University, Joondalup, Australia.

Natural Remedies That Really Work to Ease Hot Flashes

Andrea Sikon, MD, board-certified internist and director of primary care/women's health for the Medicine Institute at the Cleveland Clinic in Cleveland. She is certified as a menopause practitioner by the North American Menopause Society.

As many as 75% of menopausal women experience the sudden waves of body heat known as hot flashes. Episodes can be mild, causing just a few moments of discomfort...or intense enough to make a woman drip with perspiration.

Hot flashes and night sweats (which come on during sleep) are triggered by fluctuating levels of the hormone estrogen, affecting a woman's inner thermostat and causing blood vessels near the skin's surface to dilate. Typically, a hot flash ends after several minutes, though it can last a half-hour or more. Episodes generally abate after a few years—but some women continue to have hot flashes for the rest of their lives.

Here's what you should know about which remedies help...which are of questionable value...and which are downright dangerous.

Important: Before beginning any kind of therapy, talk to your doctor about its pros and cons and how they relate to your individual risk factors.

PRESCRIPTION DRUGS

Estrogen is the only prescription medication currently FDA-approved specifically for hot flashes, but others can be prescribed "off-label."

Most effective...

• **Estrogen therapy.** This reduces hot flashes by making up for a woman's own diminishing production of the hormone. It also eases other menopausal symptoms, such as mood swings, vaginal dryness, thinning skin and bone loss...and may reduce risk for hip fracture and colon cancer.

Caution: Estrogen therapy can increase risk for heart disease, stroke, blood clots, breast cancer and possibly Alzheimer's disease. The more time that has passed since a woman reached menopause and/or the longer she takes estrogen, the greater the risks may be.

Consider estrogen if: Hot flashes reduce your quality of life...you have additional menopausal symptoms...and your doctor says that you have no increased cardiovascular or breast cancer risk. If you have not had a hysterectomy, you also must take progestogen (a drug similar to the hormone progesterone) to guard against uterine cancer.

Sometimes helpful...

• **Antidepressants.** Selective serotonin reuptake inhibitors (SSRIs), such as *paroxetine*

(Paxil), and serotonin/norepinephrine reuptake inhibitors (SNRIs), such as *venlafaxine* (Effexor), may relieve hot flashes by stabilizing the body's temperature-control mechanism.

New: The manufacturer of the SNRI *desvenlafaxine* (Pristiq) has been given for FDA approval of the drug as a treatment for hot flashes.

SSRIs can cause weight gain, dry mouth and decreased sex drive...and may interfere with the breast cancer drug tamoxifen in some women. SNRIs can cause insomnia, dry mouth, constipation or diarrhea, and perhaps high blood pressure.

Consider an antidepressant if: You cannot or do not want to use estrogen therapy and/or hot flashes are accompanied by mood swings.

•*Gabapentin* (Neurontin). In one study, this antiseizure drug was as effective against hot flashes as estrogen. Side effects may include sedation, dizziness and mild or widespread swelling.

Consider gabapentin if: You also have insomnia and do not have additional symptoms better treated by estrogen or antidepressants.

•*Clonidine* (Catapres). This blood pressure drug affects the central nervous system. In some small studies, it reduced hot flashes. Clonidine can cause dizziness, fatigue, dry mouth and constipation.

Consider clonidine if: Other therapies have failed to relieve hot flashes, and you also require treatment for high blood pressure.

ALTERNATIVE THERAPIES

The FDA does not test herbs or dietary supplements. Nonprescription products labeled "natural" are not necessarily effective or even safe. If you try them, choose brands that have the United States Pharmacopeia (USP) seal to ensure purity.

Perhaps helpful...

•**Supplements of soy and black cohosh.** These have phytoestrogens, plant compounds with estrogen-like effects. Theoretically, they could ease hot flashes via the same mechanism as estrogen—but they also may carry similar risks.

Caution: Women who ought not take prescription estrogen (for instance, due to elevated risk for heart disease or breast cancer) should use these products only when they have their doctors' approval.

•**Flaxseeds.** One small Mayo Clinic study found that hot flash frequency was reduced by half in women who consumed two tablespoons of ground flaxseeds twice daily for six weeks.

Possible reason: Flaxseeds contain lignans, antioxidants with estrogenic effects. Get your doctor's approval before using. Drink lots of water with flaxseeds to prevent gas and constipation.

•**Acupuncture.** A few studies suggest that this is somewhat effective for hot flashes.

Best: Use an acupuncturist certified by the National Certification Commission for Acupuncture and Oriental Medicine (904-598-1005, *www.nccaom.org*).

Probably not helpful...

•**Evening primrose oil...ginseng...vitamins B, C and E.** These fared no better than placebos in studies.

Ginseng should not be used with blood thinners, stimulants or antidepressant MAO inhibitors...vitamins C and E can cause bleeding in people who take blood thinners.

•**Magnets.** Supporters claim that magnetic fields have healing powers. However, in an Indiana University study, sham magnets eased hot flashes better than real magnets.

Dangerous...

•**Over-the-counter topical progestogen cream.** Absorption varies dramatically from woman to woman—so using these without a doctor's supervision can lead to hormone imbalances.

•**Dong quai.** This herb can interfere with medications and may contain a potential carcinogen.

•**Kava.** This herb is intoxicating and can damage the liver.

•**Licorice extract.** In large doses, it can cause leg edema (swelling), high blood pressure and dangerously low potassium levels.

Hot Flashes May Signal Blood Pressure Problem

Linda M. Gerber, PhD, professor of public health and director of the biostatistics and research methodology core in the Department of Public Health at Weill Medical College of Cornell University.

Andrew L. Rubman, ND, medical director, Southbury Clinic for Traditional Medicines, Southbury, Connecticut.

Most of us women know that simply reaching midlife puts us at greater risk for heart disease, since we tend to lose the protective effects of estrogen. While previous research has linked menopause to high blood pressure (a major risk factor for heart attack), a new study links one of its most irksome symptoms—hot flashes—to high blood pressure. With hot flashes—defined as being sudden feelings of intense heat that may include sweating and a rapid heartbeat, and lasting usually from two to 30 minutes—being one of the major hallmarks of menopause and perimenopause, this study may be a "red alert" to identify a danger signal for women at risk of future heart problems.

THE RESEARCH

Researchers at Weill Medical College of Cornell University found that women who had hot flashes tended to have higher systolic (top number) blood pressure compared with the lucky ones who didn't have hot flashes. In the study, 154 women aged 18 to 65 with no previous cardiovascular disease and who either had normal blood pressure or mild hypertension (high blood pressure) wore portable monitors that recorded their blood pressure while they were awake and asleep. Women who reported having hot flashes were found to have an age-adjusted average systolic blood pressure of 141 while awake, and 129 while they were asleep, compared with 132 and 119, respectively, for women who did not report hot flashes. The blood pressure differences between these two groups remained statistically significant after controlling for high blood pressure risk factors including race/ethnicity, age and body mass index (BMI).

"One-third of the women we studied reported having had hot flashes two weeks prior to wearing a BP monitor," said Linda M. Gerber, PhD, the study's lead author, who is a professor of public health and director of the biostatistics and research methodology core in the Department of Public Health at Weill Medical College of Cornell University. "Among these women, systolic blood pressure was significantly higher—even after adjusting for whether they were pre-menopausal, menopausal or post-menopausal."

DO YOU NEED TO WORRY?

So if you are experiencing hot flashes, even only once in a while, should you worry that you may be at risk for high blood pressure? "You should keep your eye on it, but not be unduly concerned," said Dr. Gerber. "It's important to get an accurate representation of your blood pressure, but that is often difficult to get. Blood pressure varies over the course of the day. Some people get the white coat effect, in which your blood pressure is high when you go to see your doctor. I don't want people to rush to see their doctors. One way to keep an eye on it would be to get a home monitor and check it on a frequent basis."

And what about those pesky hot flashes? "You can do things that might be beneficial to limit the severity and frequency of your hot flashes," said Dr. Gerber. "Keep your weight down, exercise regularly and eat a healthy diet."

Andrew L. Rubman, ND, adds that the association between estrogen reduction and both hot flashes and increased systolic blood pressure may be due to concentrations of calcium within the tissue responsible for both. There are effective natural ways to modulate this, including black cohosh and soy isoflavones, but it's important to work with an experienced expert, such as a naturopathic physician, to ensure safety.

Most important, adds Dr. Gerber: "Be aware that if the frequency of hot flashes increases suddenly and if you have a lot of severe flashes when you didn't have them before, you should get your blood pressure checked."

Acupuncture for Female Problems

Yi Hung Chan, DPM, LAc, The Bendheim Integrative Medicine Center, Memorial Sloan-Kettering Cancer Center, New York City. *www.yourdrchan.com*

Gynecological complaints like pelvic pain, infertility, menstrual cramps and the mood swings and hot flashes of menopause are often highly responsive to acupuncture—we've heard this anecdotally from friends and, interestingly, also from doctors, both mainstream and integrative. And we are seeing more and more published research backing this up as well—most recently, a 12-week study of breast cancer patients compared acupuncture treatment to use of an antidepressant, *venlafaxine* (Effexor), for relief of severe hot flashes and other menopausal symptoms. Both treatments were effective, but with some important differences. The women in the acupuncture group reported no side effects, while the drug group suffered many unpleasant ones. The acupuncture group also reported improved energy, clarity of thinking, sexual desire and overall sense of well-being. Finally, improvement among the acupuncture patients lasted much longer—from three to four months after finishing treatment, compared with the Effexor group, in which symptoms resumed within two weeks after they stopped the drug.

WHY IT WORKS FOR WOMEN'S ISSUES

We are not surprised by this, given our many stories about acupuncture, but it prompted us to look into the therapy's use for a wider range of gynecological issues. We called acupuncturist Yi Chan, DPM, LAc, who is on staff at The Bendheim Integrative Medicine Center at Memorial Sloan-Kettering Cancer Center in New York and in private practice in West Orange, New Jersey. Dr. Chan says the basic philosophy of Chinese medicine is to maintain proper balance of energy flow (chi) in the body and that when the flow is disrupted, it creates disorders and discomfort. He likens this to the New York City subway where a breakdown of even a single train will cause widespread disruptions in the system. Acupuncture, he says, is a way to locate and correct the disruption of the chi.

Dr. Chan reports that acupuncture helps 80% of his patients—bringing "great improvement" to 60%. With acupuncture, most patients can tell by about the sixth treatment if it is helping their problem—if nothing has changed by then (as is true for about 20%), the challenge may be too great for acupuncture alone to resolve.

WHAT CAN ACUPUNCTURE HELP?

●**Menstrual cycle problems (flow, regularity, pain).** Sometimes stress, diet or excessive exercise can disrupt normal functioning of the menstrual cycle, by sending energy to the wrong places, explains Dr. Chan. Acupuncture can help repair and "smooth out the bumpy ride," whether the flow is too heavy or too little, or the cycle is shortened, delayed or irregular. Typically, the practitioner treats the patient through several cycles, with about eight to 12 weeks of treatments.

● **Fertility issues.** Acupuncture can be helpful for women having trouble conceiving, and new research shows that it improves the success rate of in-vitro fertilization. Dr. Chan suggests not waiting many months to seek acupuncture to help fertility, urging women who don't get pregnant to use acupuncture sooner rather than later, as it can "free up" their energy flow. But such women should always first have a complete physical exam by a gynecologist to be sure that everything is anatomically functional.

● **Endometriosis and uterine fibroids.** These particular problems can be stubborn and complex. While acupuncture can help ease pain and excessive bleeding, women with endometriosis and/or fibroids often require conventional treatment as well, sometimes including surgery. In those cases, acupuncture can help soothe post-surgery discomfort, supporting healing and re-establishment of the cycle. Again, it is crucial to have a gynecological examination to determine the nature and extent of the problem—if symptoms are mild to moderate, Dr. Chan says acupuncture can help right away, but for severe symptoms, he says women should first see a medical doctor and then seek out an acupuncturist.

•**Hot flashes.** As mentioned above, acupuncture can ease the frequency and severity of hot flashes as well. Dr. Chan advises his patients to keep a notebook, writing down frequency and intensity of the flashes as they occur. With acupuncture, "the frequency may abate, but the intensity remains the same—or vice-versa," he says. "By observing this carefully you will know if acupuncture is working for you." Dr. Chan also has a list of "cooling" foods advised in Chinese medicine for such patients—watermelon, mung bean, mustard greens, bitter melon and grass jelly.

FIND AN ACUPUNCTURIST

To find an acupuncturist near you, go to the Web site of the National Certification Commission for Acupuncture and Oriental Medicine at *www.nccaom.org*, which lists board certified practitioners. Word of mouth is also good, says Dr. Chan. Insurance covers treatment in many cases, though not always. Perhaps this too will change as Western medicine begins to fully embrace the benefits of acupuncture.

Natural Therapies for Endometriosis...No Surgery Needed

Victoria Maizes, MD, professor of clinical medicine, family and community medicine and public health and executive director of the Arizona Center for Integrative Medicine at University of Arizona in Tucson. She is coeditor of *Integrative Women's Health* (Oxford University). *www.integrativemedicine.arizona.edu*

With endometriosis, tissue from the endometrium (uterine lining) migrates outside the uterus via the fallopian tubes, then grows on the ovaries, fallopian tubes, rectum, bladder and/or pelvic lining.

During menstruation, this displaced tissue behaves as it would if it were in the uterus—it thickens, breaks down and bleeds. Trapped blood inflames surrounding tissues, which can lead to internal scarring. Resulting pain ranges from mild to incapacitating...scarring can impair fertility. Symptoms usually ease after menopause, though hormone therapy may lead to flare-ups.

Conventional treatment typically involves oral contraceptives, which block the effects of natural hormones on the growths outside the uterus...or the drug *leuprolide* (Lupron), which stops menstruation.

Downside: These drugs can cause weight gain and mood swings. When medication does not bring sufficient relief, patients may be advised to have endometriosis tissue surgically removed or to have a hysterectomy—but all surgery carries risks for infection and complications.

Natural approaches may help you avoid drugs and surgery. *Try...*

•**Anti-inflammatory diet.** This reduces the inflammation caused by trapped menstrual blood. To increase intake of anti-inflammatory omega-3 fatty acids, eat more fatty fish (herring, mackerel), flaxseeds and walnuts... and take a daily fish oil supplement. Every day, eat several servings of vegetables and fruits, which are rich in antioxidants. Avoid inflammation-promoting refined carbohydrates (white bread, doughnuts)...eat more whole grains (brown rice, bulgur).

•**Pelvic floor physical therapy.** Chronic muscle tension in the abdomen, legs and pelvic floor may result from a conditioned response to pelvic pain, exacerbating discomfort. Pelvic floor physical therapy from a specially trained therapist can reduce muscle tension and improve day-to-day functioning.

Also helpful: Yoga, stretching.

•**Botanical supplements.** Black cohosh, black haw and/or ginger may help by reducing the effects of inflammatory enzymes and proteins, boosting antioxidants or reducing sensitivity to painful stimuli. Supplements can cause side effects or interact with medications, so consult a holistic doctor for dosage and usage guidelines. Do not take black cohosh or black haw if you have a history of breast cancer. Do not take ginger if you have a bleeding disorder or gallstones.

• **Acupuncture.** Various studies suggest that this can ease the pain of endometriosis, though the exact mechanism is not known.

Find a practitioner: Contact the American Association of Acupuncture and Oriental Medicine (866-455-7999, *www.aaaomonline.org*).

Simplest: Use a heating pad...or take a warm bath to ease discomfort.

Reducing Breast Cancer Risk After Menopause

JoAnn E. Manson, MD, DrPH, professor of medicine and women's health at Harvard Medical School and chair of the division of preventive medicine at Brigham and Women's Hospital, both in Boston. She is one of the lead investigators for two highly influential studies on women's health—the Harvard Nurses' Health Study and the Women's Health Initiative. Dr. Manson is author, with Shari Bassuk, ScD, of *Hot Flashes, Hormones & Your Health* (McGraw-Hill).

Many postmenopausal women think their primary risk factor for breast cancer is genetics. Yet most breast cancers occur in women with no family history of the disease, and the major breast cancer genes (BRCA1 and BRCA2) account for only 5% to 10% of cases. *The primary risk factors...*

• **Age.** Average age at diagnosis is 61, and rates are highest after age 70.

• **Estrogen.** This hormone stimulates growth of breast tissues—including abnormal cells. Estrogen levels are highest during the childbearing years, so the earlier you started menstruating and the later you reached menopause, the higher your risk.

To help prevent breast cancer...

• **Guard against vitamin-D deficiency.** Vitamin D may fight formation of blood vessels that nourish tumors and inhibit division of cells that line the breast. Many experts now

recommend that all adults get 1,000 international units (IU) daily.

Sources: Sunlight (from which skin synthesizes vitamin D)...cod liver oil, fatty fish (mackerel, tuna), fortified milk and cereals...and supplements of vitamin D3 (*cholecalciferol*).

• **Get adequate folate, a B vitamin involved in DNA synthesis and repair.** Eat three one-cup servings daily of folate-rich foods—leafy green vegetables, garbanzo beans, peas, citrus fruits.

• **Avoid unnecessary hormone therapy.** Consider taking estrogen (plus progestin to guard against uterine cancer, if you have not had a hysterectomy) only if hot flashes and night sweats significantly disrupt your sleep or quality of life. Use the lowest effective dose... try to limit use to less than four or five years.

• **Watch your weight.** Obesity after menopause may double breast cancer risk, perhaps because fat cells take over the ovaries' job of producing estrogen. Nearly one-quarter of postmenopausal breast cancers in the US are due to excess weight.

• **Exercise 30 minutes or more per day.** Exercise lowers blood levels of insulin and estrogen, both of which are risk factors for breast cancer.

• **Eat less saturated fat.** In a study of 48,835 postmenopausal women, those who were accustomed to a high-fat diet reduced their breast cancer risk by adopting a diet in which less than 25% of daily calories came from fat.

• **Limit alcohol intake.** Even moderate drinking raises breast cancer risk by increasing estrogen and decreasing folate absorption. Also, alcohol can be metabolized into *acetaldehyde*, a potential carcinogen, so have no more than one drink daily.

If you're at high risk: The drugs *tamoxifen* and *raloxifene* can reduce breast cancer risk—but increase the odds of blood clots, hot flashes, uterine cancer and perhaps stroke. Ask your doctor if these drugs are right for you.

A Midwife At Menopause?

Angela Deneris, PhD, certified nurse-midwife and associate professor in the Nurse-Midwifery and Women's Health Nurse Practitioner Programs at the University of Utah, Salt Lake City.

Why would you want to see a midwife at menopause? Because they offer a uniquely personal and holistic perspective on the journey. Though historically their role has been to help women through childbirth, many modern midwives now focus on helping women to feel better and be healthier at the other end of the reproductive cycle.

It's an intriguing concept, so we spoke with Angela Deneris, PhD, a certified nurse midwife and associate professor in the Nurse-Midwifery and Women's Health Nurse Practitioner Programs at the University of Utah. According to Dr. Deneris, who has been in practice for 30 years and whose clients range in age from teens to a woman in her 80s, Certified Nurse-Midwives (CNMs) and Certified Midwives (CMs) are fully qualified to partner a woman through perimenopause, menopause and the postmenopausal years—and some actually specialize in caring for older women. All midwives are trained to provide the full spectrum of routine gynecological care—including pap smears and pelvic examinations and referrals for screening and diagnostic tests, such as mammograms and sonograms, as well as routine primary care, including annual physicals and screening for conditions such as diabetes, heart disease and declining bone health.

A MORE PERSONAL RELATIONSHIP

Midwives are trained in "whole woman care," emphasizing natural treatments and lifestyle adjustments over pharmaceutical drugs. For instance, said Dr. Deneris, for a woman complaining about hot flashes, a midwife will start by trying to ascertain whether specific situations trigger them and will also discuss dietary and lifestyle measures that might help reduce their severity or frequency. A midwife will coach patients in how to take more responsibility for the aspects of her health that she can control by eating right, exercising and keeping track of medical history and records. And for those women who really need something more, midwives are qualified to prescribe medication and hormone replacement therapy if appropriate.

MIDWIFE VS. MD— WHAT'S THE DIFFERENCE?

Education for midwives varies from state to state, with some requiring a bachelor of science and others requiring a degree in nursing prior to midwifery training. Accreditation requirements (for both Certified Midwives and Certified Nurse-Midwives) are standardized by The American College of Nurse Midwives (ACNM). An accredited midwife is able to do just about all aspects of routine care (and childbirth, of course) up to but not including surgery.

For older women in particular, midwives work closely with doctors when trying to determine whether symptoms and discomfort a patient is experiencing are caused by aging or disease—especially if serious illness, such as cancer, is suspected. In that case, the doctor will take over the patient's care, but the midwife often remains very involved.

For instance, Dr. Deneris told me she continues to provide gynecological and other care for her patients who have had breast cancer, including screening for heart disease, diabetes and depression as well as counseling for diet and exercise. "Staying involved while a woman is receiving care for a serious, chronic health issue enables us to continue to treat our patients as whole, complete women," she said.

PATIENTS GET MORE TIME

As part of their holistic perspective, Dr. Deneris said women can also expect that a midwife will devote much more time to each patient. She told me she spends about an hour with women over 40 for their annual visits. "We discuss lifestyle, diet, exercise routines, and the particular stressors in their lives, and then put the pieces together," she said. "Rather than immediately prescribing something for mood swings or insomnia, we'll look beyond such symptoms to examine the broader picture." Dr. Deneris said she routinely discusses

265

sexuality with her patients…asks about quality of life…screens for depression…and makes it a point to explore whether there are possible issues around abuse or addiction. It's all intended to provide context for understanding what is happening with a woman's health.

Most insurers cover midwife services. To locate a qualified midwife, Dr. Deneris suggested visiting *www.midwife.org*, the Web site for the American College of Nurse-Midwives, which offers a search option for locating a midwife by entering a Zip code or town.

How to (Finally!) Get Rid of Acne

Mary Ellen Brademas, MD, clinical assistant professor of dermatology at New York University Langone Medical Center and a dermatologist in private practice, both in New York City.

It's frustrating to battle pimples and wrinkles simultaneously—yet up to 15% of women do have acne breakouts in midlife and beyond.

Possible reason: Production of the hormone estrogen, a natural pimple suppressor, decreases at menopause—and may leave a relatively high ratio of acne-provoking hormones called androgens. Acne develops when pores get blocked with natural skin oils.

Acne develops when pores get blocked with natural skin oils. Products that helped when you were younger now may make acne worse because they're too drying for mature skin—and excessive dryness prompts the sebaceous glands to pump out even more pore-clogging oil. *What does help…*

• **Use anti-acne skin-care products.** Wash your face thoroughly with cold cream or a soapless product, such as Cetaphil Gentle Skin Cleanser. Exfoliate with a cream or gel containing *salicylic acid, azelaic acid* and/or *glycolic acid* to slough off dead skin cells that trap oil. Follow with oil-based moisturizer and makeup —water-based products are too drying.

• **Listen to your gut.** Stress activates the nervous system, which in turn triggers reactions in the digestive tract and skin. A churning stomach is a signal that you need to reduce stress if you want to protect your complexion.

Best: Do whatever relaxes you—listen to music, phone a friend, meditate.

• **Identify your personal pimple-provoking foods.** Chocolate doesn't cause breakouts—but the iodine in seafood may irritate pores, and some people are sensitive to dairy products and/or tree nuts (walnuts, cashews, almonds). Keep a food log for a few weeks, and look for patterns. If you discover that you always break out a day or two after eating strawberries, for instance, avoid them.

• **Try natural remedies.** Soak one-third of an ounce of witch hazel bark or white oak bark (sold in health-food stores) overnight in one cup of water. Strain liquid, then saturate a cotton ball and wipe it over your entire face. Let the skin dry before putting on your makeup.

Before bed: Beat an egg yolk, smooth it onto your face, let dry for 10 minutes, then remove it with cold water and a washcloth.

If your acne continues, see a dermatologist. *You may need to…*

• **Try prescription medication.** *Isotretinoin* (Accutane), derived from vitamin A, reduces the oil secreted by the skin…changes the shape and texture of cells that line pores so oil is less easily trapped…and restores collagen and elastin, proteins that give skin its structure. After five months, as many as three out of four patients are cured of acne.

Caution: Accutane can cause severe birth defects, so don't use it if you have any chance of getting pregnant. Accutane can raise levels of cholesterol and triglycerides (blood fats) and cause fluctuations in blood sugar—so your doctor should conduct frequent blood tests to monitor these.

• **Consider hormone therapy.** This may combat acne (and other menopausal symptoms) by raising the body's levels of estrogen. However, it can increase the risk for breast cancer and heart disease, so talk with your doctor about the potential risks and benefits.

Fight Bone Loss—And Look Better, Too

Karena Thek Lineback, certified Pilates fitness instructor and rehabilitation therapist. She is president of Pilates Teck in Santa Clarita, California and author of *OsteoPilates: Increase Bone Density, Reduce Fracture Risk, Look and Feel Great!* (New Page).

Menopause and the use of steroid drugs are common causes of the bone-thinning disease known as osteoporosis. *But few people are aware of other osteoporosis risk factors, including...*

•**Hypertension,** which can increase the amount of calcium excreted in urine, possibly resulting in loss of bone mineral density.

•**Gastrointestinal disorders,** such as colitis and irritable bowel syndrome (IBS), all of which reduce absorption of dietary calcium.

It's also a big mistake to overlook bone loss in men. While eight million American women have been diagnosed with osteoporosis, two million American men also suffer from the condition—and several million additional women and men are at risk for the disease.

Both women and men can help prevent osteoporosis with a variety of bone-protecting strategies. Among the most important are eating a well-balanced diet (including calcium-rich foods, such as low-fat dairy products ...almonds...and green, leafy vegetables, including broccoli and kale) and taking mineral and vitamin supplements (for example, calcium, vitamin D, magnesium, potassium, zinc and vitamin K).

WHAT IS OSTEOPILATES?

Most doctors recommend weight-bearing exercise, such as walking, stair-climbing and/or strength-training with hand weights, as part of an osteoporosis prevention program.

After eight years of working with women and men at risk for osteoporosis, I have developed a specialized form of the exercise technique known as Pilates to help fight bone loss. Pilates concentrates on strengthening the "core muscles" (in the abdomen and the back) that stabilize and support the spine, as well as the small muscles throughout the body.

I call my version *OsteoPilates*. The exercises of OsteoPilates are designed to stimulate bone growth in areas that are especially vulnerable to thinning (the spine, wrists and hips), while also providing the overall toning benefits of Pilates.

OsteoPilates is generally safe for people with low bone density (including those with osteoporosis) and those with normal bone density, as measured by a *dual energy X-ray absorptiometry* (DEXA) scan. Ask your doctor before starting the program.

The following basic workout, which takes about 15 minutes to complete, should be performed three times weekly, with at least one day of rest between sessions. (The floor exercises can be performed on a thin mat, such as a yoga mat.)

TOE TOUCHES

Purpose: Builds bone mass in the spine, thighs and knees.

What to do: Lie on your back with your bent legs in the air. Your knees should be positioned directly above your hips and your lower legs extended slightly higher than your knees. Point your toes. Next, while keeping your spine pressed to the floor and your legs slightly bent, move your feet forward and downward in a rainbow-like arc until the tips of your toes touch the floor. Then slowly return to the starting position. Repeat four to 12 times.

SWAN

Purpose: Builds bone mass in the spine and wrists.

What to do: Lie on your stomach with legs squeezed together and arms crossed under your head so that your forehead rests on your hands. Keeping your forehead on your hands, lift your head, shoulders and arms off the floor. As you lower them again, lift your legs off the floor, being careful to keep them straight. Imagine that you're a seesaw—as one-half of your body goes down, the other half goes up. Repeat six to 10 times.

Next, lie on your stomach with your hands under your shoulders and your palms flat on the floor. Slowly straighten your arms to lift your head and torso off the floor, while at the same time pulling your navel in toward your spine. Return slowly to the starting position. Repeat four to eight times.

MERMAID

Purpose: Builds bone mass in the spine.

What to do: While sitting on a firm chair, reach your right hand toward the ceiling, being careful to keep your shoulders level. Looking straight ahead, lean your raised arm, head and torso to the left, keeping your right hip firmly pressed down. When you've bent as far as you can, pause, then return to the starting position. Repeat three to six times on each side.

SIDE KICK

Purpose: Builds bone mass in the hips, thighs and knees.

What to do: Lie on your right side with your torso straight and your legs angled forward, so that your body is bent in a slight "L" shape. Fold your right arm under your head, rest your head on your forearm and place your left palm on the floor for support. Keeping your left hip directly above your right hip, lift your left leg about four inches. Flex your left foot and swing your left leg forward as far as you can (stopping when you feel your torso moving), giving a little extra kick at the end of the forward swing. Now swing the leg behind you, giving two small kicks at the end of the backward swing. Repeat eight times on each side.

Have Much Better Sex As You Age

Dagmar O'Connor, PhD, sex therapist in private practice in New York City. She is creator of a self-help sex book: *How to Make Love to the Same Person for the Rest of Your Life—and Still Love It* (Virgin Black Lace). *www. dagmaroconnor.com.*

Most older Americans grew up not talking about sex. Through others' silence, they were taught to believe that sex was shameful and taboo. Any men-

tion of sex between "old folks," in particular, made people shudder.

Sexual activity is a natural and healthy part of life. In fact, you can get better at sex and enjoy it more—at any age. I treat couples in their 80s and 90s who wouldn't dare tell their children or grandchildren that they're seeing a sex therapist. Typically, whatever the state of their sex life, therapy improves it.

With retirement's gift of time, you can learn how the aging body works differently from its younger self, what pleases you individually and how to please each other in new ways.

PRACTICAL MATTERS

Yes, bodies change with age. Many women start to feel old and asexual at menopause. Men may develop erectile problems. But most difficulties can be overcome.

Physical change: Chronic conditions, such as diabetes, thyroid disease, cancer, Parkinson's disease and depression, can affect sexual function. With heart disease, sex can cause chest pain, and with asthma, breathlessness.

Remember, intercourse is the equivalent of walking two city blocks. Check with your doctor first.

Physical change: Joint pain and stiffness from arthritis makes sex difficult.

Solution: Relax in a Jacuzzi or bath before sex…vacation together in a warm climate… find new positions that won't stress your sore spots.

Physical change: Many drugs—antidepressant, hypertension, heart disease and some cancer medications, as well as alcohol—can affect sexual function.

Solution: If your sex drive is down or you're having other sexual problems, ask your doctor whether your medications could be the cause and if switching might help.

Physical change: After menopause, vaginal tissue becomes less elastic, the vaginal opening becomes smaller and lubrication decreases.

Result: Discomfort during intercourse.

Solution: Don't avoid sex—increase it. The more tissue is exercised, the more it stretches and the more you relax your muscles. Using your finger or a dildo, gently widen the vaginal opening every day. If the problem persists for more than two months, see a gynecologist or sex therapist.

Meanwhile, smooth the way with a nonprescription water-based lubricant, such as Astroglide or K-Y Jelly.

Not as good: Oil-based lubricants or petroleum products such as Vaseline. They may linger in the vagina and irritate it.

Bonus: Applying lubricant may get you in the mood for sex. Or let your partner apply it as part of lovemaking. Good foreplay makes lubrication flow naturally.

Physical change: With age, men require more manual stimulation for erections, take longer to ejaculate and have a longer refractory period—the amount of time between an orgasm and the next erection.

Solution: Patience. These changes are an invitation to discover the slow, loving sex that many women, in particular, have always wanted but haven't received.

Erectile problems can be treated medically, too. Discuss the situation with your doctor. You may be referred to a urologist for medication or other treatment.

BEYOND INTERCOURSE

Couples in their 60s and 70s and older often ask me what to do about erectile problems and other issues that interfere with intercourse. I tell them to slow down—expand their sexual horizons, develop new sexual habits and start all over again. The goal is simply to feel more.

Our society fears low-level arousal—pleasurable excitement that doesn't lead to penetration or orgasm. But those who have always resisted "just touching" become gluttons for such physical connection once they realize how great it is.

Exercise: During the day or with a light on at night, one partner lies back and is touched by the other—but not on the breasts or genitals—for 15 minutes to an hour. The person being touched stipulates what's wanted in a non-verbal way. If you would like your partner to touch more slowly, put your hand over your partner's and slow it down. When the "touch-ee" is finished, switch places.

Simple interludes set a loving, sensual tone and encourage you both to overcome shyness about requesting what pleases you. Prolonged sensual touching without genital contact removes sexual anxieties...helps you become relaxed, sensitized and responsive...revives a sense of trust and well-being that you may not have experienced since you were stroked as a child.

You'll emerge from the interlude feeling wonderful about each other. Resentments and recriminations will evaporate. Making sensual, uninhibited love often follows naturally. If not, there's always next time.

LOVE YOUR BODY AS IT IS

Our society presumes that only the young and skinny are (or should be) sexually active. As a result, many older people avoid sex out of embarrassment about spotted skin, a protruding stomach, wrinkles and flab. (Do remember that while you are ashamed of your wrinkles and protruding belly, your partner's eyesight has probably also diminished!) A mastectomy or other surgery can interfere with self-esteem, too, especially with a new partner.

Your body is miraculous. Learn to love it the way it really looks. One woman attending my sexual self-esteem workshop said, "I did not learn to love my body until I lost it." But your body at any age is a gift. Value it for itself...not as it compares with anyone else's or to how you looked when younger.

Exercise: Stand together before a full-length mirror. Say what you like about your own body out loud. Do this exercise alone first, before sharing it with your partner. Then try the exercise with your partner, taking turns. Listen, but don't respond.

To learn to appreciate your body, admire it often. Come away from this event loving five things about your body.

If you look better, you'll feel better. I recommend exercise—walking, swimming, Pilates—to couples of all ages. Getting stronger makes both women and men look better and feel more powerful...more sexual.

EDUCATE YOUR PARTNER

The young body works without thought. As you grow older, you can—and may need to—benefit from learning more about your body

269

and your lover's. The key to intimacy is to express your needs—once you have learned what they are—and to insist on knowing the needs of your partner so that you can try to fulfill them.

Special note to women: If you rarely initiated sex but would like to, take baby steps. Try asking for different ways of being touched, or take his hand and show him how you like to be touched.

Exercise: Turn up the thermostat, and hang out nude together. Sleep nude in the same bed even if you haven't done so for years.

Natural Ways to Ease Menopause Symptoms

Ann Louise Gittleman, PhD, nutritionist based in Post Falls, Idaho, and author of 25 books, including *Hot Times: How to Eat Well, Live Healthy, and Feel Sexy During the Change* (Avery).

For decades, women relied on *hormone replacement therapy* (HRT) to relieve symptoms of menopause—hot flashes, sleep disturbance, anxiety and mood swings. But several large studies have linked long-term HRT with increased risk of breast cancer, dementia, heart attack and stroke.

Fortunately, there are safer, natural alternatives to HRT.

MORE THAN JUST ESTROGEN

People typically attribute menopausal symptoms to declining production of the female hormones estrogen and progesterone. But poor eating and lifestyle habits also play a role, by overtaxing the adrenal glands. For women who are going through menopause, the adrenal glands are nature's backup system. When the ovaries decrease their production of estrogen and progesterone, the adrenals have the ability to produce hormones to compensate. Poor diet and lifestyle choices put stress on the adrenals, creating an imbalance in body chemistry and contributing to the uncomfortable symptoms that we associate with menopause.

If you are a woman with menopausal symptoms, adopting healthier habits can help to even out these imbalances.

If you are a man and the woman you love is going through menopause, you can help by understanding that she is experiencing a profound physiological change. Your kindness and patience can ease her transition through a time that is confusing—for her as well as for you.

Common symptoms and natural solutions...

HOT FLASHES

As many as 80% of women experience hot flashes during menopause. One theory is that the hypothalamus, which controls body temperature, is triggered in some way by hormonal fluctuations.

• **Avoid spicy foods.** Foods containing cayenne or other peppers have a thermogenic effect, meaning that they raise your body temperature.

• **Cook with garlic, onion, thyme, oregano and sage.** These seasonings contain very small amounts of phytoestrogens (plant-based estrogens such as lignans and isoflavones that occur naturally in certain foods) and can help restore hormone balance.

• **Cut down on caffeine.** Caffeine stimulates the adrenal glands, leading to a spike in blood sugar levels followed by a plunge in blood sugar to even lower levels than before. This stresses the body and aggravates menopause woes.

If you don't want to give up coffee completely, have one cup a day with food. Don't use coffee as a stimulant between meals. Instead, eat frequent small meals for energy.

Better than coffee: Green, white and black teas have less caffeine and are high in disease-fighting antioxidants. Try substituting tea for coffee. Then transition to herbal tea or hot water with lemon.

• **Add flaxseed.** Ground flaxseed contains lignans, which seem to modulate fluctuating estrogen and progesterone levels. Aim for two tablespoons a day. Ground flaxseed has a pleasant nutty flavor—sprinkle it on cereal, yogurt and salads.

Bonus: Flaxseed reduces cholesterol, helps prevent certain cancers and relieves constipation (be sure to drink plenty of water).

• **Eat soy foods in moderation.** Some countries with diets high in soy report low rates of menopausal symptoms and breast cancer. But I'm cautious about soy. Preliminary research suggests that while isoflavones in soy appear to protect against some breast cancers, they may stimulate growth of other types of breast cancer.

I'm especially concerned about isolated soy protein, which often is added to protein powder, energy bars and supplements. This puts far more soy isoflavones into the diet than other cultures typically consume—and these high amounts may not be healthful.

If you enjoy soy foods, limit your consumption to two servings a week, and eat them in their whole-food form—as tofu, tempeh, miso and edamame.

• **Be wary of herbal remedies.** I'm cautious about black cohosh, red clover and other plant remedies with estrogenlike properties. Research has not demonstrated clearly that they help, and some can have harmful side effects if not properly monitored. However, some women do report good results from these remedies. Check with your doctor first. If you don't notice a clear change in symptoms after two to three weeks of trying a new remedy, ask your doctor about trying something else.

What men can do: Buy a dual-control electric blanket so that you both will be comfortable. Make her a cup of herbal tea. Join her in eating flaxseed—it is good for your colon and prostate.

INSOMNIA

During menopause, elevated levels of the stress hormone cortisol make it difficult to fall asleep and can trigger intermittent awakening throughout the night. *Natural sleep aids…*

• **Wild yam cream.** This topical cream extracted from yams grown in Mexico is a source of natural progesterone. It's available at most health-food stores and some pharmacies. Applying small amounts of wild yam cream daily may help to balance cortisol levels and enhance sleep. (The cream also helps reduce anxiety and hot flashes.)

Apply one-quarter teaspoon once in the morning and once at night. Gently rub the cream into areas where you see capillaries, such as the wrist, back of the knee and neck—these are the places where skin is thinnest and the cream is easily absorbed. Alternate where you apply the cream on a daily basis.

• **Magnesium.** Levels of magnesium, a natural sleep aid, are depleted when you consume too much coffee, cola, alcohol, sugar or salt. Foods high in magnesium include halibut…whole-wheat bread…leafy green vegetables such as spinach…nuts…and dried beans (soaked and cooked). If your diet is low in magnesium, take 200 milligrams (mg) to 400 mg in supplement form at bedtime.

• **Zinc.** This mineral can help quiet an overactive mind. Foods rich in zinc include poultry, red meat and nuts, but it is hard to get enough zinc from food. Take 25 mg to 45 mg in supplement form before bed.

• **Exercise.** One study found that women over age 50 who walked, biked or did stretching exercises every morning fell asleep more easily. Try to get a half-hour of exercise most mornings. Avoid working out in the evening—you may have trouble winding down. And don't go to extremes. Overexercising (more than two hours of strenuous, nonstop activity every day) can lead to hormonal imbalance.

What men can do: Exercise with her in the morning. Make sure there is a bottle of magnesium tablets by the bedside at home and when traveling.

MOOD SWINGS

Drinking less coffee and eating frequent small meals will go a long way toward balancing your moods by reducing spikes in blood sugar and stress on adrenals. *In addition…*

• **Eat a balanced diet.** The emotional and mental stress of menopause can lead to a vicious cycle in which stress depletes important mineral stores, further taxing the adrenals.

Among the minerals depleted by stress are copper, calcium, magnesium, potassium, sodium and zinc. To restore these minerals, eat an adrenal-supportive diet rich in bright-colored fruits and vegetables, legumes, lean meats and whole grains. Avoid sugar and other refined carbohydrates.

Recommended: Sea vegetables, such as nori, arame, wakame and hijiki. These are especially high in key minerals. Health-food stores sell them in dried form. They can be crumbled into soup and over fish, salad and vegetables.

●**Get the right kind of fat.** Though you should avoid saturated fats (found in pork, beef and high-fat dairy products) and hydrogenated fats (in margarine, shortening and many packaged baked goods), certain fats are necessary for hormonal regulation and proper functioning of the nervous system. Known as essential fatty acids (EFAs), these healthy fats help to stabilize blood sugar.

Strive to consume two tablespoons a day of healthy oil (use it in cooking, salad dressings, etc.). Olive, sesame, almond, macadamia and flaxseed oils are especially high in EFAs. (Flaxseed oil does not cook well.)

●**Take B-complex vitamins.** B vitamins are known as the antistress vitamins because they nourish the adrenals. Good sources of B vitamins include whole grains and dried beans (soaked and cooked). Most diets are too low in these vitamins, so supplements usually are needed to make up the deficit. Take 50 mg to 100 mg of a vitamin-B complex daily.

What men can do: Make it easy for her to avoid sugar and caffeine by cutting back on them yourself—your health will benefit, too. If she seems distant or on edge, don't take it personally. Remind yourself that it is not you—it is her biochemistry that is acting up.

WEIGHT GAIN

One reason why so many women gain weight during menopause is that the ovulation process burns calories—as many as 300 per day during the first 10 days of the menstrual cycle. When ovulation stops, fewer calories are burned and metabolism slows. *Foods to counter the slowdown…*

●**Protein.** Increasing protein intake can raise the body's metabolic rate by as much as 25%. Aim for three to four ounces of lean pro-

tein from fish, poultry, beef or lamb twice a day. Eggs and beans also are good sources.

●**Healthy carbohydrates.** Whole grains, vegetables and fruits metabolize slowly and give you energy throughout the day. Try to consume daily at least two servings of fruits, three servings of vegetables and three servings of whole grains.

What men can do: Don't nag her about her weight. Support her by not buying high-calorie foods, such as potato chips and rich desserts.

Asian Herb May Fight Urinary Infections

Soman N. Abraham, PhD, professor, department of pathology, Duke University Medical Center, Durham, North Carolina.

With their typical symptoms such as burning urination, a frequent urge to urinate and a general feeling of being unwell, *urinary tract infections* (UTIs) are an especially unpleasant problem for women. One in five women develop a UTI at some point during their lifetime and—even worse—many go on to have infection after infection, for UTIs are notoriously stubborn and often difficult to completely eliminate.

While many women rely on cranberry juice to avoid and/or ease their UTIs, there is another herbal remedy that might turn out to be even more effective—the Asian herb *forskolin*, an extract from the Indian coleus plant. The good news for all of those scientifically minded individuals in search of research studies on natural products is that researchers at Duke University in Durham, North Carolina, have found that this herbal extract, which is commonly found in weight loss aids or body-building products, may also help flush harmful bacteria from the bladder lining. Forskolin has a long history of medicinal use in Asia for ailments such as painful urination.

FLUSHING OUT
HIDDEN BACTERIA

More than eight out of 10 uncomplicated UTIs are caused by *Escherichia coli*—better known as E. coli—bacteria. Even when you take antibiotics, UTIs often hang on or return, and as many as one in five women experience another infection, with some women getting three or more in one year.

Why? According to Duke University Medical Center professor and study author Soman N. Abraham, PhD, many E. coli and other disease-causing pathogens avoid elimination from antibiotics by "hiding" within the cells of the bladder mucosa.

Dr. Abraham and his colleagues tested the effects of forskolin alone in reducing urinary tract infections in experimental mice. They discovered that the extract appeared to flush out more than 75% of hidden E. coli from their intracellular niches in mice bladders.

Once flushed out of cells, these pathogens can be eliminated in the urine and/or readily killed by antibiotics.

DON'T TRY
THIS AT HOME

Although forskolin is a common herbal extract that can be purchased over-the-counter at health-food stores, Dr. Abraham emphasizes that this should only be seen as a treatment that shows promise for the future.

It hasn't been studied for efficacy for UTIs in humans. Research is ongoing at Duke, and only time will tell if forskolin will come to play a role in eradicating UTIs.

Until we know for sure, Dr. Abraham does not advise using it for urinary tract infections. Forskolin has other effects on the body as well—for instance, it is a potent anticoagulant and a reducer of intraocular pressure and blood pressure in some. So, as always, remember "natural" and "safe" aren't necessarily the same thing.

While this finding may turn out to be important news for frequent UTI sufferers, let's wait and see what further research turns up.

Why Women Get Shorter...And How to Stand Tall

Arthur H. White, MD, retired orthopedic spine surgeon, Walnut Creek, California. He is author of *The Posture Prescription: The Doctor's Rx for Eliminating Back, Muscle, and Joint Pain* (Three Rivers). He has published more than 200 medical journal articles related to spinal health.

The cliché of the hunched-over "little old lady" may seem outdated, yet it's true—we all get shorter as we age. However, a good portion of this shrinkage can be prevented or corrected. The following steps can help you stand tall...plus reduce your risk for back pain and slim your silhouette.

PROTECT YOUR SPINE

Each vertebra (an individual segment of the spine) is separated from adjoining ones by water-filled cushions called discs. In young adults, each disc is about one inch thick.

After about age 40, these discs begin to crack and tear, which causes them to dehydrate and flatten. Over two decades or so, each disc loses about one-twelfth of an inch of thickness—and with 23 discs, that equates to a loss of nearly two inches of height.

Any uncontrolled motion that stresses your back can increase the risk for disc damage. Activities that involve abrupt twisting—racket sports, skating, roughhousing with kids—can tear the discs, hastening dehydration. There is no need to quit these activities, but do try to avoid wrenching twists.

Three other reasons we shrink as we get older are poor posture, loss of abdominal muscle tone and reduced bone density. These problems tend to worsen over time. The humpback seen in many older women is an obvious manifestation of this, but there also are more subtle warning signs that you may be aging yourself prematurely.

PERFECT YOUR POSTURE

Poor attention to posture may be to blame for height loss if you...

•**Slump forward when sitting.**

273

• **Drive, watch TV or work at a computer with your head jutting forward** (instead of centered over your torso).

• **Experience back or neck pain.**

• **Have frequent headaches.**

• **Have pain in your arms or hands (pain radiates from the spine).**

Chronic slouching weakens back and chest muscles, so you eventually may find it difficult to stand up straight even when you try. Large-breasted women are particularly prone to slouching. The extra weight they carry in front places more strain on the back muscles.

Simple steps to stand tall...

• **First, check your posture.** Have someone take your picture while you stand sideways in a doorway. Stand as you normally do—if you don't, you'll only be fooling yourself. The door frame provides a visual guide to what is straight.

• **Second, stay aware.** Whenever you pass a mirror or window, notice the position of your neck, shoulders and back. If your head juts forward, pull it back in line with your shoulders...roll your shoulders back...squeeze your shoulder blades together more...draw in your tummy...and tuck your rear end under. Even if you can't remain that straight for long, these brief moments of awareness will help to realign your spine and strengthen your muscles.

• **Third, stretch and strengthen.** When muscles are not used, they get smaller and weaker. Prevent or reverse problem posture with a few simple exercises. These are generally safe for everyone, though it is best to check with your doctor before beginning any new type of workout.

• **Secret stretch can be done anywhere.** It returns shoulders to their proper position and strengthens muscles between shoulder blades. Clasp your hands behind your back at the level of your buttocks. Push your hands down and roll your shoulders back (don't arch your back). Hold for 30 seconds. Repeat several times daily—while waiting for an elevator, watching TV or anytime you are idle.

Advanced: With hands clasped behind you and arms straight, raise arms up and away from you.

• **Doorway stretch strengthens your shoulders and back and stretches chest muscles.** Stand in a doorway, a few inches behind the threshold, feet shoulder-width apart. Place one hand on each side of the doorjamb, level with your shoulders. Keeping your back straight, lean forward, feeling the stretch across your upper chest as your back muscles work to draw your shoulder blades together. Hold for 30 seconds...repeat five times. Do every other day or whenever you feel upper-back tension.

FABULOUS ABS HELP

When tightened, abdominal muscles act as a muscular corset, supporting the vertebrae and protecting them from injury. Strong abs allow you to stand tall by preventing your rib cage from slumping down toward your pelvis.

Women generally have a more difficult time maintaining abdominal strength than men because pregnancy overstretches the belly muscles. A little effort goes a long way, however, in restoring the strength of the abs. *To try...*

• **Isometric crunch and hold.** Lie with knees bent and feet flat on the floor. Cross arms across your chest. Tuck chin slightly... then raise your head and shoulders (not your entire back) off the floor by tightening your belly muscles. Keep your head in line with your shoulders, and leave enough space to fit a tennis ball between your chin and chest. Hold the position as long as possible, then slowly lower down to the starting position. Repeat, continuing for three to five minutes. At first, you may be able to hold the pose for only a second or two and may need to rest between each crunch. Keep at it daily—soon your abs will get stronger.

BUILD STRONGER BONES

Osteoporosis is a disease in which bones become so fragile that even the jolt of slipping off a curb can fracture the spine. In severe cases, the weight of the person's own body can slowly crush vertebrae, producing a rounded humpback that steals as much as four inches of height.

Because estrogen helps to build bone, women are susceptible to osteoporosis after menopause, when estrogen levels drop. Ask your doctor about taking supplements of calcium and vitamin D. *Also...*

• **Go for a walk.** Every time your foot hits the ground, the impact sends a vibration through your bones. This produces an electrical force (the *piezoelectric effect*) that strengthens bones by encouraging calcium deposits throughout the skeleton.

Alternatives: Running builds even more bone density but may injure joints—so stick to brisk walking unless you're already an accomplished runner. Weight lifting also builds bone through similar forces, but the effect is less because there is no impact or vibration.

The Strange, Bone-Saving Power of Prunes

From Bottom Line's *Breakthroughs in Drug-Free Healing* by Bill Gottlieb. Bottom Line Books. *www.bottomlinepublications.com.*

D ried plums—known to scientists as *Prunus domestica*, and to the rest of us as prunes—are loaded with powerful natural compounds that fight cell-damaging oxidation and inflammation. Could they protect bones?

In a recent study, postmenopausal women who ate nine to 10 prunes a day for three months had big boosts in two biomarkers that indicate bone growth. A group that ate dried apples didn't have an increase.

In 2005, female rats that had eaten a bone-eroding diet were given diets rich in prunes, and bone mass returned. The animals had incurred a type of bone damage that scientists up to then thought was irreversible—but prunes reversed it, says Bahram H. Arjmandi, PhD, RD, a professor at Florida State University and the lead researcher on all the prune studies.

In 2006, Dr. Arjmandi and his colleagues showed that prunes prevent bone loss in male rats.

In 2007, a study showed that prunes strengthen the structure of bone in male and female laboratory animals.

And recently Dr. Arjmandi launched another study with postmenopausal women, who will eat nine or 10 prunes a day for one year. At the start of the study, the women had their bone density measured; similar measurements will be taken at the end of the study.

Of course, you don't have to wait until the study is concluded to begin snacking on prunes.

Try this: The California Dried Plum Board (which calls prunes dried plums) offers the following ideas for putting more prunes in your diet...

• **Snack on prunes.**

• **Sprinkle prunes on oatmeal or ready-to-eat cereal, or into pancake batter as a complement to sliced bananas.**

• **Add chopped and pitted prunes to apple butter, orange marmalade, peanut butter or low-fat cream cheese.**

• **Add halved and pitted prunes to turkey or chicken salad.**

More Information: You can find dozens of prune recipes at *www.californiadriedplums.org.* Address: California Dried Plum Board, 3840 Rosin Court, Ste. 170, Sacramento, CA 95834, 916-565-6232.

21

Natural Remedies For Men

Breakthrough Treatments for Hair Loss

Why do some men go bald in their 30s while others have a full head of hair until their final days? Why do some women have ever-thinning hair, while others never seem to lose a single strand?

Blame your genes, first of all. If your mom, dad or a grandparent had hair loss, chances are greater that you will, too. Even so, there are ways to slow hair loss and stimulate growth.

THE HORMONE FACTOR

You grow and shed hair all the time. Of the 100,000-plus strands of hair on your head, it is perfectly normal to lose 50 to 100 every day. Once a hair is shed, a new hair grows from the same follicle. Hair grows at a rate of nearly one-half inch per month (faster in warm weather, slower when frost is on the vine).

Baldness results when the rate of shedding exceeds the rate of regrowth.

Hair loss usually accelerates when you're over age 50. One hormone, *dihydrotestosterone* (DHT), seems to be the chief culprit. DHT is a derivative of testosterone (the sex-determining hormone that is more abundant in men than women). In both men and women, DHT increases in the presence of the enzyme *5-alpha reductase*, which is produced in the prostate, adrenal glands and the scalp. 5-alpha reductase is more likely to proliferate after age 50. When DHT is overproduced, hair follicles are damaged. Some follicles die, but most shrink and produce thinner, weaker hairs—and the weak hairs are the ones that fall out.

Mark A. Stengler, NMD, licensed naturopathic medical doctor in private practice, Stengler Center for Integrative Medicine, Encinitas, California...adjunct associate clinical professor at the National College of Natural Medicine, Portland, Oregon...author of many books, including *The Natural Physician's Healing Therapies* and coauthor of *Prescription for Natural Cures* (both from Bottom Line Books)...and author of the *Bottom Line/Natural Healing* newsletter. *www.drstengler.com*

276

An oily skin substance called *sebum*—produced by the sebaceous glands—makes matters worse. Excess sebum clogs follicles and contributes to high 5-alpha reductase activity, which stimulates production of DHT.

STRESS

Among my own patients, stress is a factor for both men and women. I have found that highly stressed women, in particular, have higher-than-normal levels of cortisol, a stress hormone that can contribute to hair loss.

A study published in the *Journal of Clinical Biochemistry* confirms that cortisol is indeed elevated in some women who suffer hair loss—and that when they learn to cope better with stress, hair growth improves.

For stress relief, I recommend daily exercise, such as brisk walking, as well as relaxation techniques, including deep breathing and meditation. B vitamins and ashwagandha (a stress-reducing herb from India) also can help counteract the effects of cortisol.

A regular daily dose of 100 mg of a B-vitamin complex and 250 mg to 500 mg of ashwagandha can help control cortisol levels. Look for Sensoril Ashwagandha, a patented extract formula by Jarrow Formulas, available at many health-food stores or by calling 800-726-0886 or at *www.jarrow.com*.

A PROMISING FORMULA

Taking a daily multivitamin and mineral supplement as well as the herbal remedy saw palmetto also can help slow hair loss. A daily scalp massage with essential oils is beneficial, too.

Saw palmetto helps block the effects of DHT on hair follicles, strengthening hair. In a study in the *Journal of Alternative and Complementary Medicine*, researchers used a product containing saw palmetto and a plant compound called beta-sitosterol that is found in saw palmetto and other plants. The study included 19 men between ages 23 and 64 who had mild-to-moderate hair loss. Men in one group were given a placebo daily...and men in the other group received the saw palmetto/beta-sitosterol combination (none of the participants knew which group they were in). After five months, researchers found that 60% of the men who received the saw palmetto/beta-sitosterol combination showed improvement, while only 11% of the men receiving a placebo had more hair growth.

In my clinical experience, saw palmetto is helpful for both men and women. I recommend 320 mg to 400 mg daily of an 85% liposterolic extract. It is safe to use long term but should not be taken if you are pregnant or nursing.

For a more aggressive approach, you should also take beta-sitosterol. Source Naturals (800-815-2333, *www.sourcenaturals.com*) offers a 113-mg tablet that can be taken daily. It is available at health-food stores and at *www.iherb.com*.

The essential oils of rosemary and lavender have been shown to improve hair growth when applied to the scalp. My own belief is that they improve blood flow to the scalp, ensuring that nutrients get to the sites where they're needed.

You can purchase these essential oils in separate containers. Pour some of your regular shampoo into the lid of the shampoo bottle, then add five to 10 drops of each essential oil. Massage into the scalp and leave on three to five minutes before rinsing thoroughly.

OTHER SUPPLEMENTS

If you have tried these approaches for two to three months and still aren't satisfied with the growth of your locks, here are some other supplements that can help both men and women...

Biotin, a nutrient that is required for hair growth, is particularly good for brittle hair. Food sources of biotin include brewer's yeast, soybeans, eggs, mushrooms and whole wheat. For supplementation, take 3,000 micrograms daily for at least two months or use a biotin-enriched shampoo daily.

A great source of sulfur, *methylsulfonylmethane* (MSM) is an integral component of the amino acids that are the building blocks of hair protein. MSM improves the strength, sheen and health of hair. In one study, 21 adults (16 men and five women) who were assessed by a certified cosmetologist under the direction of a medical doctor were given MSM or a placebo and then were reassessed at the end of six weeks. The participants did not know who was given MSM and who was given a placebo.

Those given MSM showed significant improvement in hair health, while those taking a placebo showed few or no changes.

I recommend a 3,000-mg daily dose of MSM. Look for Opti-MSM or Lignisul MSM, available from many manufacturers and at health-food stores.

Essential fatty acids keep hair from becoming dry and lifeless by decreasing inflammation. Inflammation worsens the quality of hair follicles, and essential fatty acids are needed for the proper development of hair.

Food sources include walnuts, eggs, fish, olive oil, flaxseed and hempseed and flax oils. Or you can take a formula like Udo's Choice Oil Blend, produced by Flora (800-446-2110, *www.florahealth.com*). Follow directions on the label. The formula contains both omega-3 fatty acids (from flax oil or fish oil) and omega-6 fatty acids from evening primrose oil or borage oil.

Don't expect immediate results, however. It can take four to six weeks to see improvement.

Fight Hair Loss by Getting More Iron

You normally shed about 100 hairs a day, but if hair comes out in clumps, get screened for iron deficiency. Getting more iron (through diet or supplements) may limit shedding and promote regrowth.

Caution: Do not take supplements without consulting a physician—too much iron can lead to heart disease, liver disease and diabetes.

Leonid Trost, MD, resident physician in dermatology at Cleveland Clinic Foundation, Cleveland, and co-author of a research review published in *Journal of the American Academy of Dermatology.*

The Secret Recipe for Hair Growth

Jane Buckle, RN, PhD, president, RJ Buckle Associates LLC, Hazlet, New Jersey.

When you hear the word "aromatherapy," you probably think of a scented bath or a fragrant candle. But medical practitioners in the United States and around the world are using distilled oils of aromatic plants medicinally. Essential oils activate the parasympathetic nervous system, causing relaxation, which speeds healing.

AROMATHERAPY IN ACTION

Plant oils can be used in a warm bath...in a "carrier oil"—such as almond or sesame oil—for massage...or in a lotion.

The aromas can be sniffed from a bottle... a cotton ball...or a diffuser—a machine that emits the aroma into the air.

Clinical and scientific studies support the use of aromatherapy as an adjunct to medical care for treating...

• **Anxiety.** Essential oils that were inhaled for three minutes relieved anxiety in men and women, according to research published in the *International Journal of Neuroscience.* Use rosemary, Roman chamomile or patchouli.

Typical treatment: Sniff one to three drops when anxious.

Caution: Avoid using rosemary if you have high blood pressure.

• **Bronchitis.** Use spike lavender.

Typical treatment: One drop of spike lavender in a bowl of three cups of boiling water. Drape a towel over your head and inhale the steam. Do this for five minutes, four times a day.

• **Hair loss.** In people with hair loss due to *alopecia areata*, essential oils helped restore hair growth, notes an *Archives of Dermatology* study. A carrier oil contained a mixture of thyme (two drops), rosemary (three drops), lavender (three drops) and cedarwood (two drops).

Typical treatment: Massage the mixture into the scalp for two minutes daily.

• **Headache.** Use peppermint. If pain isn't gone in five minutes, try Roman chamomile or true lavender.

Typical treatment: Five drops in one teaspoon of carrier oil. Apply to temples or sniff.

• **Hot flashes.** Use clary sage, fennel, geranium or rose.

Typical treatment: Ten drops in two cups of water in a spray bottle. Spray on face during hot flash.

• **Insomnia.** Use ylang-ylang, neroli or rose.

Typical treatment: Five drops in a diffuser placed in the bedroom.

• **Low-back pain.** Use lemongrass. If you feel no relief in 20 minutes, try rosemary or spike lavender.

Typical treatment: Five drops in one teaspoon of carrier oil. Apply to the painful area every three hours.

• **Menstrual cramps.** Use geranium.

Typical treatment: Five drops added to one teaspoon of carrier oil. Rub on the lower abdomen and lower back every three hours.

• **Muscle spasms.** Use clary sage, sage or try lavender.

Typical treatment: Five drops added to one teaspoon of carrier oil. Apply to the affected muscles at least every three hours.

• **Osteoarthritis.** Use frankincense, rosemary or true lavender.

Typical treatment: Five drops added to one teaspoon of carrier oil. Apply to the painful area every three hours.

WHAT TO BUY

Aromatherapy is most effective when the essential oils are prepared with no extraneous ingredients. One good brand includes Scents & Scentsibility (*www.scentsandscentsibility.co. uk*). Its products are also available in health-food stores.

USING AROMATHERAPY SAFELY

Some essential oils are irritating if applied undiluted. Always dilute with a plain carrier oil (scentless organic vegetable oils such as sunflower or safflower are good choices) be-fore using topically. If skin stings or becomes red, wash with unperfumed soap.

Essential oils are flammable. Store them away from candles, fires, cigarettes and stoves. Don't pour oil on lightbulbs to scent a room.

Caution: Essential oils can be lethal if they are ingested—even in tiny doses. Keep away from children and pets. People with asthma or epilepsy and pregnant women should consult their doctors before using aromatherapy.

"Natural" Treatment for Prostate Enlargement: Hope or Hype?

Kevin T. McVary, MD, professor of urology, Northwestern University Feinberg School of Medicine, Chicago. He is chairman of the American Urological Association's Benign Prostatic Hyperplasia Guidelines Panel. *www. auanet.org.*

Besides saw palmetto, which has been proven ineffective, there is an array of natural supplements that are reputed to relieve symptoms of *benign prostate enlargement* (BPH). While none of these supplements is believed to be unsafe, that doesn't necessarily mean that they're all effective. *A quick report card on the most popular natural BPH treatments...*

PROMISING

• **Lycopene.** There's evidence that this antioxidant compound—found in red tomatoes and in processed tomato products, such as tomato sauce, tomato paste and ketchup—may lower the risk for prostate cancer. It's currently an area of active investigation as a potential treatment for BPH as well.

• **Omega-3 fatty acids** (taken in food, such as fish or avocados, or in flaxseed or fish oil supplements) have a beneficial impact on the vascular system, which is good for general health—including the health of the prostate gland. Their vascular effects may improve erection quality (which can be impaired by some

BPH medications) and may also hold benefits for certain urinary disorders.

- **Pygeum africanum.** This bark extract is a promising medication based on preliminary data from human and laboratory studies, but at this point, no specific mechanism of action has been identified and no proven impact on BPH has been demonstrated. Further investigation is needed.

NOT PROMISING

- **Rye grass pollen extract.** No sound studies have found convincing evidence of its effectiveness.

- **Stinging nettle.** No sound studies have found convincing evidence of its effectiveness.

- **Zinc** (taken in food, such as pumpkin seeds, or in supplement form). Studies have found that zinc has no impact on BPH.

Natural Help for Men's Urological Problems

Geovanni Espinosa, ND, MS., LAc, director of clinical trials, clinician and co-investigator at the Center for Holistic Urology at Columbia University Medical Center in New York City (*www.holisticurology.columbia.edu*). He is author of the naturopathic section in *1,000 Cures for 200 Ailments* (HarperCollins).

If you've ever had an acute infection of the prostate, you may know that antibiotics often clear up the problem in just a few days. But as the antibiotics eliminate infection-causing bacteria, these powerful drugs also wipe out "healthy" organisms that aid digestion and help fortify the immune system. You may experience diarrhea, upset stomach or a yeast infection while taking the medication.

What's the answer? Holistic medicine uses alternative therapies, such as dietary supplements, nutritional advice and acupuncture, to complement—or replace—conventional medical treatments, including prescription drugs.

For example, probiotic "good" bacteria supplements help replenish the beneficial intestinal bacteria killed by antibiotics. Ask your

doctor about taking 10 billion to 20 billion colony forming units (CFUs) of probiotics, such as *lactobacillus* or *acidophilus*, two to three hours after each dose of antibiotics.*

Holistic treatments for other urological problems that affect men…**

IMPOTENCE

For stronger, more reliable erections, conventional medicine offers several medications, such as *sildenafil* (Viagra) and *vardenafil* (Levitra). But these drugs can have side effects, including painful, prolonged erections and sudden vision loss. *Holistic approach…*

- **Maca** is a root vegetable from South America. In supplement form, it has been shown to increase libido in healthy men.

Recommended dosage: 500 mg to 1,000 mg three times daily.

- **Niacin,** a B vitamin, widens blood vessels when taken in high doses (500 mg to 1,000 mg daily) and may help promote erections in some men who do not improve with the impotence remedy described above. A doctor should monitor high-dose courses of Niacin.

CHRONIC PROSTATITIS

Pain and swelling of the prostate (prostatitis) may be caused by inflammation that develops for unknown reasons or by an infection. The prostate enlargement that characterizes BPH, on the other hand, is likely due to hormonal changes that occur as men age. Symptoms of chronic prostatitis, such as pelvic pain and pain when urinating, can linger for months. Conventional medicine has little to offer other than antibiotics. *Holistic approach…*

- **Fish oil and quercetin** (a plant-based supplement) are both anti-inflammatories. The fish oil supplements should contain a daily total of about 1,440 mg of *eicosapentaenoic acid* (EPA) and 960 mg of *docosahexaenoic acid*

*To find a doctor near you who offers holistic therapies, consult the American Holistic Medical Association, 216-292-6644, *www.holisticmedicine.org*. Holistic doctors can help you choose high-quality supplements—these products may contain impurities.

**Because some supplements can interact with prescription drugs, raise blood sugar and cause other adverse effects, check with your doctor before trying any of the therapies mentioned in this article.

(DHA). Take 500 mg of quercetin twice daily. Fish oil and quercetin can be combined.

INCONTINENCE

Because incontinence can be caused by various underlying problems, including an infection, a neurological disorder (such as multiple sclerosis) or an enlarged prostate, any man who suffers from incontinence should first be evaluated by a urologist.

Holistic approach…

•**Buchu,** cleavers and cornsilk are herbal remedies that often help when overactive bladder (marked by a sudden, intense need to urinate) causes incontinence. Some products contain all three herbs. For dosages, follow label instructions.

•**Bromelain,** an enzyme derived from pineapple, acts as an anti-inflammatory to help treat incontinence caused by an inflamed prostate. Take 500 mg to 2,000 mg daily in two divided doses.

•**Pumpkin seed oil extract** may ease incontinence in men when overactive bladder is related to an enlarged prostate. Typical dosage: 160 mg of pumpkin seed oil extract, taken three times daily with meals. Pumpkin seed oil extract can be combined with saw palmetto. Ask your doctor for advice on combining pumpkin seed oil extract with any of the other incontinence remedies described above.

Promising Study

Beta sitosterol is found in wheat germ, rice bran, corn oil, soybeans and other plants. Several human studies have shown that it reduces the urinary symptoms of benign prostate enlargement, including nighttime urination. Beta sitosterol also may help to shrink an enlarged prostate—animal studies show that it inhibits activity of the enzyme that causes the prostate gland to swell. The herb saw palmetto, commonly used by men with enlarged prostate, also contains beta sitosterol. Studies of beta sitosterol have used 60 mg to 130 mg

daily. Take it two hours or more away from any vitamins or medications you take, because it may prevent them from being properly absorbed. Otherwise, side effects are rare.

Mark A. Stengler, NMD, licensed naturopathic medical doctor in private practice, Stengler Center for Integrative Medicine, Encinitas, California…adjunct associate clinical professor at the National College of Natural Medicine, Portland, Oregon…author of many books, including *The Natural Physician's Healing Therapies* and coauthor of *Prescription for Natural Cures* (both from Bottom Line Books)…and author of the *Bottom Line/ Natural Healing* newsletter. *www.drstengler.com*

Eating Fish Helps Prostate Cancer Survival

Mark A. Stengler, NMD, licensed naturopathic medical doctor in private practice, Stengler Center for Integrative Medicine, Encinitas, California…adjunct associate clinical professor at the National College of Natural Medicine, Portland, Oregon…author of many books, including *The Natural Physician's Healing Therapies* and coauthor of *Prescription for Natural Cures* (both from Bottom Line Books)…and author of the *Bottom Line/Natural Healing* newsletter. *www.drstengler.com*

A 22-year Harvard School of Public Health study of 20,167 men found that fish intake did not reduce the incidence of prostate cancer but did improve survival rates among men who had prostate cancer. Men with prostate cancer who ate fish five or more times weekly had a 48% lower risk of dying from the disease than those who ate fish less than once a week.

My view: Several animal studies have shown that omega-3 fatty acids found in fish inhibit prostate cancer growth. One component of omega-3 fatty acids, known as *eicosapentaenoic acid* (EPA), and one of its metabolites have been shown to suppress the proliferation of prostate cancer cells. I recommend consuming five weekly servings of fish, especially those with the least mercury and other contaminants, such as sardines, trout and wild Alaskan salmon. Or take a fish oil supplement that supplies a combined daily total of 1,000 mg of EPA and *docosahexaenoic acid* (DHA).

Natural Ways to Fight Prostate Enlargement

Mark A. Stengler, NMD, licensed naturopathic medical doctor in private practice, Stengler Center for Integrative Medicine, Encinitas, California...adjunct associate clinical professor at the National College of Natural Medicine, Portland, Oregon...author of many books, including *The Natural Physician's Healing Therapies* and coauthor of *Prescription for Natural Cures* (both from Bottom Line Books)...and author of the *Bottom Line/Natural Healing* newsletter. *www.drstengler.com*

If you're a man approaching age 45, you have a nearly 50% chance of having an enlarged prostate. By age 70, the chances are almost nine in 10 that you'll have it. Called *benign prostatic hyperplasia* (BPH), the condition involves an enlarged prostate that compresses the urethra and partially blocks urine flow. BPH is the most common prostate problem among men. While it's not life-threatening—it is not, for example, related to the development of prostate cancer—symptoms can be troublesome. Fortunately, there are natural ways to prevent and treat it.

THE PROSTATE PRESSURE POINT

The job of the prostate is to produce fluid that nourishes and transports sperm. This walnut-sized gland weighs approximately 20 grams, about as much as two Fig Newtons. Located in front of the rectum and below the bladder, the prostate surrounds the urethra, the passageway that carries urine away from the bladder and into the penis.

A swollen prostate can compress the urethra like a clamp on a garden hose, restricting urine flow. It also may press upward, irritating the outer wall of the bladder. This irritation makes the bladder wall thicker and even more easily irritated. A man with BPH might start having bladder contractions, making him feel the need to urinate frequently even when there's not much urine. Over time, the bladder may lose the ability to completely empty, increasing discomfort.

POSSIBLE CAUSES

There remains a lot to be answered when it comes to the causes of BPH. One thing researchers can agree on is that hormonal factors play the largest role.

Research has focused on the hormone testosterone and a related substance called *dihydrotestosterone* (DHT). Some researchers believe that testosterone, an anabolic (growth-promoting) hormone, is the main culprit. Others disagree because prostate growth tends to be a problem later in a man's life, while the amount of testosterone is at its highest when males are in their late teens or early 20s.

The conversion of testosterone to DHT increases as men get older—and DHT is very potent. It stimulates the proliferation of new prostate cells and slows the death of older ones. But if DHT is a cause, why do some men with prostate enlargement have normal DHT levels? Could another hormone be involved?

Now researchers are looking at the effect of the hormone estrogen (especially the kind called *estradiol*) on prostate growth. Estrogen isn't just a "female" hormone. Men have it as well, and as they age, estrogen levels increase. High estrogen-to-testosterone ratios could increase the effects of DHT on prostate cells.

LOOKING FOR TROUBLE

The most common test to diagnose BPH and other prostate-related problems is a digital rectal exam. Your physician inserts a gloved finger into the rectum and feels the part of the prostate next to the rectum for any enlargement or hardness. All men over age 40 should have this test once a year.

A variety of pharmaceuticals can help relieve BPH symptoms, but each has potential side effects. Many doctors prescribe alpha-blockers, such as *terazosin* (Hytrin) or *doxazosin* (Cardura), which relax the neck of the bladder, making urination easier—but these can cause fatigue, weakness, headaches and dizziness. Another prescription drug, *finasteride* (Proscar), relieves symptoms by shrinking the prostate gland, but it can cause impotence and reduced sexual desire.

For men who have very serious BPH problems that are interfering with their lifestyle, some doctors recommend surgical procedures—but surgery can also lead to impotence or incontinence.

I find that drugs and surgery usually are unnecessary. As long as a man is getting his prostate checked at least once a year and there are no signs of tumor growth or urinary blockage, BPH can be treated with natural therapies. These include improved diet and supplements. Also, 30 minutes of daily exercise has been shown to reduce BPH symptoms quite significantly.

HEALING FOODS

Avocados contain beta sitosterol, a phytonutrient that protects against prostate enlargement by inhibiting growth factors that cause prostate swelling. Avocados also are a good source of oleic acid, a monounsaturated fatty acid that is thought to reduce inflammation, which can contribute to BPH. Have at least two weekly servings (one-fifth of a medium avocado per serving). If you don't like avocados, you can have three half-cup servings a week of peanuts, rice bran or wheat germ.

Fish is a good source of *eicosapentaenoic acid* (EPA), a powerful omega-3 fatty acid that helps reduce swelling and inflammation. Eat at least two three-ounce servings of trout, salmon or sardines each week.

Ground flaxseed has been shown to reduce estrogen levels, and it contains anti-inflammatory omega-3 fatty acids. I advise men to take one or two tablespoons daily along with 10 ounces of water (to prevent constipation). Ground flaxseed has a mild, nutty flavor and can be added to salads, cereals, yogurt, smoothies and protein shakes or just eaten plain.

Pumpkin seeds are natural sources of zinc. This mineral helps keep your prostate healthy by reducing the activity of the enzyme *5-alpha-reductase*, which produces DHT. Sprinkle a tablespoon or two of pumpkin seeds—raw or roasted, with or without the hulls—on salad, yogurt, cereal, etc. four times weekly.

Soy contains a number of phytoestrogens (plant chemicals that balance estrogen), including *genistein*, which can help control prostate enlargement. I prefer fermented soy foods, such as miso, tempeh and fermented soy protein powder, which provide a form of genistein that can be readily absorbed by the body. Have at least one-half cup serving daily.

Tomatoes are rich in the disease-fighting antioxidants known as carotenoids. Preliminary scientific research has suggested that tomatoes and tomato products help prevent prostate cancer. They also may have a beneficial effect on prostate enlargement. Consume two servings of fresh tomatoes and two servings of cooked tomatoes (e.g., tomato paste/sauce) weekly (one serving equals one-half to one cup of tomatoes and/or tomato sauce). If you don't like tomatoes, eat watermelon or cantaloupe.

Foods to avoid: Men with BPH should avoid caffeinated beverages and alcohol—they irritate and inflame the prostate. Also reduce your intake of foods that contain harmful fats, such as hydrogenated or partially hydrogenated oils, that promote inflammation. Stay away from packaged foods that are high in sugar, which also can worsen inflammation.

NATURAL SUPPLEMENTS

The following supplements are listed in order of importance—start with the first and move down the list until you find what works best for you. Many formulas contain a blend of two or three of the ones listed.

Saw palmetto berry extract is a mainstay in the natural treatment of BPH and alleviates most symptoms. It was first used medicinally by Native Americans for prostate and urinary tract problems. Recently, researchers have found that saw palmetto helps the prostate by reducing activity of the DHT-producing enzyme 5-alpha-reductase. A review of 18 randomized, controlled trials involving 2,939 men found saw palmetto to be as effective as the BPH drug *finasteride*.

It can take six to eight weeks before this natural prostate protector begins to fully take effect. I recommend a product that is standardized to contain 80% to 95% fatty acids (check the label) and a total daily dosage of 320 mg, which can be taken all at once. Two brands I recommend are Nature's Way Standardized Saw Palmetto Extract and Enzymatic Therapy Super Saw Palmetto, which are widely available at health-food stores. It is best to take it on an empty stomach. A small percentage of men get stomach upset from saw palmetto. If this occurs, try taking it with meals.

Pygeum africanum, an extract that comes from the bark of the African plum tree, decreases the need to urinate at night and improves urine flow during the day. I prefer a formula that combines pygeum with saw palmetto, such as Ultra Saw Palmetto and Pygeum by Jarrow Formulas (800-726-0886, *www.jarrow. com*). The daily pygeum dosage is 100 mg.

Nettle root can provide modest benefits. The nettle-containing product from Nutrilite, Saw Palmetto with Nettle Root, produced good results in a UCLA study. Over six months, the 44 men in the study showed modest improvements in BPH symptoms. The Nutrilite formula includes saw palmetto, nettle root, beta-carotene, pumpkin seed oil and lemon bioflavonoid concentrate (Nutrilite, 800-253-6500, *www.quixtar. com*). Take one softgel three times daily.

Rye grass pollen extracts seem to relax the muscles of the urethra and improve the ability of the bladder to contract. Take three 63-mg tablets twice daily for a total of 378 mg.

Fish oil can help reduce prostate swelling and inflammation. Take 3,000 mg to 5,000 mg daily in addition to two weekly servings of fish. If you prefer a vegetarian source of omega-3 fatty acids, use one to two tablespoons of flaxseed oil.

Caution: Fish oil should not be used by anyone who takes blood-thinning medications such as *warfarin* (Coumadin).

Exercise for Better Sex

Men who exercise vigorously at least three hours a week are 30% less likely to suffer from *erectile dysfunction* (ED) than men who are sedentary.

A daily walk is also beneficial. It lowers the risk for ED by 15%.

The Medical Post.

Soy Protection?

Soy seems to protect against localized prostate cancer—but it may fuel more advanced cases.

Recent study: Men who ate the most soy—in miso soup, tofu and other forms—had up to 50% less risk for developing prostate cancer over a 10-year period than men who consumed the least.

The effect was especially pronounced among men over age 60.

However: The study also showed that among the men who did develop cancer, those who ate two bowls of miso soup daily had twice the risk for developing advanced prostate cancer as men who ate less than one bowl a day.

More research is needed before recommendations can be made about the use of soy supplements.

Shoichiro Tsugane, MD, chief of epidemiology and prevention, National Cancer Center, Tokyo, Japan, and coleader of a study of 43,509 men, published in *Cancer Epidemiology, Biomarkers & Prevention.*

Good News About Omega-3 Fatty Acids

Omega-3 fatty acids may cut prostate cancer risk in men with a family history of the disease.

Omega-3s—found in fish-oil capsules and certain fish—slowed disease progression in mice genetically engineered to develop prostate cancer.

Yong Q. Chen, PhD, researcher, Wake Forest University School of Medicine, Winston-Salem, North Carolina, and leader of a study published in *Journal of Clinical Investigation.*

Vegetables Protect The Prostate

Recent study: In a 14-year analysis of the diets of 32,000 men, researchers found that men who ate the most vegetables—six one-half cup servings daily—had an 11% lower risk for *benign prostatic hyperplasia* (BPH), or enlarged prostate, than men who ate the least—an average of 1.5 servings daily.

Theory: Antioxidants in vegetables may reduce the negative effect of free radicals on prostate cells.

Sabine Rohrmann, PhD, MPH, researcher, German Cancer Research Center, Heidelberg, Germany.

Common Symptoms Of BPH

Here is a list of the seven most common symptoms of *benign prostatic hyperplasia* (BPH).

- **A need to urinate frequently**
- **Urination that is hard to start or stop**
- **Weak urination or "dribbling"**
- **Sensation of an incompletely emptied bladder**
- **Increased need to urinate at night**
- **Burning pain accompanying urination**
- **Recurring bladder infections**

Red Wine Cuts Prostate Cancer Risk

The fermentation process concentrates *resveratrol*, the compound in grapes that is believed to protect against prostate cancer. This natural antibiotic also is a strong antioxidant and anti-inflammatory agent. To benefit, men need at least four four-ounce glasses of red wine a week. White wine, grapes and grape juice contain little resveratrol.

Janet L. Stanford, PhD, director of the prostate cancer research program, Fred Hutchinson Cancer Research Center in Seattle. Her study of prostate cancer patients and healthy men was published in the online edition of *International Journal of Cancer.*

Sunshine May Protect Against Prostate Cancer

Men with high sun exposure were 49% less likely to have prostate cancer than men with the least exposure. Sun helps the body manufacture vitamin D, which may protect against prostate cancer.

Downside: Frequent exposure still puts people at risk for skin cancer.

Best: Spend 10 minutes a day in the sun without sunscreen.

Esther M. John, PhD, MSPH, epidemiologist at Cancer Prevention Institute of California, Fremont, and principal investigator and lead author of a study of 905 men, published in *Cancer Research.*

22

Breakthroughs for Better Sex

Maca: The Super Food That Helps with Everything from Memory to Arthritis and Even Sex Drive

Super foods are foods and herbs considered to be especially healthful due to their hefty nutritional content. The list includes familiar favorites, such as blueberries, broccoli and beans. Now a more exotic super food you may never have heard of is generating excitement in the world of natural health—a Peruvian root vegetable called *maca* (*Lepidium meyenii* or *peruvianum*), pronounced MACK-ah.

The root of the maca is shaped like a large radish. It is a cousin to other cruciferous plants, such as cauliflower and brussels sprouts. Peruvians traditionally boil or roast the maca root or grind it into flour for baking. However,

despite maca's popular description as a "super food," you won't see it in food form in this country. Instead, the root is dried and ground into a fine powder. It then is distributed primarily in capsules, although you also can buy the powder to blend into beverages or sprinkle on foods.

I began looking into maca for my patients about seven years ago. In addition to its healthful fiber, complex carbohydrates and protein, maca provides numerous minerals, including calcium, magnesium, phosphorous, potassium, sulfur, iron, zinc, iodine and copper...vitamins B-1, B-2, C and E...nearly 20 amino acids, including linoleic acid, palmitic acid and oleic acid...as well as various plant sterols, which

Mark A. Stengler, NMD, licensed naturopathic medical doctor in private practice, Stengler Center for Integrative Medicine, Encinitas, California...adjunct associate clinical professor at the National College of Natural Medicine, Portland, Oregon...author of many books, including *The Natural Physician's Healing Therapies* and coauthor of *Prescription for Natural Cures* (both from Bottom Line Books)...and author of the *Bottom Line/Natural Healing* newsletter. *www.drstengler.com*

are natural cholesterol-lowering agents. All of these nutrients have been shown to promote health in a multitude of ways.

Here is what this super food can do for you...

BOOST SEX DRIVE

Legend holds that in the era of the Inca empire, battle leaders provided maca to warriors to enhance their strength—then cut off the supply after the fighting ended to protect women from the warriors' maca-heightened libidos.

Modern research has suggested that maca does indeed increase sex drive in men. One double-blind, randomized study published in the journal *Andrologia* examined the effect of maca on sexual desire in 57 men, ages 21 to 56. Participants took either placebos or 1,500 mg or 3,000 mg of maca daily. After four, eight and 12 weeks, they reported on their sex drive levels. Placebo users experienced no change in libido, while the men taking either quantity of maca reported heightened sexual desire starting at eight weeks and continuing throughout the study.

How it works: Maca's libido-enhancing powers are attributed primarily to its amino acids and sterols, among other properties. Blood tests indicated that maca did not affect the men's levels of the hormones testosterone or *estradiol* (a form of estrogen present in women and men). This is just one of maca's virtues—it does not change hormone regulation in men.

A small study published in the *Asian Journal of Andrology* yielded some interesting results, indicating that maca also improves male fertility. Nine men, ages 24 to 44, received either 1,500 mg or 3,000 mg of maca per day. Compared with tests done at the outset of the study, semen analysis performed at the end of the four-month research period demonstrated that maca increased semen volume, sperm count and sperm motility at both dosage levels. Again, maca achieved these results by unknown mechanisms that were not related to increases in testosterone or other hormones.

SOOTHE MENOPAUSAL SYMPTOMS

For women, maca has a long-standing reputation for soothing menopausal symptoms. A study published in the *International Journal of Biomedical Science* details research at five sites in Poland, focusing on 124 women, ages 49 to 58, in the early stages of menopause.

During the study, the women took varied combinations of either a placebo or 2,000 mg of maca every day.

Results: Compared with placebo users, those taking maca experienced significant reductions—84%, on average—in the frequency and severity of menopausal symptoms, particularly hot flashes and night sweats. The participants also reported that maca reduced nervousness, mood swings, fatigue, stress, headaches and depression, as well as improved sleep patterns and libido.

Bonus: In a substudy of the trial, researchers found that the women taking maca had a notable increase in bone density.

How it works: Blood tests showed that maca reduced follicle-stimulating hormone, which normally increases during menopause and is thought to be one cause of troublesome symptoms, such as hot flashes and night sweats. Study authors speculate that maca stimulates the regulatory mechanism responsible for optimizing ovarian function and estrogen secretion, significantly increasing the level of estradiol in a woman's body.

It appears, then, that maca offers a safe and effective way to reduce menopausal symptoms —and it is unlikely to increase a woman's risk for breast cancer, heart disease and stroke, as can non-bioidentical hormone replacement therapy.

We don't know this for certain, but the fact that breast cancer is not among the leading causes of death in Peruvian women, despite a diet rich in maca, supports the assumption. In addition, increases in estradiol as a result of taking maca supplements may be safer than adding a hormone to a woman's system because maca appears to stimulate the body's natural estrogen production.

Historically, maca also has been used to improve libido in women. The National Institutes of Health (NIH) conducted a study to determine if maca effectively addresses female sexual dysfunction caused by antidepressant drugs.

The result: "It appears maca root may alleviate SSRI-induced sexual dysfunction and there may be a close-related effect. Maca may also have a beneficial effect on libido.

FIGHT STRESS AND DISEASE

Any kind of stress—from work, personal problems, illness, injury, toxins, hormonal imbalances or any other source—can negatively affect how our bodies function. Maca is what holistic doctors call an *adaptogen*, a plant or herb that boosts the body's ability to resist, deal with and recover from emotional and physical stress.

Practitioners of traditional medicine from China and India have known about and made use of adaptogens for centuries, though the term itself was not coined until the middle of the 20th century. Well-known adaptogens include the herbs ashwagandha, ginseng, rhodiola and licorice root, all of which I have prescribed to my patients with much success over the years.

How it works: To be classified as an adaptogen, a natural substance must meet specific criteria. It must be nontoxic...normalize levels of chemicals raised during periods of stress...and produce physical, chemical and/or biological responses that increase the body's resistance to stress.

Although all adaptogenic plants contain antioxidants, researchers do not believe that antioxidants alone account for adaptogens' normalizing powers. Rather, it is thought that a variety of phytochemicals helps balance the dozens of endocrine, digestive and neural hormones that operate throughout the body—including insulin (which regulates blood sugar levels) and dopamine (which enhances and stabilizes mood). Many adaptogens also stimulate immune system components, leading to better immune function.

MORE OF MACA'S SUPER POWERS

In addition to its documented beneficial effects on the human reproductive system, laboratory tests and animal studies suggest that maca may reduce the risk for...

•**Arthritis**—by promoting cartilage growth.

•**Blood toxicity**—by improving the function of the liver.

•**Diabetes**—by allowing for better control over blood sugar levels and body weight.

•**Digestive health**—by combating ulcers.

•**Fatigue**—by increasing energy and by increasing endurance.

•**Heart disease**—by lowering levels of LDL "bad" cholesterol and triglycerides (a type of blood fat).

•**Infertility**—by stimulating production of estrogen and other hormones in women and boosting sperm count in men.

•**Memory and mood**—by enhancing certain brain chemicals.

•**Osteoporosis**—by increasing your bone density.

•**Premenstrual syndrome (PMS)**—by regulating hormone levels.

•**Prostate problems**—by reducing prostate enlargement.

THE SAFEST WAY TO START

Maca generally appears to be safe, given its long history of use by Peruvians...but there are a few guidelines to bear in mind. Women who take estrogen to ease menopausal symptoms should talk to their doctors about using maca. They may be able to wean off hormone therapy or at least lower the estrogen dosage under a doctor's supervision.

Breast cancer patients taking tamoxifen or other estrogen blockers and women who have had breast cancer must not use maca, because it raises estrogen levels. Women in a family with a strong history of breast cancer should discuss maca use with their doctors first. People who take thyroid medication should be monitored by their doctors because maca may increase thyroid activity. Women who are pregnant or breast-feeding should not take maca, as a general precaution.

Since its long-term effects have not been scientifically studied, I recommend taking a break from maca now and then in order to give the body's cell receptors a break from any hormone stimulation. People who want to try maca to see if it is a "super food" for them should take supplements for three months (six months for women with severe menopausal symptoms), then stop using maca for one or two weeks. They may then continue this regimen as needed for symptom relief.

HOW MUCH TO TAKE

Maca is available in supplement and powder form.

The average dose of maca supplements is 1,000 mg to 2,000 mg daily—which you can take with or without food at any time of day.

Or you can get your maca by adding powder to your favorite foods and drinks. It has a slightly nutty flavor, so you may enjoy mixing it with almond milk. *Other ways to incorporate maca into your diet…*

• **Sprinkle on cereal (hot or cold).**

• **Mix into your favorite smoothie or protein shake.**

• **Add to yogurt or applesauce, perhaps with a little cinnamon.**

• **Stir into tea**—especially chai blends, as the flavors complement each other.

• **Use in baking**—substitute maca powder for one-quarter of the flour in any recipe (no more, or it might affect texture or consistency).

Be aware: Maca powder has a high fiber content and may initially cause gassiness. I suggest beginning with one teaspoon a day, then gradually increasing your intake by one teaspoon every five days until you find your comfort zone. The optimum dosage is three to six teaspoons daily.

HOW TO GET YOUR MACA

I recommend organically grown maca products from Natural Health International, or NHI (888-668-3661, *www.naturalhi.com*, available online or through naturopathic doctors). The company sells a blend for women called Femenessence MacaPause (the same blend used in the study of Polish women, who experienced significant improvement in their menopausal symptoms) and another for men, Revolution Macalibrium, formulated to enhance energy and vitality in men as they age.

Cost: $35 for 120 capsules of 500 mg each. The average dosage of maca supplements is 1,000 mg to 2,000 mg daily, which you can take anytime.

You can also sprinkle maca powder into your favorite foods and drinks. The powder costs about $17 for a 16 oz bag and is available online from *www.macaweb.com*.

Why Men Never Remember and Women Never Forget

Marianne Legato, MD, FACP, physician and professor of clinical medicine at Columbia University, New York City, and founder of Columbia's Partnership for Gender-Specific Medicine. She is author of several books, including *Why Men Never Remember and Women Never Forget* (Rodale).

Neither men nor women can claim that their brains are "better." While men's brains are 10% larger on average, women's brains have more elaborate connections that make them more efficient. Male and female brains unquestionably are different, in terms of both structure and chemistry, and that can cause problems when we try to communicate with one another.

Most of us speak to our spouses just as we would speak to members of our own sex—then wonder why they don't seem to understand us.

Here's how to communicate more effectively with the opposite sex…

NONVERBAL CUES

The female brain is good at decoding nonverbal signals, including facial expressions and tone of voice, perhaps because mothers must understand the needs of children too young to speak. When women send nonverbal signals to men, women are often dismayed to find that these signals are ignored.

Women don't realize that the typical male brain is not skilled at interpreting nonverbal communications. Men are particularly bad at identifying signs of sadness in women—though men are pretty good at spotting signs of anger and aggression.

Women: Tell him verbally when something is bothering you. A sad expression or the silent treatment won't get you anywhere. It's not that he is ignoring your feelings—he is just unaware of them.

If a man asks you what he can do to make you feel better, tell him. If you say "nothing," he'll assume that you mean nothing and he'll do nothing. He isn't trying to hurt you—men's brains just work in a more linear, literal manner. Because men often like to be left alone when they're upset, he might conclude that he is doing you a favor by giving you some space.

Men: Search for clues beyond her words when she seems unusually quiet or terse. She might be sending signals that you're not picking up. If you can't figure out the signals and she won't tell you what she needs, remind her that you really want to help, but it's hard for you to pick up her nonverbal cues.

LISTENING

The female brain seems to be better at listening than the male brain—women have more nerve cells in the areas known to process language and put a larger percentage of their brains to work when they hear someone speak.

The more elaborate wiring of the female brain also makes women better multitaskers than men. Evolution likely made women this way so that mothers could keep an eye on the children and still get other things done. Evolution shaped the male brain to focus on one very difficult task at a time. Tiger hunts were more successful when the hunters could focus all their attention on the tiger.

Add men's inferior listening ability to their superior focus, and the result is a phenomenon most wives know well. Tell a man something important while he's watching a ball game, and he might not remember a word of it. He isn't purposely ignoring you—his brain simply isn't wired to hear what you said.

Women: Put him on alert that what you're about to say is important. If it's particularly vital information, begin with a gentle "I need you to look me in the eyes." If there are too many distractions in your present location, ask him to go with you for a walk or out to a very quiet restaurant.

Men: Don't be insulted if she doesn't stop what she is doing when you want to talk. Chances are that she can pay attention to you even if she's occupied. If you want her undivided attention, ask for it.

PROBLEM SOLVING

The structure of the male brain makes men straight-ahead thinkers—when they see a problem, their instinct is to try to solve it.

Women are more likely to ruminate over decisions. They'll verbalize a problem and talk though all the implications and issues before they proceed. When women try to talk through their problems with men, they're often dismayed and insulted that the men try to tell them what to do. This confuses the men, who thought they were being asked for a solution to the problem.

Women: Tell a man the specific type of response you want before you share a problem. Are you asking the man for a solution, or do you just want to talk through the issue so it's clear in your mind? If you don't specifically tell him that it's the latter, he'll assume it's the former. If he tries to solve your problem anyway, understand that this is just how his brain responds.

As for how to respond to a man's problems, this rarely comes up. Men tend not to share their problems with anyone.

Men: Understand that women like to verbalize their thinking and don't always want you to solve their problems.

Instead, wait for a question before providing an answer. Ask what you can do to help rather than assume you know. And if your wife starts crying, holding her quietly works better than telling her she's being too emotional.

DIFFERENT INTERESTS

Women tend to expect their male partners to be interested in every subject they wish to discuss. That isn't fair. A woman wouldn't expect her female friends to chat about a subject that she knows bores them.

Women: Tailor your conversation to your partner's interests. (Men should do this, too, but because men talk less, it isn't as often an issue.) Find other conversation partners for topics that don't interest him.

Men: Encourage your partner to spend time with female friends so there's another outlet for the conversations that don't interest you.

Don't get upset if she's busy with friends when you want to see her.

BETTER ARGUMENTS

During an argument, women are more likely to bring up past events. Estrogen increases the amount of cortisol, a memory-boosting hormone, released by the adrenal glands during stressful moments. Because the female brain has more estrogen, memories of old fights remain fresher in a woman's mind. The male brain finds it easier to forget emotional situations and move on. Maybe forgetting a close call on a tiger hunt made it easier for men of the past to continue to hunt.

Women: Use simple, declarative sentences, and state what you want in outline form when imparting important information to men. Leave out anecdotes and unnecessary adjectives. Take advantage of your ability to read his emotions to spot the signs of boredom. When you see them, sum up your argument with a closing statement and end the conversation. Try not to rehash old arguments.

Men: Try to keep women focused on the point under discussion. If during an argument she brings up a fight you had five years ago, tell her, "We've discussed that already and it isn't going to help to go over it again. Let's focus on the current problem."

Gender Bender

Men and women view their fitness levels differently.

Recent study: Men and women who practiced strength training for 12 weeks all felt better about themselves in the end—but men based their new body image on feeling thinner, while women were more focused on their strength and the size of their muscles.

Kathleen Martin Ginis, PhD, professor of kinesiology, McMaster University, Hamilton, Ontario, and leader of a study of body image changes in 44 men and women in a strength-training program, published in *Body Image*.

Diseases Strike Men and Women Differently

Women who don't smoke may be more susceptible to lung cancer than male nonsmokers...women are more likely to get autoimmune diseases, such as rheumatoid arthritis and lupus...heart attacks in women often don't involve chest pain, but instead produce vague, flu-like symptoms.

Catherine DeAngelis, MD, MPH, editor in chief, *Journal of the American Medical Association*, 515 N. State St., Chicago 60610.

Is Your Marriage Making You Sick?

Theodore Robles, PhD, assistant professor of health psychology in the department of psychology at the University of California, Los Angeles. Robles' research focuses on the effects of marital conflict on endocrine and immune functioning in healthy adults. He was lead author of "Positive Behaviors During Marital Conflict: Influences on Stress Hormones," *Journal of Social and Personal Relationships*.

Researchers have long known that marriage can improve one's health. But only recently has scientific evidence emerged indicating that serious health consequences can result from a chronically stressful marriage.

Important new findings...

• **Increased heart disease risk.** Negative marital interactions have been convincingly linked by studies at the University of Utah to increases in heart rate and blood pressure, coronary artery fatty deposits (plaques) and decreased elasticity in the arteries—all of which contribute to heart disease.

• **Weakened immunity.** Married couples who were more hostile or angry during a single interaction were found to have decreased function of infection-fighting natural killer cells in a study at Ohio State University and, in a later study, slower rates of wound healing.

As a health risk, marital stress is on par with social isolation, high cholesterol, poor diet and lack of exercise, according to these and other findings. For unknown reasons, women seem to be particularly hard hit by marital woes—studies consistently show that wives experience stronger cardiovascular, hormonal and immunological reactions to marital stress.

Good news: While virtually all marriages endure some degree of conflict, studies suggest that it's how we deal with disagreements—not just whether we have them—that largely determines the effects on our health. For example, University of Utah researchers have shown that a couple's demeanor during disputes—warm, hostile, controlling, submissive—is as good an indicator of underlying heart disease as cholesterol levels.

To minimize the health impact of marital stress...

• **Break the tension.** Ohio State University researchers recently measured blood levels of the stress hormones *cortisol* and *adrenocorticotropic hormone* (ACTH) in 90 newlywed couples before, during and after a 30-minute discussion about sensitive marital issues. When both partners were consistently negative, the wives' cortisol and ACTH levels escalated.

However, when one or both partners were supportive and constructive—even during heated discussions—the wives' stress hormones declined throughout the discussion. (Men's hormone levels were unaffected by both the negative and supportive behaviors.)

What both spouses can do: Agree with your partner on some points...accept responsibility for your shortcomings...and propose compromises.

Research involving women with high blood pressure suggests that more hostile behaviors during marital discussions are associated with elevated blood pressure during the exchanges, and more supportive behaviors are associated with lower blood pressure during the discussions.

• **Watch your words.** While husbands appear less physiologically affected by their wives' hostility, they do react—with increased heart rate and blood pressure—to perceived challenges to their competency or skills.

What both spouses can do: Avoid controlling statements such as "You're never on time...why don't you wear your watch?" or "Why can't you just do what I ask?"

Replace comments such as: "You're spending us into bankruptcy!" with: "I know you love to shop for the grandkids, but we need to stick to a budget."

Helpful: Because we cannot control everything about our spouses, look for something to value even in those things you may not readily admire. For example, if you resent your spouse's messiness but value his/her easygoing nature, try viewing these qualities as flip sides of the same coin. You may find you have greater tolerance for—and less need to control—the clutter.

• **Trust your spouse.** In a University of Utah study involving 300 middle-aged and older couples, researchers found no correlation between self-reports of anger or antagonism and calcium buildup in their coronary arteries (a risk factor for cardiovascular disease). However, partners whose spouses had rated them high on scales of anger and antagonism were more likely to have significant calcium buildup.

What both spouses can do: Pay attention if your partner says you are being angry, hostile, unreasonable or cold. While you may be unaware of your negativity, your arteries could be paying the price.

• **Speak your mind.** In a University of Michigan study involving 192 older couples, those in which both spouses clammed up to avoid confrontation were much more likely to experience the death of one or both partners over a 17-year period. In fact, among 26 such "dual-suppressor" marriages, 27% suffered the loss of one spouse, and 23% experienced the death of both partners, while among the 166 more communicative couples, a significantly lower 19% experienced one death, and only 6% experienced the death of both partners.

Shocking new finding: In a recent study involving nearly 4,000 married adults from Framingham, Massachusetts, women who reported regularly stifling themselves during marital disagreements were four times more likely than outspoken wives to die during a 10-year period.

The culprit could be stress—when husbands respond with silence to their wives' anger, studies show that wives' cortisol levels go up and stay up for the day. Chronically elevated cortisol has been linked to impaired cognitive and immune functioning, heart disease, diabetes and other ills.

What both spouses can do: Communicate openly.

• **Relax.** Studies have shown that the higher a woman's levels of stress hormones before she and her husband engage in a discussion about their relationship, the more likely she and her husband are to be critical, defensive or hostile to one another during conflict. Unfortunately, these negative behaviors only exacerbate the wife's already elevated ACTH and cortisol levels.

What both spouses can do: Make time daily to relax, whether with exercise, meditation, hobbies or spending time with friends. By lowering stress, women, in particular, may be able to keep hostility—and their stress hormones—from escalating during marital conflict.

Men, Women and Weight

Men who weigh too much are likely to have poor sperm quality. Overweight women have trouble conceiving naturally—and are less likely to become pregnant even when embryos are fertilized in the lab and implanted.

David Ryley, MD, clinical fellow, reproductive endocrinology and infertility, Beth Israel Deaconess Medical Center, Boston, and leader of a study of more than 5,800 attempts at in vitro fertilization, published in *Fertility and Sterility.*

To Cut Calories, Dine With a Man

When eating out, whom you are with can influence how much you eat.

Recent study: Women consumed, on average, about 665 calories when eating with one other woman and about 800 calories when eating with three other women—but just 552 calories when eating with a man. Men ate about the same amount regardless of the sex or number of companions.

Theory: Women want to look attractive and in control when with a date or mate.

Lesson: There's no need to skip a night out with the girls—just be mindful of how much you are eating.

Meredith E. Young, PhD, assistant professor of cognitive psychology, Centre for Medical Education, McGill University, Montreal, Canada, and leader of a study of 469 people.

Libido Boost

In order to wake up your libido, try combining and drinking equal parts of the tincture form of the herbs *damiana* and *Panax ginseng* to stimulate arousal and increase levels of the hormone testosterone. Works for women and men. Consult a health-care professional knowledgeable in herbal medicine to determine if the formula is right for you and what dosage you should use.

If that doesn't work: Ask your doctor to check you for a deficiency in *dehydroepiandrosterone* (DHEA). The steroid hormone is available at health-food stores and is a precursor to such hormones as estrogen and androgen. Ask your doctor if this is right for you.

Jane Guiltinan, ND, dean of Naturopathic Medicine, Bastyr University, Seattle.

Eastern Practices for Better Sex

Women with low libido who began a regular practice of mindfulness (a meditative focus on the moment) reported improved sexual arousal. Women with a genital pain disorder who received a varying number of acupuncture treatments in areas linked to the liver, spleen and kidneys reported reductions in pain. Both groups reported increased vaginal lubrication and sexual satisfaction.

Lori A. Brotto, PhD, assistant professor, department of obstetrics and gynecology, University of British Columbia, Vancouver, Canada, and co-reviewer of 48 studies.

Sex Can Ease Migraine Pain

Women who have sex when they feel a migraine coming on experience less head and neck pain, fatigue and moodiness. Nearly one-third of women who had sex at the start of a migraine reported reduced symptoms…and for 12%, sex stopped the migraine completely.

Possible reason: Sex and orgasm boost levels of the pleasure hormone *serotonin*—which is known to be low in migraine sufferers.

James R. Couch, MD, PhD, professor of neurology, University of Oklahoma Health Sciences Center, Oklahoma City, and leader of a study of 82 women with migraines, published in *Headache: The Journal of Head and Face Pain.*

23

Natural Weight-Loss Remedies

Your Lucky 13—The Best Secrets for Losing Weight Without Feeling Hungry!

When your stomach is sending out insistent, incessant "feed me!" messages, it makes it almost impossible to stick to a strict diet. That's why the real key to weight-loss success is to shut down hunger and short-circuit food cravings—because then it is easier to cut down on calories. *Here are 13 simple strategies for slimming down without making yourself feel deprived…*

1. Have two servings of protein at breakfast. Proteins are natural appetite suppressants. This means that even if eating more protein ups your usual morning calorie count, you will feel fuller longer—so over the course of the day, you'll wind up eating less.

Breakfast combinations: An egg scrambled with an ounce of shredded cheese…or eight ounces of low-fat yogurt mixed with an ounce of slivered almonds. Do not just have coffee for breakfast—you'll feel ravenous later.

2. At lunch and dinner, consume items in order of least-to-most calories. Start the meal with your salad and vegetables…eat the grains next…and then work your way around the plate to the heavier foods, such as meat. By the time you get there, you're already starting to feel full—so it is easier to control your portions of those calorie-dense items.

Interactive tool: Gauge proper portion sizes based on your weight, height and exercise level at *www.mypyramid.gov* (click on "Get a personalized Plan").

3. Don't think of snacking as cheating. Wisely chosen snacks keep hunger pangs at

Keith T. Ayoob, EdD, RD, nutritionist and associate clinical professor, Department of Pediatrics, at Albert Einstein College of Medicine, Bronx, New York. He is coauthor of *The Uncle Sam Diet: The 4-Week Eating Plan for a Thinner, Healthier America* (St. Martin's).

bay, so you won't overindulge later in the day. Have a midafternoon and an evening snack every day, combining two food groups.

Examples: Pair a vegetable with a whole grain (hummus or salsa with whole-wheat pita or crackers)…or pair fruit with dairy (pineapple with low-fat cottage cheese, a smoothie made with blueberries and low-fat yogurt). Prepare healthful snacks ahead of time so you'll reach for them—not candy or chips—when your stomach grumbles.

4. Choose foods that you can't eat quickly. Labor-intensive foods—pistachios in the shell, edamame in the pod, peel-and-eat shrimp—force you to savor each bite instead of shoveling everything down. This leisurely pace fools your brain into thinking that you're consuming much more than you actually are.

5. Drink water to squelch the munchies. People often mistake thirst for hunger—so downing eight ounces of water may quickly quell food cravings.

Also helpful: Make sure your diet includes high-water–content foods—cucumbers, lettuce, zucchini…oranges, peaches, strawberries, watermelon…low-fat broth and tomato-based soups.

6. Cut down on caffeine. Yes, caffeine gives a short-term energy buzz—but it also contributes to hunger.

Reason: Caffeine stimulates insulin secretion…which reduces blood sugar…which tells your brain that it's time to eat. Limit caffeinated coffee, tea and cola to two cups daily, consumed with meals, to see if this eases food cravings. Cut back further if you have insomnia.

7. Chew sugarless cinnamon gum. Of course, when there's gum in your mouth, you won't be tempted to put food in there, too—but there's more to this strategy. Chewing gum helps improve mental focus, so that you stay engaged in your activity and are less apt to hear the call of the refrigerator. Also, chewing gum helps relieve the stress that can lead to overeating. Why choose cinnamon? It retains its flavor longest.

8. Fill up on fiber. Soluble and insoluble fibers hold water and expand in your stomach, making you feel fuller longer.

Daily goals: Four cups of fruits and vegetables (assuming foods are small, such as berries, or chopped)…one-half cup of beans (which are highly nutritious yet underappreciated) or other legumes…and three servings of whole grains (brown rice, oatmeal, whole-wheat bread).

Party trick: Eat half an oat-bran muffin before you go out. Those 100 calories will save you hundreds more because you'll feel less enticed by the hors d'oeuvres.

9. Indulge in chocolate for dessert. One ounce of dark chocolate with 70% or more cocoa content has only about 150 calories. Savor it with a cup of decaf coffee or herbal tea—its big taste belies its relatively modest calorie count.

Delectable brands: Scharffen Berger (866-972-6879, *www.scharffenberger.com*)…and Valrhona (888-682-5746, *www.valrhona.com*).

10. Fool the hunger hormone. *Ghrelin*, a hormone that stimulates hunger, drops about a half-hour after you eat—so nibble on a half-ounce of nutrient-rich nuts 30 minutes before dinner to make it easier to keep meal portions modest. If you're going out, carry nuts in your purse. (Recycle an Altoids mint tin—it's the perfect size for your portable nut stash.)

11. Shake your booty—or just take a brisk walk. Aerobic exercise lowers hunger-triggering ghrelin…increases levels of the appetite-suppressing hormone *peptide YY*…burns calories…and relieves stress.

Goal: At least 30 minutes of aerobic exercise (such as quick-paced walking) every day.

12. Retrain your palate. When you habitually consume lots of sugar, salt or fat, your taste buds become desensitized. Like addicts, they need a bigger and bigger "fix" to feel satisfied. But when you cut back on those three troublemakers, within a few weeks you regain the ability to detect and enjoy subtler flavors—and sugary, salty and fatty foods lose their appeal.

13. Move up your bedtime. People who sleep less than five hours a night have higher ghrelin levels—causing them to feel near-constant hunger. Sleeping for about eight hours per night helps normalize ghrelin levels. Also, fatigue increases stress and impairs judgment—so by getting more rest, you become better able to make sensible decisions about food.

Bonus: An early bedtime means that you won't be tempted to have a midnight snack, so you're likely to wake up weighing less—and feeling proud.

Diet Personality— What's Your Secret To Getting Slim and Staying Slim?

Heather K. Jones, RD, nutritionist and journalist in private practice in Seattle. She is coauthor of *What's Your Diet Type?* (Hatherleigh) and a nutrition consultant for *The Best Life Diet* (Simon & Schuster) by Bob Greene, Oprah Winfrey's personal fitness trainer. *www.MyDiet Type.com.*

If you struggle over and over again to lose weight (or at least to avoid gaining more), yet seldom have much success, you probably chide yourself for being weak-willed. Stop that! The problem isn't your flawed character—it's that your dieting strategies are out of sync with your personality.

Just as you are born right- or left-handed, you come into the world with a distinct personality type. Though you continue to evolve physically, emotionally, mentally and spiritually throughout your life, your inborn personality type doesn't change much.

What this means: Rather than trying to force yourself to fit the mold of a preconceived diet plan, you'll have better results if you customize your dieting approach to suit your personality.

Here are the four distinct "Diet Types"... clues that help you determine which type you are...and the corresponding tactics that will help you lose weight and keep it off.

THE DIET PLANNER

Security and stability are of utmost importance for this type of person. *You're a Diet Planner if you...*

- **Have a strong sense of right and wrong**
- **Value your traditions and enjoy your regular routines**
- **Take your various duties and responsibilities very seriously**
- **Are organized, disciplined and hardworking.**

Your trouble spot #1: When life throws you a curveball (for example, your mother breaks her hip), you move your own needs to the bottom of your priority list so that you can get everything else done. Caught up in your duties (doctor appointments, insurance claims), you have no time left to plan your meals and instead eat haphazardly.

Solution: To stay organized, devise a week's worth of menus so you know exactly what to buy at the grocery store. Keep healthful snacks (baby carrots, an apple) in your purse so you needn't resort to the vending machine if you are delayed (for instance, at your mother's physical therapy appointment). Make a backup plan for missed workouts, committing to an evening aerobics class if you miss your usual morning class.

Your trouble spot #2: You're nostalgic—so it's hard to give up that customary buttered popcorn at the movies or ham-and-cheese quiche for Sunday brunch.

Solution: Go ahead and eat your traditional favorite treats—but make small modifications that cut big calories.

Examples: Leave the popcorn unbuttered ...make a veggie quiche for brunch.

THE DIET PLAYER

This personality type is characterized by spontaneity and adaptability. *You're a Diet Player if you...*

- **Focus on today rather than worrying about tomorrow**
- **Seek fun, variety, stimulation and also excitement**
- **Trust your impulses**
- **Dislike rules and regulations.**

Your trouble spot #1: You get bored eating the same diet foods day after day. So when the impulse to eat strikes, instead of having yet another ho-hum salad, you reach for something fun—and fattening—instead.

Solution: Clear your kitchen of all high-calorie, low-nutrition items, then stock up on healthful foods you actually enjoy—exotic fresh fruits, five different flavors of yogurt, a sampler of imported nuts.

Your trouble spot #2: You feel burdened by rules, so you rebel against regimented diet plans.

Solution: Forget about following a by-the-book diet, and simply focus on paring down portions. Make whatever type of sandwich suits your fancy today, but save half of it for tomorrow…try the black squid ink pasta in cream sauce if it intrigues you, but order the appetizer size, not the entrée.

THE DIET FEELER

Relationships and unity are top priorities for this type of person. *You're a Diet Feeler if you…*

• **Value family and friends far more than money or prestige**

• **Are very conscious of your own and other peoples' emotions**

• **Enjoy the role of teacher, counselor or confidant**

• **Are concerned with personal growth and development.**

Your trouble spot #1: You are a classic emotional eater. Because relationships are so important to you, interpersonal conflict often makes you reach for comfort foods—even though the comfort is only temporary and does nothing to resolve underlying issues.

Solution: Keep a food/mood journal, writing down everything you eat and how you feel before and after. Look for patterns. Do you long for macaroni and cheese when you're mad or crave chocolate cake à la mode when you're sad? Make a list of food-free activities to turn to when you need an emotional boost—such as phoning a friend when you're lonely or practicing yoga when you feel worried.

Your trouble spot #2: You love feeling connected to the people around you, so you fall prey to peer pressure to eat.

Example: If your friends all order pie at the restaurant, so do you—even if you're not hungry and don't particularly like pie.

Solution: You can share fun without sharing food. Meet up with friends at a bowling alley instead of a bistro. When the family lingers over dinner, let them pick at what's left on the serving platters while you sip a cup of coffee or tea and focus on what really matters—the conversation.

THE DIET THINKER

This type of personality centers on knowledge and accomplishment. *You're a Diet Thinker if you…*

• **Are a lifelong learner who strives to understand the world**

• **Look for logical answers for everything**

• **Enjoy discovering new and different ways of doing things**

• **Hate to fail and are your own worst critic.**

Your trouble spot #1: You take a scholarly approach to weight loss, researching and contemplating various diet plans and exercise routines—but you're so busy thinking that you don't actually do anything.

Solution: Consider why you are procrastinating. Because you haven't found the "perfect" plan? Because you're afraid you'll fail at losing weight? Give yourself a deadline of two weeks to research your options (for instance, the various online calorie-monitoring plans or the latest high-tech pedometers), then commit to a specific approach.

Your trouble spot #2: Your keen analytical abilities let you rationalize diet-sabotaging behaviors.

Example: You justify eating potato chips because they provide more potassium than a banana.

Solution: Instead of finding excuses for indulgences, do what you do best—seek knowledge from reliable sources. Once you are convinced of the many benefits of weight control, it is easier to make healthful decisions based not on twisted logic but on irrefutable facts.

Foods that Boost Your Mood...And Help You Lose Weight

Susan M. Kleiner, PhD, RD, Mercer Island, Washington–based nutritionist who has worked with Olympic athletes, professional sports teams and Fortune 500 company executives. She is the author of *The Good Mood Diet: Feel Great While You Lose Weight* (Springboard), *www.goodmooddiet.com*, and *Power Eating* (Human Kinetics).

It's long been known that our eating habits can have a dramatic effect on our overall health.

Now: A growing body of scientific evidence shows that the foods we eat can either improve—or harm—our mood.

Bonus: Mood-boosting foods will help you lose weight if you have some extra pounds to shed. They can give you the mental and physical energy to be active as well as the nutrition that best supports physical activity, muscle growth and fat burning. People of normal weight can adapt these food recommendations to their daily calorie needs.

FEEL-GREAT BUILDING BLOCKS

The basic nutrients in the food we eat each play a role in optimizing our mood and energy levels...

•**Carbohydrates are viewed negatively by most people who are trying to eat healthfully.** But, in fact, these nutrients—when eaten in the proper form—are crucial to maintaining mood.

Here's why: Your mood is largely determined by a proper balance of brain chemicals (neurotransmitters). One key neurotransmitter, *serotonin*, is strongly linked to positive feelings.

Surprising fact: The brain uses the amino acid *tryptophan*, which is contained in most dietary proteins, to manufacture serotonin. But to cross from the bloodstream to the brain, tryptophan must compete against other amino acids. Carbohydrates help displace the other amino acids, thus increasing the amount of tryptophan that gets through—and the amount of serotonin that is produced.

A steady stream of carbohydrates will help your brain reach ample levels of tryptophan.

Best carbohydrate sources: Fruits (such as bananas, blueberries, mangoes, oranges, pomegranates and strawberries) and vegetables (such as broccoli, spinach, yams and carrots). These foods not only supply carbohydrates, but also contain water and fiber that slow the rate at which the carbohydrates are digested and absorbed into the bloodstream.

Helpful: When your favorite fruits and vegetables are out of season, frozen versions (without added sauces) are economical and convenient.

•**Fats, like carbohydrates, have been pegged as "no-nos."** But dietary fats should not be eliminated altogether—they make foods filling and satisfying.

Surprising fact: Fats are essential in keeping brain-cell membranes supple and well-functioning. For example, the omega-3 fatty acids found in certain fish (such as salmon, mackerel and sardines) have been shown to improve mood in people who are depressed.

Best fat sources: In addition to fish, try olives (any type), nuts, seeds, avocados, extra virgin olive oil and cold-pressed canola oil.

•**Proteins can be converted into blood sugar (glucose)**—but slowly, to keep glucose on an even keel. These nutrients also help keep metabolism (the rate at which you burn calories) high.

Surprising fact: Proteins are the raw materials from which neurotransmitters, including serotonin, are manufactured.

Best protein sources: Lean organic meat (beef, pork or lamb) or poultry...fish...low-fat or fat-free dairy products...eggs...and legumes (such as pinto beans or lentils).

GOOD MOOD MEALS

After three hours of not eating, glucose levels fall and so do your spirits and energy levels. To avoid "panic eating," have a meal or substantial snack every two to three hours. *For example...*

Breakfast: ½ cup of shredded wheat cereal...2 tablespoons of raisins...1 cup of fat-free milk...1 egg (cooked without butter or margarine).

Mid-morning snack: 1 cup of fat-free milk...omelet from 4 egg whites or 2 ounces of sliced turkey.

Lunch: 1 cup of bean soup (low-sodium canned soup is okay)...tuna salad (without mayonnaise, but with reduced-fat salad dressing made with olive oil and vinegar)...and mixed greens.

Afternoon snack: Orange...mini-carrots with 1 tablespoon of natural-style peanut butter.

Dinner: 1 cup of whole-wheat pasta tossed with 1¼ tablespoons of pesto (homemade or store-bought)...4 ounces of chicken (grilled, broiled, baked or roasted)...2 cups of sliced cucumber...at least 1 cup total of carrots and cherry tomatoes...and 1¼ cups of fresh strawberries with 1 tablespoon of full-fat dairy whipped topping (it has only a few more calories than a "lite" version).

Evening snack: 1 cup of hot cocoa made with fat-free milk, 1 to 2 rounded teaspoons of unsweetened cocoa powder and Splenda (one packet or to taste) or another sweetener, such as agave nectar (a syrup derived from a desert plant). It is sold in health-food stores.

EXERCISE-MOOD CONNECTION

Exercise not only helps control your body weight, but also has been shown to improve mood and reduce depression (as effectively as medication, in some studies). At a minimum, get 30 minutes of activity (at the level of brisk walking) five to six days a week.

Yoga May Slow Midlife Weight Gain

People in their 50s who regularly practiced yoga lost about five pounds over 10 years, while those who did not practice yoga gained about 13 pounds. Most yoga exercises do not burn enough calories to account for the weight loss, but some practitioners believe that yoga keeps people aware of their bodies and their eating habits.

Alan Kristal, DrPH, researcher, Fred Hutchinson Cancer Research Center, Seattle, and leader of a study of 15,550 people, published in *Alternative Therapies in Health and Medicine*.

A Better Way to Walk— Boost Calorie Burn by Nearly 20%

Timothy S. Church, MD, MPH, PhD, professor of preventive medicine research at Pennington Biomedical Research Center in Baton Rouge, Louisiana. He has coauthored a number of journal articles on pole-walking and the role of exercise in health.

You can turn a walk into a whole-body workout with a pair of Nordic fitness poles—long, handheld poles modeled after cross-country ski poles. Pole walking (or Nordic walking) is a low-impact aerobic activity that strengthens the upper body... improves posture...minimizes back and leg strain...and boosts your calorie burn during a walk by almost 20%.

•**Picking poles.** One-piece poles are safest, especially for seniors and people with balance problems, because they won't collapse the way adjustable-length telescoping or twist-locking poles might.

Test for size: Grasp the pole handle and place the tip on the ground a few inches in front of you, elbow bent and tucked into your side. If your elbow makes a 90-degree angle, the pole is the proper length.

Or: Multiply your height in centimeters by 0.68—the resulting number is your pole size. Choose poles with interchangeable tips— metal for trails, grass, sand or snow...rubber for pavement and mall walking. Poles are sold at sporting-goods stores and online (check 877-754-9255, *www.skiwalking.com*).

Cost: $70 to $160.

•**Correct technique.** To get started, swing your arms normally as you walk—left arm moving forward as the right foot takes a step and vice versa. As the right foot lands, bend your left elbow to 90 degrees and plant the left pole tip across from your right heel...then push the pole against the ground to help propel yourself forward. Keep poles angled rearward—they should never be farther forward than the front foot.

Goal: Walk at a moderate to brisk pace for at least 30 minutes five times a week. Pole-walking is safe for just about everyone—but it's best to check with your doctor before starting any exercise program.

Money Motivates Weight Loss

Overweight people offered $14 for every 1% decrease in body weight lost more weight than those offered $7 for the same amount of weight loss. People offered no financial incentive lost the least weight.

Eric Finkelstein, PhD, director, Public Health Economics Program, RTI International, a research organization, Research Triangle Park, North Carolina, and author of a weight-loss incentive study, published in *Journal of Occupations and Environmental Medicine.*

Rice Cakes Can Cause Weight Gain

Even though they are low in calories, they boost blood-sugar and insulin levels, causing the body to store extra sugar as fat.

Other products to avoid for the same reason: Mashed potatoes, instant rice, dried dates, fruit roll-ups and jelly beans.

Men's Health, 33 E. Minor St., Emmaus, Pennsylvania 18098.

Medical Scams, Cons And Rip-Offs

Chuck Whitlock, journalist whose work exposing scams has been featured on many television programs, including *Inside Edition* and *Extra.* He is author of several books about scams, including *MediScams: Dangerous Medical Practices and Health Care Frauds* (St. Martin's Griffin). *www.chuckwhitlock.com*

Bogus "miracle cures" and quack physicians probably have been around as long as the health-care profession. Con artists prey upon the unhealthy because sick people may be so desperate to find a cure that they will try any possible treatment, however expensive and farfetched.

These snake oil salesmen have been on the rise in recent years, as our aging population has more medical problems...millions of underinsured and uninsured Americans search for health-care options that they can afford... and the surging popularity of "alternative medicine" makes unscientific treatments seem more mainstream.

Sometimes it's obvious when a claim is fraudulent—but certain scams and unethical practices are difficult to spot...

SCAMS

•**Cheap health insurance.** Many of the more than 45 million Americans who are without health insurance are desperate to find affordable coverage. Disreputable insurance companies offer these people exactly what they want—health insurance at a low price, sometimes as little as $50 per month.

Most buyers are so thrilled to find insurance they can afford that they don't pay attention to the fine print. Many of these policies have huge deductibles, scant benefits and other restrictions that make them virtually worthless.

Most policyholders do not discover the problems until they have a serious health condition and receive the bill.

What to do: Look for a policy that covers doctor visits and protects against a major medical expense. A way to spot-check the quality of a policy is to look at the benefits for hospital stays. A good policy should pay $500 or more per day for the hospital room, with additional coverage for other hospital costs. An inadequate policy might provide only $100 a day.

Wise: Contact your state's insurance commissioner to find out if complaints have been filed against the company. Blue Cross/Blue Shield offers many reputable plans, and Kaiser Permanente has a good reputation for a health maintenance organization (HMO).

• **Natural appetite suppressants.** Unscrupulous marketers claim that there are natural supplements that help you lose weight—but these supplements don't work or have dangerous side effects. The most heavily promoted "appetite suppressants" include *ephedra, garcinia cambogia* and *hoodia*.

• Ephedra is an herbal stimulant, and like other stimulants, it does suppress appetite but at the price of increased heart rate, nervousness and agitation. In large doses, ephedra has killed people, and the FDA has pulled it off the market, though it's still available on the Web.

• Garcinia cambogia (a fruit from Asia) and hoodia (from a succulent African plant) are not stimulants and seem to be safe—but they don't work. No studies have shown them to be effective in suppressing one's appetite.

What to do: The only reliable cures for excess weight are consuming fewer calories and getting more exercise.

• **Organ transplants in developing countries.** America's organ donation program can't keep pace with the demand for transplants. For patients languishing on waiting lists, flying to a developing country where organs can be purchased on the black market might seem viable. Before you board a plane to India, the Philippines, Hungary or Russia and agree to pay $1,000 to $100,000 for an organ, consider that you're putting yourself in the hands of people who are more interested in taking your money than saving your life.

These people might find an organ for you—but you might not receive it until you've been milked for many times the agreed-upon price. Some patients are told at the last minute that someone else will pay more for the organ, which might or might not be true. To get the organ, you have to top this other offer. Even

when patients do get their organs, their transplants often are performed according to medical standards that are not as strict as they are in the US.

What to do: Talk to your doctor about the best options.

UNETHICAL PRACTICES

• **Bonuses from HMOs and PPOs to doctors who skip useful tests.** HMOs and preferred provider organizations (PPOs) often give cash bonuses to doctors who don't perform pricey tests—even when those tests are in the patient's best interest. They are essentially bribing doctors to scam their patients.

Example: Your HMO or PPO doctor tells you that he/she is going to spare you the invasive thallium stress test (where radioactive dye is injected into your bloodstream) and perform a routine treadmill test without thallium, though the thallium test is warranted.

What to do: When your HMO or PPO doctor tells you that you have a particular health condition, research that condition on a reliable Internet Web site, such as *WebMD.com* or *MayoClinic.com*. If the site mentions a test that your doctor has not performed, ask him why it was skipped. If the doctor's response seems evasive, consider getting a second opinion.

• **Unqualified plastic surgeon.** Many doctors have switched to plastic surgery in recent years, drawn by the lucrative nature of the specialty and its lower reliance on insurance payments. (Most plastic surgery procedures are elective and not covered by insurance.) No law or regulation prevents doctors from changing their specialty to plastic surgery—even if they have no background or training in this field. Patients likely have no idea that they are trusting their lives and appearances to what are essentially unqualified, untrained novices.

What to do: If you're considering plastic surgery, ask the surgeon…

• **Are you board-certified in plastic surgery?** He/she should be.

• **At what hospital do you have physician's privileges?** A general hospital is fine, but a university hospital is even better—university hospitals tend to have very high standards.

• **Who will be handling my anesthesia?** Don't trust a plastic surgeon who says he'll handle it himself. He may be trying to cut corners and putting your health at risk in the process.

Natural Alternative To Sugar

Mark A. Stengler, NMD, licensed naturopathic medical doctor in private practice, Stengler Center for Integrative Medicine, Encinitas, California...adjunct associate clinical professor at the National College of Natural Medicine, Portland, Oregon...author of many books, including *The Natural Physician's Healing Therapies* and coauthor of *Prescription for Natural Cures* (both from Bottom Line Books)...and author of the *Bottom Line/Natural Healing* newsletter. *www.drstengler.com*

Artificial sweeteners and the chemical processes used to create them have been making headlines recently. The controversy focuses primarily on the fact that the sugar in Splenda is converted to a sweetener using *chlorine*. Little information has been published about all the truly natural alternatives to sugar.

The result is that most Americans remain unfamiliar with healthy, natural options like *Luo Han Guo*, also referred to as *Lo Han*. A rare fruit found in China, Luo Han yields a powder 250 to 300 times sweeter than sugar.

And that's just the tip of the iceberg when it comes to the benefits of Luo Han.

As a sweetener, Luo Han Guo has no calories, does not elevate blood sugar, and is heat stable—which means it can be added to both hot and cold foods. It also helps prevent cavities and has no after-taste. These attributes make it an ideal, versatile option as a natural sweetener for tea, coffee or other beverages, and for use in making desserts.

ITS ORIGINS

While Westerners may have much to learn about Luo Han, the fruit has been used in a variety of ways, for thousands of years in China. The Lo Han Guo is a round, green perennial vine fruit in the melon family that grows wild throughout the mountainous terrain of Southwest China. Historic Chinese writings describe Song Dynasty monks brewing the fruit for medicinal beverages more than 800 years ago.

Luo Han, which is typically dried and sold in Chinese medicinal herb shops, has long been used in China and other Asian countries as a food and beverage, and also treats colds, coughs, sore throats, stomach distress, heat stroke, constipation and diarrhea.

The dried fruit is sold in a variety of forms, including whole, liquid, powdered or in a tea.

Often, in Chinese households, Luo Han is cooked with pork as a remedy for lung congestion. In fact, the *Encyclopedia of Traditional Chinese Medicine* recommends 10–15 grams—or one fruit—boiled in water per day, to address lung complaints, as Luo Han is a natural expectorant and helps clear the lungs of airborne pollutants.

The move toward using Luo Han as a sweetening agent is a more recent development.

THE VERSATILITY OF LUO HAN

In 1995, Procter & Gamble Company patented a process for making a sweetener from the fruit. Now, many sugar substitutes derived from Luo Han are available for manufacturing and home use.

The Luo Han fruit, which is sold mostly in Chinese grocery stores in the United States, can be simmered into a thick, sweet juice and used during food preparation.

There are many benefits to using the Luo Han extract as a sweetening agent and sugar substitute—chief among them is the fact that the fruit contains sweet compounds called glycosides, specifically *triterpene glycosides*. The body does not break glycosides down like other simple sugars, which means blood glucose or insulin levels do not rise like they do with other sugars—making it ideal for diabetics.

Luo Han also contains high amounts of amino acids, vitamins, minerals and potent antioxidant properties, which benefit immune function and the body's ability to maintain healthy balance.

Why the French Don't Get Fat

Will Clower, PhD, president and founder of PATH Healthy Eating Curriculum, an educational and consulting program based in Pittsburgh that teaches weight-control strategies in corporate and academic settings, and founder of Mediterranean Wellness, LLC, also in Pittsburgh. He is a neurophysiologist and former neuroscience historian at University of Pittsburgh and author of *The Fat Fallacy: The French Diet Secrets to Permanent Weight Loss* (Three Rivers). *www.willclower.com.*

The fad diets that sweep America are almost unheard of in France. The French don't count carbs or fill their pantries with low-fat snacks. They eat foods that make diet-conscious Americans cringe—buttery croissants, rich cheeses, fat-laden pâtés. Few belong to health clubs.

Yet the French don't get fat. In France, the obesity rate is only about 8%—while about 30% of Americans are obese. The French are three times less likely than Americans to get heart disease. And they live longer—men live an average of two years more…women, three years more. Why are the French trimmer and healthier?

Americans focus on what they should not eat. They look at a piece of pie and say to themselves, "I shouldn't eat that—it will make me fat." Eating becomes less about pleasure than avoiding hazards. That's a key reason why many people don't stick with a diet. A Tufts University study showed that 22% of people on low-carb or low-fat diets abandoned them after two months. After a year, the drop-out rate was almost 50%.

The French have a healthier relationship with food. They don't have to diet because they're not overweight. *And they're not overweight because they…*

•**Choose quality over quantity.** A Frenchman would rather have 10 perfect pommes frites than a plateful of soggy French fries or a small dish of creme brûlée rather than a mass of store-bought cookies. Also, the stomach stretches and demands more food if you take big servings on a regular basis.

Helpful: Take a little less than you think you want. Studies show that people typically overestimate the amount of food they need—and once it's on the plate, they tend to eat it even if they have had enough. If you're going out to eat, share an entrée or just have an appetizer as your main course.

•**Savor each bite.** It's common in France to linger for hours over meals. Eating quickly almost guarantees that you'll take in excess calories. It takes 15 to 20 minutes for the stomach and small intestine to signal the brain that you're full.

Helpful…

Make a conscious effort to take small bites. Give yourself time to appreciate the aroma, texture and flavors.

Set down your fork between bites. Don't pick it up until you have chewed and swallowed your food. Americans often fill their forks for the next bite before they have finished the previous one.

Make time for conversation…and only talk when your mouth is empty. This naturally slows the pace of meals and reduces the calories you consume.

•**Plan on seconds.** Knowing that you can have a second helping is psychologically reassuring—you're more likely to take a smaller portion the first time around if you know that you can have more. By the time you're ready for seconds, you may not want them—or you may choose to have a small dessert instead.

•**Don't combine eating with other activities.** This means not nibbling in front of the TV or while driving. The French make eating a special occasion, and they rarely snack.

•**Forgo "faux" foods.** A lot of things we eat are little more than an accumulation of chemicals. If you look at the labels on chips, sodas and other snacks, you'll see *partially hydrogenated oils, sodium stearyl lactylate, polysorbate 60,* etc. Also because these products lack flavor, they're often loaded with corn syrup.

The French rarely eat processed foods or have soft drinks. Most of their diet consists of grains, legumes and fresh fruits and vegetables. They get fewer sugar calories…and the fiber that is in natural foods slows digestion and increases feelings of satiety.

• **Get enough healthy fat.** The French don't worry about fat. About 35% to 45% of their daily calories come from fat. Some comes from the saturated fat in butter, cheese and red meat, though the French eat red meat only about once a month. They mainly eat fish or game meats, such as rabbit or pheasant, which are naturally low in saturated fat. Most of the fat the French consume comes from nuts, fish and olive oil—healthy fats that cause you to feel full without elevating cholesterol or heart disease risk. (The French also drink wine regularly, and wine—in particular, red wine—has been shown to improve cardiovascular health.)

Adequate fat intake increases metabolism—by as much as 15%, compared with diets that are very low in fat and calories. Eating fat causes you to burn more calories…and promotes the absorption of beta-carotene and other fat-soluble nutrients.

• **Exercise daily.** Even though the French don't work out in gyms as often as Americans, they're not sedentary. They ride bikes. They go for long walks.

I usually advise people to try dance classes, yoga or tai chi. These activities burn calories and are more enjoyable for most people than lifting weights or running on a treadmill.

Too Busy to Go to the Gym? Get Fit in Just a Few Minutes

Joan Price, certified fitness instructor and motivational speaker based in Sebastopol, California, and author of six books, including *The Anytime, Anywhere Exercise Book* (iUniverse). *www.joanprice.com*

Lack of time is a primary reason people give for failing to get the recommended 30 to 60 minutes of moderate-intensity exercise most days of the week. Admittedly, it can be tough to find such a big chunk of time in your busy schedule.

What helps: Instead of feeling compelled to cram an entire day's worth of exercise into a single block of time, commit to fitting in little bursts of physical activity—two minutes, five minutes, 10 minutes—throughout the day. The more these "fitness minutes" add up, the more you reap the benefits of exercise, including improved health, better weight control, increased energy and a sense of well-being.

IN THE MORNING

• **When your alarm clock rings**—instead of pressing the snooze button, get up and use those extra minutes to do some gentle yoga poses.

• **While brushing your teeth**—do calf raises. Standing, slowly rise onto the balls of your feet…hold for several seconds…return to the starting position. Repeat, continuing for two minutes.

• **In the shower**—give your upper back muscles a workout. Squeeze your shoulder blades together…hold for five to 10 seconds…rest for a moment. Repeat 10 to 15 times.

• **While you style your hair**—squeeze your buttocks muscles as hard as you can for 10 seconds…rest for several seconds…repeat five to 10 times.

• **When going down stairs**—turn around at the bottom of the stairs and go back up, making one or more extra up-and-down trips.

• **As the coffee is brewing**—hop on your right foot 10 times…then hop on the left foot. Repeat twice.

• **When letting the dog out**—go with him for a short walk.

OUT AND ABOUT

• **At the gas station**—walk inside to pay rather than swiping a credit card at the pump. Instead of sitting in your car as the gas flows, clean all your windows, alternating the hand that holds the squeegee.

• **At every red light**—do shoulder shrugs and roll your shoulders…repeatedly tighten and release your thigh muscles…rotate one wrist, then the other wrist.

• **When parking**—instead of finding a spot close to your destination, get one a few blocks away.

• **Upon entering a store**—if all the items you need will fit in a shopping basket, choose a basket instead of a cart.

• **As you shop**—if you need a cart, do 10 bicep curls with weightier items—soup cans, juice jugs—before placing them in your cart. (If you feel silly doing this in public, do your bicep curls at home as you put the items in the pantry.)

• **While waiting in line**—work your abdominal muscles. Suck in your belly and tighten your abs…hold for 10 seconds…relax. Repeat five to 10 times.

• **On a long car trip**—stop every 50 miles or so, and take a walk around a rest stop or scenic area.

• **When traveling by bus, plane or train**—walk up and down the aisle for at least five minutes every hour.

AT YOUR DESK

• **While on the phone**—march in place or pace around your office.

• **As you read e-mail**—lift your right foot several inches off the floor…rotate your ankle clockwise several times, then counterclockwise…lower the foot. Repeat on the left side.

• **If you need to talk with a coworker**—walk over to her office instead of phoning. When you get back to your own desk, before sitting down, hold your arms out to the side and circle them forward 15 times, and then backward.

• **Each time you finish a task**—do "chair dips." With feet flat on the floor, place your hands on the armrests and push your body up (so your rear end hovers above the seat)…hold for several seconds…lower yourself back into the chair. Repeat 10 times. (Skip this if your chair has wheels.)

• **During your lunch break**—take a walk through the office complex.

• **In the restroom**—stand and reach for the sky for 30 seconds…then do 10 jumping jacks.

• **If you drop a pencil (or at least once a day)**—do a variation on toe touches. Stand up, bend down, pick up the pencil, straighten up…drop the pencil again. Repeat 10 times.

IN THE EVENING

• **Before starting dinner**—take a quick ride around the neighborhood on your bicycle.

• **At the dinner table**—do leg lifts. Sit with feet flat on the floor. Straighten your right leg to hold your right foot out in front of you…lift your right thigh a few inches off the chair and hold for several seconds…lower the foot. Repeat 10 times, then switch to the left leg.

• **Doing laundry**—when you grab a basket of clothes, tighten abdominal muscles and, with your back straight, lift the basket from hip height to chest height five times.

• **Listening to the radio or a CD**—dance around the room for one entire song. Repeat several times.

• **While watching TV**—pop an exercise video or DVD in your player. Every time the TV show cuts to a commercial break, turn on the player and follow along with the workout for several minutes.

• **Climbing the stairs**—take the steps two at a time. (Do not do this if you have balance problems.)

• **After washing your face**—tilt your head slowly from side to side, feeling a good stretch along your neck…try to touch your chin to your chest to stretch the back of your neck.

• **Before climbing into bed**—raise your arms overhead…tilt gently to the right, feeling the stretch along the left side of your torso…then tilt to the left. Repeat five times.

• **When you lie down**—do knee hugs. Lie on your back with your knees bent, feet flat on the mattress. Raise one leg, place your hands behind the thigh and draw the leg toward your chest. Hold for 30 seconds…return to starting position. Repeat with the other leg.

• **Closing your eyes**—breathe in and out deeply 10 times, feeling grateful for all that your body was capable of doing during the day.

A Drink a Day May Keep The Pounds Away

People who drink one alcoholic drink a day, including wine, beer and mixed drinks, are 54% less likely to be obese than those who don't drink at all. Those who have two drinks are 41% less likely to be obese.

But: Don't overdo it—people who drink four or more drinks a day are 46% more likely to be obese than nondrinkers. Binge drinkers, who sometimes have five or more drinks per day, are 80% more likely to be obese.

Ahmed A. Arif, PhD, associate professor, Department of Public Health Sciences, College of Health and Human Services, The University of North Carolina at Charlotte, Charlotte, NC, and leader of a study of the link between obesity and alcohol consumption in 8,236 nonsmokers, published in *BMC Public Health.*

Dieting? Don't Drop Dairy

Dieters don't have to skip dairy products. Thirty-four overweight men and women drank 20 ounces of skim milk or a fruit drink with breakfast (two slices of toast with jam and margarine), followed by lunch (a sandwich) four hours later.

Result: The skim milk group ate 50 fewer calories, on average, at lunchtime compared with the fruit-drink group, and reported feeling fuller.

Theory: Milk's high protein content, lactose (natural sugar) and/or thickness may contribute to feelings of fullness.

If you are trying to manage your weight: Consider drinking skim milk with your breakfast.

Emma R. Dove, MD, research associate, School of Medicine and Pharmacology, University of Western Australia, Perth.

Vitamin C Helps Burn More Fat When You Exercise

People who took 500 milligrams (mg) of vitamin C daily burned 39% more fat while exercising than people who took less. Since it is difficult to get enough vitamin C just from fruits and vegetables, take a vitamin C supplement to be sure you get at least 500 mg per day.

Carol S. Johnston, PhD, RD, professor and director, department of nutrition, Arizona State University in Mesa, Arizona. She has published more than 80 research papers and book chapters on nutrition subjects and received the 2004 Grace A. Goldsmith Award from the American College of Nutrition in recognition of her research.

Inadequate Sleep May Lead to Weight Gain

Lawrence J. Epstein, MD, instructor in medicine at Harvard Medical School in Boston, medical director of Sleep HealthCenters, based in Brighton, Massachusetts and author of *The Harvard Medical School Guide to a Good Night's Sleep* (McGraw-Hill).

If a busy schedule prevents you from getting the full seven-and-a-half to eight hours of sleep per night that the vast majority of adults require, it's no wonder that you often feel drowsy during the day.

But what if you spend plenty of time in bed yet still never feel fully rested? Something in your sleep environment may be keeping you up or creating disturbances that, even without waking you fully, interfere with the normal progression of sleep stages that you need to feel truly rested.

Concern: Chronic sleep deprivation negatively affects virtually every aspect of life—energy, alertness, work performance, mood, sex drive.

New finding: Sleep deprivation also contributes to weight problems. Studies show that losing sleep for just a few nights raises levels of hormones linked with overeating and weight gain and makes a person more likely to reach for fattening comfort foods instead of nutritious fare.

Even worse: Sleep deprivation increases the risk for diabetes and heart disease as well as car crashes and other accidents.

What to do: Speak to your doctor—sleep problems sometimes signal a potentially serious condition, such as sleep apnea (repeated cessations in breathing during sleep) or depression. If you still have trouble sleeping well even after underlying medical problems are ruled out or treated, chances are that your bedroom is not offering an optimal sleep environment.

Vinegar to Lose Weight (Lower Blood Sugar, Too)

Mark A. Stengler, NMD, licensed naturopathic medical doctor in private practice, Stengler Center for Integrative Medicine, Encinitas, California...adjunct associate clinical professor at the National College of Natural Medicine, Portland, Oregon...author of many books, including *The Natural Physician's Healing Therapies* and coauthor of *Prescription for Natural Cures* (both from Bottom Line Books)...and author of the *Bottom Line/Natural Healing* newsletter. *www.drstengler.com*

Vinegar has been used as a folk medicine for such things as headaches and indigestion. Now several studies reinforce its benefit for weight management and blood sugar control. Researchers believe that it is the *acetic acid* in any type of vinegar (apple cider, balsamic, white or red wine) that produces this effect, interfering with enzymes involved in the digestion of carbohydrates and those that alter glucose metabolism (so that insulin does not spike).

One recent study found that mice fed a high-fat diet—and given acetic acid—developed up to 10% less body fat than those not given acetic acid. Another study found that having small amounts of vinegar at bedtime seemed to reduce waking blood glucose levels in people.

More studies need to be done on vinegar, but it does seem that people can benefit from sprinkling vinegar on salads...adding a teaspoon to marinades...and adding a few drops to mustard. For blood sugar balance (for those with diabetes or on diabetes medication) or weight loss, dilute one to two tablespoons (some people start with teaspoons) in an equal amount of water—and drink it at the beginning of a meal.

The Pen and Paper Diet

Jack F. Hollis, PhD, senior investigator, Center for Health Research at Kaiser Permanente Northwest, Portland, Oregon.

Losing weight and keeping it off remains at the top of the list of difficult challenges for most people in America, with about 65% of adults in this country currently overweight or obese. Research shows that between 20% and 40% of Americans are currently trying to lose weight...sadly, without much success. Now a recent study from the Kaiser Permanente Center for Health Research in Portland, Oregon, has identified what weight strategies appear to be most highly associated with successful weight loss. One of the most effective is also one of the easiest to do.

ABOUT THE RESEARCH

Researchers enrolled 1,685 overweight or obese adults in a weight loss program that included 20 group training sessions over six months. During that time, participants were given instructions on how to follow a calorically appropriate diet, low in sodium and high in fruits and vegetables and containing low-fat dairy. According to Jack Hollis, PhD, lead researcher, participants were also instructed to engage in 30 minutes of moderate exercise each day, including a 30-minute brisk walk held during the weekly group meeting. They were also taught how to keep a food diary, in which they were to write down everything they consumed, and were strongly encouraged to do so.

After six months, 69% of the participants had lost at least 8.8 pounds of body weight, an amount considered to be clinically significant. The mean amount lost was 13 pounds after 20 weeks. Researchers then analyzed what behaviors were most correlated with success.

A particularly striking finding was that participants who kept daily records of what they ate lost twice as much weight as those who kept no records. "The act of writing down what you eat makes you more conscious of what you're eating," Dr. Hollis says calling it "a powerful self-management tool." Other behaviors that correlated with weight-loss success were number of minutes per week spent exercising and how many group meetings a member attended.

HOW TO DO IT

Dr. Hollis offered some tips for those interested in getting this good habit going...

• **Measure, as much as possible.** Use tablespoons, measuring cups or a food scale to get an approximation of quantity. In the study, the participants were taught to estimate using common visual reference points—for instance, a serving of mashed potatoes the size of a computer mouse is four ounces, while a three-ounce portion of chicken, fish or steak is about the size of a deck of cards.

• **Estimate how many calories you're eating.** Use a calorie book or look up your food online. This is easier than it sounds, says Dr. Hollis, since most people eat the same foods often.

• **Simple notes are fine.** Keeping a food diary doesn't have to mean lugging around a notebook—you can jot intake down on a Post-it and it will still help you be more attentive to what you're eating.

• **If you miss a day...start again.** Those who kept the most consistent food records lost the most weight in the study, but even those who kept some records regularly lost more than those who kept none.

24

Hearing/Tinnitus Cures

Everyday Vitamins May Prevent Common Hearing Loss

How about a "morning after" pill for loud concerts? Researchers recently identified supplements so helpful at preventing and healing noise-induced hearing loss that we may very well see pills and snack foods marketed with that premise in the not-too-distant future. Long viewed as a hazard for people exposed to prolonged high-decibel sound (such as workers around jet engines or jackhammers, battlefield soldiers and rock stars), excess noise contributes to more than one-third of the 28 million Americans suffering from some degree of hearing loss.

RESEARCH RESULTS SOUND PROMISING

We spoke with scientist Colleen Garbe Le Prell, PhD, to find out more about the research her team recently conducted, which showed that a simple blend of common nutrients may help reduce hearing loss. In the study, four groups of guinea pigs were exposed to five hours of 120 decibel sound, which is as loud as a jet engine at takeoff. One hour before exposure, each group received either a nutrient blend or placebo. Thereafter, each group continued receiving the treatment regimen once daily for five days. One group was fed the synergistic blend of vitamins A, C and E with magnesium...a second group received magnesium alone...a third group was given A, C and E without magnesium...and a fourth group received a placebo.

The result: Using electrodes to test the animals' threshold hearing sensitivity before and after noise exposure, the group receiving the blend of vitamins A, C and E with magnesium had significantly less hearing loss than any of the three other groups.

Colleen Garbe Le Prell, PhD, associate professor, department of speech, language, and hearing sciences, and director, The Hearing Research Center, University of Florida, Gainesville.

Why should these extremely common supplements make such a big difference in hearing protection? Loud noise causes the over-stimulation of inner ear sensory cells, which drives the production of free radicals even after noise exposure. The free radicals and a resulting constriction of blood flow ultimately damages the outer hair cells. The blend of vitamins A, C and E with magnesium binds with the free radicals in the inner ear, helping to prevent this damage.

YOU HEARD IT HERE FIRST...

According to Dr. Le Prell, the upper limit for intake of vitamins A, C and E and magnesium has been well defined by the US Institute of Medicine (IOM), and should not be exceeded. As with any dietary supplement, moderation and supervision by a physician trained in natural medicine is important. Clinical trials to confirm safety and efficacy of this micronutrient blend for humans, at levels that adhere to IOM limits are underway and soon, says Dr. Le Prell, we may see products marketed to be taken around the time of noise exposure or daily as a preventive measure. For now though, Dr. Le Prell suggests checking with your physician to maintain (but do not exceed) recommended daily doses of vitamins A, C, E and magnesium—and turning down the volume.

Quiet the Ringing in Your Ears

Aaron G. Benson, MD, otolaryngologist in private practice at Toledo Ear, Nose and Throat in Maumee, Ohio. He specializes in hearing disorders, *www.toledo ent.com.*

Perhaps you hear a high-pitched ringing...perhaps a buzzing, chirping, whistling or whirring. Nobody else can hear it—but the quieter it gets around you, the worse the noise in your head. This bothersome condition, *tinnitus*, afflicts an estimated 10% to 16% of Americans.

Tinnitus most often develops when a person has hearing loss caused by nerve damage from prolonged or extreme exposure to loud noise. It also can be a side effect of antibiotics, aspirin, diuretics and some cancer drugs. Tinnitus usually appears after age 50 but is increasingly common in younger people due to high-volume use of personal music players (i.e. iPod). It can occur during pregnancy due to increased blood volume—and may or may not go away after delivery.

Tinnitus usually is not a serious health problem, but it should be evaluated—so consult an otolaryngologist.

Referrals: American Tinnitus Association, (800-634-8978, *www.ata.org*).

There is no cure, but various strategies can ease symptoms and help you cope...

• **Cut caffeine and salt.** Caffeine (in coffee, tea, cola and chocolate) constricts blood flow to the ear...and salt can raise blood pressure, aggravating tinnitus.

• **Keep ears clean.** Excessive earwax can muffle outside noises and amplify internal ringing.

Home remedy: Mix hydrogen peroxide with an equal amount of water, and place two drops in each ear weekly. Or see your doctor to have your ears irrigated.

• **Reduce stress.** Muscle relaxation, meditation, biofeedback, exercise and other stress-reducing techniques may alleviate symptoms.

• **Fill the room with white noise.** A constant low-level background sound masks the inner ringing. In a quiet room and at bedtime, turn on a fan or tabletop fountain, or use a white-noise machine (about $30 to $60 at home-products stores).

• **Wear a tinnitus masker.** This miniature white-noise device resembles a hearing aid and fits behind or in the ear.

Cost: About $2,000.

To obtain one, ask your doctor for a referral to an audiologist.

• **Try a hearing aid.** This eases tinnitus for about half of people with significant hearing loss. It amplifies outside sounds, which obscures inner sounds.

• **Retrain your brain.** A new treatment provided by trained audiologists, *tinnitus retraining therapy* (TRT) may help up to 80% of patients. Sometimes improvement is noticed after just a few sessions. Typically, you attend weekly or monthly hour-long sessions during which you wear a special hearing aid programmed with a facsimile of your particular tinnitus sound. You are shown how to train your brain to be less sensitive to the ringing.

Rarely, tinnitus may be caused by a tumor. Call your doctor without delay if your tinnitus sounds like a pulsing or whooshing...is heard on only one side of your head...or is accompanied by dizziness or a sudden decrease in ability to discriminate between similar words, such as cat and hat.

and Neck Surgery Foundation. *Most important ones...*

• **Use body-temperature water in an ear syringe to dissolve cerumen buildup.** You do not need expensive wax-dissolving drops.

• **Do not clean your own ears if you have diabetes or your immune system is weakened—this may occur during steroid use, cancer therapy or with certain infections.** Syringing with water can trigger a serious outer-ear infection that may require hospitalization. Instead, a physician can safely remove excess cerumen with a microscope and specialized instruments.

• **If you use a hearing aid, get your ears checked twice a year.** The repeated removal and replacement of hearing aids increases the risk for impaction.

The Ears Have It!

Rebecca Shannonhouse, editor *Bottom Line/Health,* Boardroom Inc., 281 Tresser Blvd., Stamford, CT 06901. *www.bottomlinepublications.com*

About one in 20 adults—and up to one-third of older adults who are cognitively impaired—have impacted earwax (*cerumen*). The symptoms are reversible, but not all doctors are paying enough attention to the problem.

Normally, jaw movements—from chewing, for example—cause excess cerumen to gradually migrate out of the ear canal and fall out unnoticed. If this doesn't occur, a feeling of fullness and hearing loss are among the most common symptoms, but *tinnitus* (ringing in the ears) also may occur, explains Richard Rosenfeld, MD, MPH, a professor and chairman of otolaryngology at SUNY Downstate and chairman of otolaryngology at Long Island College Hospital both in Brooklyn, New York.

It's a bad idea to dig out earwax with cotton swabs or other implements—this often pushes earwax deeper into the ear canal. For the first time, there are now evidence-based guidelines for treating earwax impaction, released by the American Academy of Otolaryngology–Head

Do-It-Yourself Tinnitus Treatment

Sujana S. Chandrasekhar, MD, director, New York Otology, associate clinical professor of otolaryngology, Mount Sinai School of Medicine, New York City. *www.newyorkotology.com*

Tinnitus can be like the soundtrack to a scary movie—a constant, high- or low-pitched drone, whistling, clicking, even roaring sound in your ear that never stops. There's no medicine or procedure that can be relied upon to make it go away. Nor is there a single specific cause—tinnitus can be brought on by loud noise or a head injury, it is sometimes a side effect of medication and sometimes can arise seemingly out of nowhere.

It's common, too: According to the Cleveland Clinic, 12 million people in the US suffer from persistent tinnitus that interferes with daily life.

What I'm about to tell you may come as music to your ears, then, if you or someone you know suffers from tinnitus: A new treatment shows great promise—though it is important to note that the initial research was done on a very small group. That said, this is a simple, straightforward technique that can actually be enjoyable (and if you're good with computers, you might even be able to do it on your own). It's called "notched music," and it's a technique that lets you change your favorite music and then use it as treatment for your tinnitus. That's it—no drugs, no complicated procedures.

When you "notch" music, you remove a one-octave frequency range, in this case it would be the range that is centered on the tone of your own tinnitus.

The treatment is very simple: After you have found the tone and removed that frequency range from your favorite music, you just listen to it often. How does it work? Over time, the brain begins to respond differently to frequencies that it is not regularly exposed to—therefore, the loudness of your tinnitus gradually subsides (it typically takes six months or so) though it is unlikely to disappear altogether.

This therapy was tested on 23 patients at the University of Munster in Germany. Researchers found that after one year of listening to notched music for approximately 12 hours per week, patients reported a significant reduction in the loudness of their tinnitus. In comparison, there was no change at all in the two control groups used in the study, one of which listened to randomly notched music, the other to unnotched music.

HOW TO DO IT

To notch music, you'll need a "tone generator" to pinpoint the frequency of your tinnitus and music-editing software to notch your digital music files. Examples I found online are ToneGenerator ($80) and WavePad ($80), both offering free demonstrations at *www.nch.com. au*. From there, it's easy—just listen to the music you love and see how it helps. It's a low-cost, non-invasive solution that sounds to me like a treatment worth trying.

Cures for Tinnitus

Mark A. Stengler, NMD, licensed naturopathic medical doctor in private practice, Stengler Center for Integrative Medicine, Encinitas, California...adjunct associate clinical professor at the National College of Natural Medicine, Portland, Oregon...author of many books, including *The Natural Physician's Healing Therapies* and coauthor of *Prescription for Natural Cures* (both from Bottom Line Books)...and author of the *Bottom Line/Natural Healing* newsletter. *www.drstengler.com*

Tinnitus is the medical term for noise or ringing in the ears. While many cases have no known cause, the disorder can result from a loud noise that causes damage to the ear...changes to the bones of the inner ear...or circulation problems within the inner ear. I find that the herb ginkgo biloba, which can improve circulation to the inner ear, helps some patients, although studies have shown mixed results. Take 120 mg daily of a ginkgo biloba extract (it should contain 24% *flavone glycosides* and 6% *terpene lactones*). Since ginkgo biloba is itself a blood thinner, don't take it if you are on blood-thinning medication. One product that contains both homeopathic remedies and Chinese herbs is Clear Tinnitus from Clear Products Inc. (888-257-2532, *www.clearproductsinc.com,* which was shown in a small trial to benefit most people with tinnitus. Follow the instructions on the label.

Hearing Loss

Barbara McLay, MA, clinical associate professor of communication science and disorders and head of the hearing conservation program, University of Missouri, Columbia.

Whether hearing loss can be reversed depends on where in the ear it occurs and what causes it.

Inner ear: Damage to the inner ear from aging, hereditary factors, disease (such as meningitis) and exposure to a sudden loud sound can be irreversible. Some medications (for example, certain antibiotics and chemotherapy drugs) also can cause irreversible hearing loss.

Middle ear: Upper respiratory infections can lead to fluid buildup and difficulty hearing. Treating the infection will restore hearing.

Abnormal bone growth around the tiny bones in the middle ear also can cause hearing loss and can be corrected with surgery.

Outer ear: The most common reason for outer-ear hearing loss is wax buildup.

Have earwax removed at the doctor's office or try an over-the-counter wax-removal product to help restore hearing.

To prevent hearing loss...

•**Maintain your general health by eating right, not smoking, etc.**

•**Protect ears from loud noises.**

•**Do not put cotton-tipped swabs or other objects in your ears.**

•**See your doctor immediately if you experience sudden hearing loss in one or both ears.**

Melatonin May Help Symptoms of Tinnitus

Melatonin may improve symptoms of *tinnitus* by allowing sufferers to sleep better. About 15 million Americans have severe tinnitus, the sensation of a ringing, roaring or humming sound. Sleep disturbance is common among tinnitus sufferers.

Recent study: Researchers gave people with tinnitus 3 milligrams (mg) of melatonin every night for one month to help them sleep, then tracked them for a second month when they did not take the supplement. By the end of the study, tinnitus symptoms had been reduced by nearly 30%. Participants slept best while taking melatonin, but the improvement in their sleep and tinnitus symptoms continued through the month when they were not taking it. Patients with the greatest sleep disturbances improved the most.

Jay F. Piccirillo, MD, professor, otolaryngology, head and neck surgery, Washington University School of Medicine, St. Louis, and lead author of a study of tinnitus sufferers, published in *Otolaryngology—Head and Neck Surgery.*

25

Natural Ways for Healthy Vision

8 Simple Steps That Keep Your Eyes Young

If you are holding this article at arm's length or had to reach for your reading glasses to make out the words, you are well aware that aging affects the eyes. But farsightedness is just one of the vision problems brought on by the passage of years.

Diet and lifestyle choices, genetic risk factors, exposure to sunlight and the gradual deterioration of eye tissue all combine to make eyes increasingly vulnerable to various diseases and disorders. *Examples...*

•**Macular degeneration,** a deterioration of the retina (the light-sensing lining at the back of the eye), is the leading cause of blindness in the US.

•**Glaucoma,** the second most common cause of blindness, results from increased fluid pressure inside the eye.

•**Cataract,** a clouding of the eye's normally clear lens, obscures the vision.

Fortunately, there's a lot you can do to protect yourself against these and other types of age-related vision loss. *Starting today...*

1. Get treated for any other health problems. Sleep apnea is a common condition that has been linked to glaucoma. People with apnea periodically stop breathing during sleep, which leads to a buildup of carbon dioxide and a shortage of oxygen circulating to various parts of the body—including to the optic nerve. As a result, fluid pressure could increase and cause nerve cells to die. If you have been told that you snore (a sign of apnea), get evaluated at a sleep center.

Diabetes also can affect eye health. Poorly controlled blood sugar levels contribute to *diabetic retinopathy* (blockage, bleeding or fluid

J. James Thimons, OD, clinical professor of optometry at Pennsylvania College of Optometry in Philadelphia and an optometrist in private practice in Fairfield, Connecticut. He is chairman of the National Glaucoma Society and a member of the national board of directors of Prevent Blindness America.

315

leakage in the retinal blood vessels) and loss of vision.

Best: Work with your doctor and a nutritionist to stabilize blood sugar levels.

2. Eat foods that protect eye cells. The retina, lens and eye fluid require large amounts of antioxidants to fight cell damage from oxidation. Numerous studies show that the antioxidants *lutein, zeaxanthin,* and vitamins A, C and E promote better overall vision and reduce the risk for macular degeneration, cataracts and possibly glaucoma.

Good food sources of antioxidants: Fortified whole-grain hot and cold cereals…nuts and peanut butter…cantaloupe and citrus fruits… avocado, broccoli, carrots, collard greens, corn, kale, peppers, spinach and turnip greens. Have at least five to seven servings of these foods weekly.

3. Consider supplements to slow macular degeneration. Once an eye disease develops, larger doses of antioxidants are needed than can be obtained just from foods.

Study: A six-year trial of nearly 4,000 people showed that taking a supplement combination of vitamin C (500 mg), vitamin E (400 IU), beta-carotene (15 mg) and zinc (80 mg as zinc oxide) slowed the progression of early macular degeneration by about 25%. In other studies, daily supplementation with both lutein and zeaxanthin also delayed vision loss from macular degeneration.

4. Boost night vision with bilberry extract. Similar to the blueberry, bilberry contains antioxidant *anthocyanosides.* The extract may improve circulation in the eyes and protect against retinal damage, helping you to see better when driving in the dark or reading in low light.

Dosage: Three times per week, take 80 mg to 100 mg of a bilberry extract containing 20% to 25% anthocyanosides.

5. Increase omega-3s to relieve dry eye. Dry eye syndrome (a lack of tears) is more than a nuisance—it can lead to pain, infection and blurred vision. The problem results from age-related eye inflammation and a decrease in oil production. Changes in hormone levels also may play a role.

A study that evaluated the diets of more than 32,000 women found that those who consumed the least fish (and thus got the least omega-3 fatty acids) had the highest risk for dry eye. Consuming omega-3–rich fish (anchovies, mackerel, salmon, tuna) several times a week is smart—but if you already have dry eye, you also need supplements.

Bonus: Fish oil may delay macular degeneration.

Dosage: Each day, take 1,000 mg of fish oil (which reduces eye inflammation)…and 1,000 mg of flaxseed oil (which improves the quality of oil in the eye gland). It takes about a month to notice the effects of omega-3s on dry eye. If discomfort doesn't ease within six to eight weeks, ask your eye doctor about the prescription eyedrop medication *Restasis,* which increases tear production.

6. Wear sunglasses—especially if your eyes are blue or green. Exposure to bright sunlight, particularly during childhood but also accumulated over a lifetime, significantly increases the risk for cataracts and macular degeneration. Compared with dark-eyed people, those with light-colored eyes have less eye pigment— allowing more light to enter the lens—which increases sensitivity to sunlight and glare.

Important: When outdoors, wear high-quality sunglasses that do not cause optical distortion and that block both UVA and UVB rays. Polarized lenses, which have special glare-blocking filters, are best for driving or whenever there is glare from snow, water or pavement. Use wraparound-style sunglasses if your eyes are very sensitive to light or if you've had cataract surgery.

7. Stop smoking. Compared with a non-smoker, a pack-a-day smoker is significantly more likely to go blind from macular degeneration by age 65. Smoking damages blood vessels throughout the body, including in the eyes…depletes antioxidants…and greatly increases cataract risk. It takes about 10 years for the effects of nicotine to clear from the eyes—so quit now rather than later.

8. Have an annual eye exam—even if you see as well as ever. Your eye doctor checks not only for changes in vision, but also for eye problems that may not be evident to you.

Example: Glaucoma causes no symptoms until permanent damage has been done.

Referrals: American Optometric Association, 800-365-2219, *www.aoa.org.*

Arugula and Other Salad Stars Help Your Vision

Leo Galland, MD, director, Foundation for Integrated Medicine, New York City. He is author of *The Fat Resistance Diet* (Broadway). *www.fatresistancediet.com.* Dr. Galland is a recipient of the Linus Pauling award.

Peppery arugula...crisp endive and romaine...crunchy green peppers. Stars of restaurant menus, these vegetables can turn an ordinary salad into an extraordinary treat. They are power-packed with surprising nutritional benefits, according to Leo Galland, MD, author of *The Fat Resistance Diet*, including the ability to help fight the effects of aging, preserve vision and build bone strength.

Dr. Galland notes that salads are an excellent example of the high nutrient density foods he uses in his "fat resistant" diet program. "The vegetables in garden salad have a high ratio of nutrition to calories—I believe eating foods with high nutrient density is the key to healthy weight loss." *Here are some of the best...*

ARUGULA

The taste of arugula is distinctively sharp with an earthy aroma. Arugula is not only an excellent source of bioflavonoids, but it also contains vitamin A, which helps build immunity...potassium, important for muscles... and calcium, with 32 mg of calcium per one cup. Plus the body absorbs calcium in arugula (along with kale and broccoli) more readily than from milk. For those cutting back on milk-based dairy products, this makes arugula a very nice vegan source of calcium.

ENDIVE

Endive is widely used in Northern Europe, especially Belgium, Holland and France. It is a potent source of vitamin K, helping to maintain bone strength, as well as vitamin A. Endive packs a big appetite-satisfying crunch for super-low calories...there are only eight calories in one cup of chopped endive! This amount of Belgium endive also contains 1.6 grams of fiber.

ROMAINE LETTUCE

In spite of its light taste, fresh romaine lettuce is a big source of antioxidants, which are higher after consumption of fresh lettuce than after consumption of packaged lettuce. Romaine is also a good source of vitamin A, folate and vitamin K.

GREEN, RED AND ORANGE PEPPERS

Sliced bell peppers are an appetizing addition to any garden salad and enhance your body's levels of anti-inflammatory carotenoids. With bell peppers, the color is key to the special nutrients found in each. For example, green bell peppers are an excellent source of the carotenoids *lutein* and *zeaxanthin*, which help to preserve vision. Sweet orange peppers are also high in zeaxanthin and reduce the risk of macular degeneration, the leading cause of vision loss in older Americans. Red bell peppers are very high in the carotenoids *beta carotene* and *beta cryptoxanthin*. These antioxidants can help protect the body against free radical damage and fight the effects of aging.

EASY TIPS ON MAKING THE BEST SALAD

When shopping for salad, freshness comes first. Select vegetables that are vibrant, brightly colored, firm and crisp. When buying romaine lettuce and arugula, look for deep green leaves that appear fresh-picked. Skip anything that is wilted or waterlogged. Buy fresh greens, rather than the packaged products and plan to eat as quickly as possible—they taste better and are more nutritious, too. For Belgium endive, look for leaves that are firm, mostly white with green-tinged edges. Don't buy endive that has browned or softened. Same idea for bell peppers—these should be very firm to the touch when you buy them, with no soft areas.

All vegetables should be washed carefully, even fresh-picked organic ones.

Here is another surprising tip: To get the most nutrition from salad, don't use fat-free dressing, Dr. Galland told me. "You have to consume a bit of healthy oil with vegetables to absorb carotenoids, so I recommend eating salad with dressing made with olive oil, for example."

Pecans for Vision and Other Healthy Nuts

Joy Bauer, MS, RD, CDN, nutrition expert for the *Today* show and Yahoo.com, with offices in New York City and Westchester, New York. She is a nutrition columnist for *Woman's Day* magazine and coauthor, with Carol Svec, of *Joy Bauer's Food Cures* (Rodale). *www.joybauer.com*

Nuts are among the most healthful foods you can eat. Rich in nutrients, they can help prevent some of the most common—and most serious—diseases.

Example: In a long-running health study conducted by researchers at Loma Linda University, participants were asked what foods they ate most often. Those who ate nuts five or more times a week were about 50% less likely to have a heart attack than those who ate them less than once a week.

FORGET THE FAT

Many Americans avoid nuts because they want to cut back on fat and calories. It's true that a single serving of nuts can have 20 grams (g) or more of fat and 180 to 200 calories, but most of the fats are healthful fats, such as omega-3 fatty acids and monounsaturated fat. Americans need to get more, not less, of these fats. As long as you limit yourself to a small handful of nuts daily—the recommended amount, unless otherwise noted—you don't need to worry about the "extra" calories.

Each type of nut contains a different mix of nutrients, fats and protective antioxidants, which can "neutralize" cell-damaging free rad-icals. People who eat a variety of nuts will get the widest range of benefits. Raw, toasted or roasted nuts are fine as long as they are unsalted.

Here's what nuts can do…

NUTS FOR THE HEART

All nuts are good for the heart, but the following nuts are especially beneficial…

• **Macadamia nuts.** Of the 21 g of total fat in a serving of macadamias, 17 g are monounsaturated—the kind of fat that lowers a person's levels of harmful LDL cholesterol without lowering levels of beneficial HDL cholesterol. Both the antioxidants and the monounsaturated fat in macadamias have anti-inflammatory effects—important for curtailing arterial damage that can lead to heart disease.

• **Peanuts.** Actually a type of legume, not a true nut, peanuts contain 34 micrograms (mcg) of folate per one-ounce serving, a little less than 10% of the recommended daily amount. Folate is a B vitamin that lowers levels of homocysteine, an amino acid that damages arteries and increases the risk of heart disease.

Peanuts also are high in *L-arginine*, an amino acid that is converted by cells in blood vessels into nitric oxide. Nitric oxide improves circulation and may inhibit fatty buildups in the arteries.

• **Pistachios.** A study conducted by Penn State University found that pistachios lower blood pressure. Men who added 1.5 ounces of shelled pistachios to their daily diets had drops in systolic pressure (the top number in a blood pressure reading) of 4.8 points. The antioxidants and healthy fats in pistachios relax blood vessels and allow blood to circulate with less force.

ALMONDS FOR BONES

Just about everyone needs more calcium, the mineral that strengthens bones and reduces the risk of osteoporosis. The recommended daily amount is 1,000 milligrams (mg). Almonds have more calcium than other nuts, with about 80 mg in 20 to 25 nuts. For people with lactose intolerance, who have trouble digesting dairy, a daily dose of almonds helps raise calcium to bone-protecting levels.

Blood pressure bonus: One serving of almonds has 98 mg of magnesium, about one-fourth the recommended daily amount. Magnesium, along with potassium and calcium, controls the relaxation and contraction of blood vessels and can help control blood pressure.

BRAZIL NUTS FOR PROSTATE

Brazil nuts are a superb source of selenium, with about 155 mcg in just two nuts. The recommended daily amount is 55 mcg. They're also high in vitamin E. One study—the Selenium and Vitamin E Cancer Prevention Trial—found that men getting selenium and vitamin E, alone or in combination, reduced their risk of prostate cancer by up to 60%. Selenium improves the ability of the immune system to recognize and destroy cancer cells in the prostate. Vitamin E is an antioxidant that also has been linked to reduced cancer risk.

Caution: People who get too much selenium may have decreased immunity. Because Brazil nuts are so high in selenium and calories (50 calories in two nuts), don't have more than two nuts daily. If you take a multivitamin that has more than 50% of the daily value of selenium, opt for one nut.

PECANS FOR THE EYES

The most serious eye diseases, including cataracts and macular degeneration, are caused, in part, by free radicals. The antioxidants in nuts and other plant foods fight free radicals to keep the eyes healthy.

A study conducted by the US Department of Agriculture (USDA) found that pecans are particularly rich in antioxidants. The National Eye Institute's Age-Related Eye Diseases Study reported that patients with macular degeneration who had adequate intakes of antioxidants were 29% less likely to experience disease progression than those who got lower levels.

Bonus for heart health: The vitamin E in pecans reduces the tendency of LDL cholesterol to oxidize and stick to artery walls. Pecans also are high in phytosterols—plant compounds that are similar to the active ingredients in cholesterol-lowering margarines, such as Benecol.

WALNUTS FOR MOOD

A part from fish and flaxseed, walnuts are one of the best sources of omega-3 fatty acids. They're the only nut that contains *alpha linolenic acid* (ALA), a polyunsaturated fat that is converted to omega-3s in the body.

The omega-3s appear to help maintain healthy brain levels of serotonin, a neurochemical involved in mood. People who eat walnuts and/or two to three fish meals a week may experience a reduction in symptoms of depression.

Bonus for heart health: Omega-3s lower LDL cholesterol and triglycerides, another type of blood fat…increase HDL good cholesterol… inhibit blood clots in the arteries…and reduce arterial inflammation.

The "Clothing Cure" for Glaucoma

Robert Ritch, MD, professor of clinical ophthalmology, New York Medical College, Valhalla, and chief, Glaucoma Services, The New York Eye and Ear Infirmary, New York City.
British Journal of Ophthalmology.

Ties that bind the neck may raise the risk of the eye disease glaucoma. So says a controversial study that found snug neckwear can increase intraocular pressure (IOP) in the eyes, possibly leading to glaucoma.

"If men wear tight neckties when their IOP is measured, it can raise their IOP," says Robert Ritch, MD, lead author of the study and a professor of clinical ophthalmology at New York Medical College.

DOUBLE TROUBLE

That double Windsor knot may be double trouble. If a person has moderate or severe glaucoma damage, the increase in IOP caused by a tight tie may make it worse. What's more, patients without glaucoma whose tight tie falsely increases IOP might end up being treated for glaucoma when they don't need to be.

Although there are no reported cases of glaucoma being caused by a tight necktie, Dr. Ritch says it's theoretically possible.

Dr. Ritch became aware of the issue during his regular practice. "I noticed that some patients had tight neckties. When I loosened the neckties, their IOP would go down several points," he says.

To quantify his observation, Dr. Ritch and his colleagues looked at 20 healthy men and 20 men with open angle glaucoma, the most common form of the disease.

The researchers measured IOP first while the men weren't wearing neckties, then three minutes after they put on a tight necktie, and once again three minutes after the tie was loosened.

Dr. Ritch's team found that in 70% of the healthy men, a tight necktie increased mean IOP, as it did in 60% of those with glaucoma.

Increases in IOP while wearing a tight necktie ranged from more than 2 mmHg to more than 4 mmHg (millimeters of mercury, a measure of pressure), compared with IOP readings when no ties were worn and after ties were loosened. This is a clinically important increase.

Dr. Ritch speculates that when a necktie exerts too much pressure on the jugular vein located in the neck, pressure is increased in the entire venous system, including in the eyes.

To learn more about glaucoma, visit the Glaucoma Research Foundation at *www.glaucoma.org*.

Reverse Cataracts Without Surgery

Marc Grossman, OD, LAc, optometrist in private practice in New Paltz, New York.

More than 50% of Americans over 65 and 70% over 75 have a vision-blurring (and sometimes vision-dimming, vision-clouding and vision-yellowing) cataract. That's why cataract surgery is the most frequently performed operation among seniors, with about 400,000 procedures a year.

And cataract surgery works very well, says Marc Grossman, OD, LAc, an optometrist in private practice in New Paltz, New York, and medical director of the Web site, *www.natural eyecare.com*.

In about 15 minutes, the surgeon removes the damaged lens and inserts a clear artificial replacement. You recover in about a day, with your eye adjusting to the new lens over the next few weeks. Piece of cake!

However: If you have a cataract, it's a myth that cataract surgery is always a must, says Dr. Grossman. You can reverse a cataract without surgery. *And it might not take any longer than squeezing an eye drop or two out of a bottle…*

•**NAC**—the super-antioxidant that can prevent, stop or reverse cataracts. Cataracts are caused by the same process that scientists now understand contributes to and causes a range of age-related diseases, such as heart disease and Alzheimer's—oxidation, a kind of biochemical rust. Oxidation is carried out by molecular bad guys called free radicals, hyperactive compounds that damage the delicate outer lining (membranes) of cells and the DNA inside them, leading to cell mutation and death. Free radicals are generated by many factors, including sunlight (think age spots, wrinkles and skin cancer), smoking (think lung cancer) and diets high in fat and sugar (think heart disease and diabetes).

Fortunately, there are antiaging antioxidants such as vitamin C and vitamin E that can neutralize free radicals. And a particularly powerful antioxidant is *carnosine*, a combination of two amino acids, the building blocks of protein.

Now, scientists have found that a form of carnosine—*N-acetyl-carnosine*—is uniquely effective at stopping the aging process in the eyes.

"Research shows that N-acetyl-carnosine eyedrops can help improve cataracts—and possibly enable the patient to keep their natural lens, avoiding the need for cataract surgery," says Dr. Grossman.

Study: Researchers in Russia studied 49 people (average age 65) with "minimal to advanced" cataracts, dividing them into three groups. One received twice-daily eye drops with N-acetyl-carnosine, one group received placebo drops, and one group didn't receive any treatment.

After six months, 90% of the group receiving the drops had an improvement in glare sensitivity (a common symptom of cataracts), 42% had an improvement in the light transmission through the lens and 90% had an improvement in "visual acuity" (they could see better). Those not using the drops had negative changes in all those parameters.

"As shown by this study, the N-acetyl-carnosine drops can help the aging eye to recover from cataract, by improving its clarity, glare sensitivity, color perception and overall vision," says Dr. Grossman.

"I recommend a minimum six-month period of use to evaluate the benefits."

Product: Can-C Eyedrops, available at *www. naturaleyecare.com*, or call 845-255-8222. Address: Natural Eye Care, 3 Paradies Lane, New Paltz, NY 12561.

How to use: "You can also use the drops to prevent cataract," says Dr. Grossman.

For prevention, he suggests one to two drops in each eye, one to two times per day. For treatment, he suggests two drops in the affected eye, two times per day.

"To apply the drop, lean your head back and look up. Put one drop into your eye, blink a couple of times and then gently close the eye. Do not blink again or reopen for sixty seconds. If you use a second drop, repeat this procedure. This allows each drop to be absorbed into the eye tissue."

As with all natural remedies, use these eyedrops only with the approval and supervision of a qualified health professional, such as an optometrist or ophthalmologist.

• **Eat "The Vision Diet."** "If you're thinking about cataract surgery, try following these dietary recommendations for several months first," says Dr. Grossman. "You may find that your vision has improved enough to skip the surgery."

• **Cut back or eliminate sugar.** "High levels of sugar in the blood contribute to cataract formation," says Dr. Grossman. "People with diabetes, for example, are at three to four times the risk of cataracts. That's because blood sugar interferes with the lens' ability to pump out excess sugar from the eye and maintain its clarity."

• **Drink lots of water.** Dr. Grossman recommends eight to ten, 8-ounce glasses a day. "This maintains the flow of nutrients to the lens and the release of waste and toxins from the tissues."

• **Eat foods high in beta-carotene, vitamins C and E, and sulfur-bearing amino acids.** "These are antioxidants that combat free radicals," says Dr. Grossman.

Foods rich in these factors include garlic, onions, beans, yellow and orange vegetables, spinach and other green, leafy vegetables, celery, seaweed, apples, carrots, tomatoes, turnips and oranges.

• **Watch out for "congesting" foods.** "For many people, dairy, wheat and soy foods create sinus congestion, which impairs lymph and blood drainage from the area around the eyes—speeding the development of cataracts," says Dr. Grossman. "Try avoiding these foods for a month to see whether you are less congested," he says. "Then reintroduce them one at a time to help you identify your specific problem foods."

• **Wear (the right) sunglasses.** Maybe you routinely wear sunscreen to protect yourself from skin-damaging UV radiation. But UV radiation can also damage your eyes.

Fact: Eighty percent of Americans know that UV exposure from the sun can cause skin cancer, but only 5% know it can harm the eyes, causing cataracts.

"Whenever you're outdoors, you should wear sunglasses with UV coating," says Larry Jebrock, OD, a behavioral optometrist in Novato, California.

What most people don't realize: The degree of UV protection has nothing to do with the darkness of the lens of the sunglasses, says Dr. Jebrock.

Look for a pair with at least UV 400, which you should find listed on the product label or a sticker on a lens.

Miracles Do Happen

Joan Borysenko, PhD, cofounder and former director of the mind-body clinical programs at two Harvard Medical School hospitals, now merged as Boston's Beth Israel Deaconess Medical Center. Based in Boulder, Colorado, she runs workshops and conducts lectures on mind-body healing. *Minding the Body, Mending the Mind* (Da Capo). *www.joanborysenko.com*

O n occasion, a health problem that was expected to be permanent or fatal instead disappears without medical intervention. The limited research that has been done suggests that the reason why one person recovers when most others do not might have as much to do with the mind as the body.

We interviewed Joan Borysenko, PhD, a former Harvard medical scientist who is a renowned expert in the field of mind/body healing. *She relayed this true story of spontaneous healing…*

A VISION IN LOURDES

Nearly 150 years ago, a teenage girl in Lourdes, France, reported seeing a vision of the Virgin Mary. Ever since, the waters in that area have been credited with healing powers. Most of these incidents involve cancer, multiple sclerosis and other diseases that occasionally go into remission, even without a visit to Lourdes.

The 1908 case of Marie Bire is more interesting. The 41-year-old French woman was blind as a result of optic atrophy—the degeneration of her optic nerve. According to medical science, it should not have been possible for optic nerves to recover from such a condition.

At Lourdes, the blind Bire attended Mass and received Holy Communion. Then, as the Blessed Sacrament in procession was passing the place where she sat, she suddenly regained her sight. Ten doctors examined Bire. They all found that her optic nerves were still withered but that she could see.

What may have happened: We do not have to believe in divine miracles to believe that Bire's faith might have played a role in her recovery. Studies have found that depending upon the medical condition, between 30% and 50%

of people respond to placebos. If you tell these people that you have given them painkillers, their brain activity will show that they actually feel less pain.

Does MSG Cause Glaucoma?

Marc Grossman, OD, LAc, optometrist in private practice in New Paltz, New York.
Marc R. Rose, MD, and Michael R. Rose, MD, ophthalmologists at the New Institute for Visual Wellness in Costa Mesa, California, and authors of *Save Your Sight!* (Grand Central Publishing).

I f you have glaucoma, you should avoid the food additive *monosodium glutamate*, popularly known as MSG, says Marc Grossman OD, LAc, an optometrist in private practice in Rye and New Paltz, New York. Why?

The amino acid glutamate in MSG targets receptor sites on nerve cells, creating *excitotoxicity*—overstimulation and destruction of the cells. Including the cells in the optic nerve. That fact led an international team of ophthalmologists to conclude, in the journal *Experimental Eye Research* that "a diet with excess [MSG] over a period of several years…may cause retinal cell destruction."

But MSG isn't always called MSG on food labels, say Marc R. Rose, MD, and Michael R. Rose, MD, ophthalmologists at the New Institute for Visual Wellness in Costa Mesa, California, and authors of *Save Your Sight!* (Grand Central Publishing).

Watch out for foods with the following ingredient or ingredients listed on the label, which may indicate the presence of MSG: hydrolyzed vegetable protein, hydrolyzed protein, hydrolyzed plant protein, plant protein extract, textured protein, sodium caseinate, calcium caseinate, yeast extract, autolyzed yeast, hydrolyzed oat flour, malt extract, malt flavoring, bouillon, broth stock, flavoring, natural flavoring, natural beef or chicken flavoring, seasoning or spices.

Thyroid Disorders May Increase Glaucoma Risk

When researchers reviewed health data for 12,376 adults, they found that those diagnosed with glaucoma were 38% more likely to have had a thyroid disorder, such as *hypothyroidism* (underactive thyroid) or *hyperthyroidism* (overactive thyroid).

Theory: Thyroid disease causes chemical deposits to develop in the blood vessels that circulate blood to the eye, causing increased pressure within the eyeball (a hallmark of glaucoma).

If you are diagnosed with a thyroid condition: See an ophthalmologist to be screened for glaucoma, which can be treated if detected at an early stage.

Gerald McGwin, Jr., PhD, professor, department of epidemiology, surgery and ophthalmology, University of Alabama at Birmingham.

Lower Blindness Risk

In a study of 4,170 people, those who ate the most foods rich in beta-carotene, vitamins C and E and zinc were 35% less likely to develop age-related macular degeneration (the leading cause of blindness in people over age 65) than those who ate less of these nutrients.

Theory: The antioxidants in these foods help protect against free radical damage to the retina.

Self-defense: Eat generous amounts of foods that contain the above nutrients, such as whole-grain cereal, eggs, poultry and olive oil.

Redmer van Leeuwen, MD, PhD, resident in ophthalmology, Erasmus Medical Centre, Rotterdam.

B Vitamins for Vision Protection

For about seven years, study participants took a daily supplement that included 50 mg of vitamin B-6, 1 mg of vitamin B-12 and 2.5 mg of folic acid (another B vitamin). Compared with women who took a placebo, supplement users were 34% less likely to develop age-related macular degeneration, the most common cause of vision loss among seniors.

Best: Ask your doctor if B-vitamin supplements are right for you.

William G. Christen, ScD, associate professor, division of preventive medicine, Harvard Medical School, Boston, and leader of a study of 5,205 women.

26

Anti-Aging Strategies And More

Why Vitamin C Gets A's from the Experts

Practically everyone "knows" vitamin C is good for you...but not many people really understand how good. Identification of its import dates back to early explorers crossing the ocean by ship who suffered from something called *scurvy*—caused by a deficiency of vitamin C.

For a long time now, the recommended daily allowance of vitamin C has been at levels that prevent such a deficiency—but decades ago, some scientists, including Nobel Prize-winner Linus Pauling, began to argue that much higher doses of vitamin C are needed for optimal health. There is now a continual stream of research on vitamin C and its related health benefits—which include antioxidant, anti-inflammatory and anti-aging properties, along with the fact that it has been shown to be a heart-health booster. We spoke with naturopathic medical doctor Mark Stengler, NMD, author of *Bottom Line/Natural Healing* newsletter for the latest thinking on the many positive attributes of vitamin C, along with guidelines on how much we need to reap its benefits.

HEART HEALTH

Much of the new buzz on vitamin C relates to its value in reducing risk for cardiovascular disease, Dr. Stengler told me, citing numerous research studies showing its protective role in heart health. Among these is research based on the Nurses' Health Study which followed more than 85,000 women for up to 16 years, and that demonstrated that a higher intake (in this case, more than 359 mg/day from dietary sources and supplements) reduced car-

Mark A. Stengler, NMD, licensed naturopathic medical doctor in private practice, Stengler Center for Integrative Medicine, Encinitas, California...adjunct associate clinical professor at the National College of Natural Medicine, Portland, Oregon...author of many books, including *The Natural Physician's Healing Therapies* and coauthor of *Prescription for Natural Cures* (both from Bottom Line Books)...and author of the *Bottom Line/Natural Healing* newsletter. *www.drstengler.com*

diovascular risk by 27%...and an analysis of nine other studies tracking more than 290,000 adults that showed a 25% reduction in risk in those who took more than 700 mg of supplemental vitamin C, compared with those who took none.

In addition, a Finnish study examining the health of middle-aged men who had no evidence of pre-existing heart disease found that those who were deficient in vitamin C were 3.5 times more likely to suffer heart attack.

Not only has vitamin C been shown to decrease risk for heart attacks, it also seems to reduce damage following one. In a study called the *Myocardial Infarction and Vitamins* (MIVIT) trial, researchers found that patients who suffered an acute heart attack and then supplemented for one month with 1,200 mg of vitamin C (along with 600 mg of vitamin E) after an initial IV infusion of vitamin C had a reduced rate of complications from the heart attack. The supplemented group also had fewer additional heart attacks and deaths, reducing by nearly 20% the combined rate of death, new heart attack and other severe complications. "This doesn't surprise me," Dr. Stengler said, "since vitamin C has so many protective functions, including increasing blood vessel flexibility (so they do not rupture as easily) and preventing the oxidation of LDL cholesterol." Cholesterol becomes problematic when it oxidizes—and vitamin C helps prevent that, he said.

IMMUNE BOOSTING

In addition to acting as a powerful antioxidant and helping protect the body from free radical damage, vitamin C also supports immune function. It enhances the activity of white blood cells, the body's first defense against pathogens. And it improves immune response partly by activating an antiviral chemical produced by the body called *interferon*.

Additionally, vitamin C helps to regenerate other antioxidants, including vitamin E, by acting as a "recycling service" for antioxidants in the body, causing them to re-circulate in the bloodstream and thus delivering "double duty" protective action.

Inflammation is a component of major degenerative diseases and other conditions including diabetes, Alzheimer's, obesity and heart disease—and C-reactive protein is one effective measure of inflammation levels. "Vitamin C as a supplement has been shown in studies to reduce C-reactive protein," Dr. Stengler said.

AND YET MORE HEALTH BENEFITS

"Vitamin C has powerful healing effects on many other systems in the body as well," Dr. Stengler added. "I'd say it's one of the most versatile, multi-factorial nutrients for our bodies."

In particular, vitamin C is...

• **A collagen builder.** Collagen is an important structural component of bones and tissues—and Dr. Stengler notes that vitamin C plays a critical role in the human body's synthesis of collagen, helping replace what is degraded by normal wear and tear.

• **A detoxifier.** "Vitamin C is involved in the production of bile acids, which carry toxins out of the liver," Dr. Stengler explained.

• **An agent for longevity.** Two major studies have associated vitamin C status with longevity. In a study of more than 19,000 adults, those with the highest blood levels of vitamin C had about half the risk for mortality compared with those with the lowest levels of vitamin C in their blood. Also, a decade-long study from UCLA of more than 11,000 adults showed that men with high vitamin C intake (at least 50 mg daily from their diet and regular vitamin C supplement) had a total death rate that was 41% lower than the rate among the men with low intake (less than 50 mg daily).

WHAT YOU NEED TO KNOW ABOUT VITAMIN C SUPPLEMENTATION

Recently, there's been reason to worry about the safety of food and other products imported from China, and it is distressing to hear that about 80% of the ascorbic acid—vitamin C—made in the world originates in that country. We asked Dr. Stengler if we should be concerned. He noted that there is little reason to fear toxicity. "American companies import the raw ingredients but the reliable manufacturers verify quality," he said. "They're doing their own tests before putting their labels on the products. If you stick with the big name brands when buying vitamin C, you have very little to worry about."

Though the current recommended dietary allowance (RDA) for vitamin C is only 90 mg for men and 75 mg for women (add an extra 35 mg for smokers), Dr. Stengler believes a far higher intake is beneficial. "For general prevention and overall health, studies suggest 400 to 500 mg daily," he said. For those with heart disease he recommends 500 mg to 1,500 mg daily. "For my patients with existing disease, such as cancer, I prescribe oral (or sometimes intravenous) doses that are much higher. These should be taken only under supervision—especially when undergoing chemotherapy or radiation."

The Truth About Aging

Mark A. Stengler, NMD, licensed naturopathic medical doctor in private practice, Stengler Center for Integrative Medicine, Encinitas, California...adjunct associate clinical professor at the National College of Natural Medicine, Portland, Oregon...author of many books, including *The Natural Physician's Healing Therapies* and coauthor of *Prescription for Natural Cures* (both from Bottom Line Books)...and author of the *Bottom Line/Natural Healing* newsletter. *www.drstengler.com*

The myth about longevity is that we have no control over how long we live. We do have some control—even though we all know some people who lived healthfully but died suddenly...and others who didn't take care of themselves and lived on and on.

It is easy to fall back on the idea that we can't escape our heredity, but our parentage isn't as important as you might think. Having long-lived ancestors and siblings does increase your odds of living to old age, but it doesn't guarantee longevity.

Reason: Your genes, the biological programs that govern the activity of your body's 70 trillion cells, may influence only half of the factors involved in aging, according to the Okinawa Centenarian Study. That means we can have a direct effect on our aging process by focusing on the other factors.

Proof: Americans are living longer than ever, although not as long as people in other countries. The number of centenarians (people who are 100 years old or older) in the US is at an all-time high of about 50,000!

Surprise: Centenarians often are in better health than younger seniors. About 20% of centenarians are "escapers," people who have entirely avoided serious diseases, and 40% were escapers until at least age 85, according to a *Journal of the American Medical Association* (*JAMA*) article.

While there is no one secret to longevity, we can adopt aspects of healthful aging into our lives and improve our chances of reaching the century mark. I have seen many patients improve their health and add years to their lives. You can do the same by following these recommendations. You'll feel better and have greater vitality right away.

ADD YEARS TO YOUR LIFE BY...

• **Protecting your genes.** A strong nutritional foundation safeguards our genes. Crucial to this protection is vitamin B, which can help repair genes and slow gene damage.

Advice: I recommend that most adults take a high-potency multivitamin each day that contains at least 50 milligrams (mg) each of vitamins B-1 and B-2, 400 micrograms (mcg) of folic acid and 50 mcg to 100 mcg of vitamin B-12. If your multivitamin is low in B vitamins, take an additional B-complex supplement so that you get the amounts listed above. These amounts are safe for everyone except those taking *methotrexate* for rheumatoid arthritis and for certain types of chemotherapy patients because high amounts of B supplements can interfere with these treatments.

• **Eating healthfully.** Nutrients serve as the building blocks of our biochemistry. Vitamin and mineral deficiencies can impair our normal biochemistry and increase the formation of age-promoting free radical molecules.

A study in *Journal of the American Geriatrics Society* found that centenarians consume, on average, about two-and-a-half times more antioxidant-packed vegetables than seniors ages 70 to 99. Incredibly, the centenarians ate five times more veggies than typical 40-year-olds.

All those antioxidants help protect against the types of cell damage involved in aging. Similarly, studies of Seventh Day Adventists in California—who do not smoke or drink but do eat lots of vegetables—have found that they have higher levels of antioxidants and tend to live longer.

Bottom line: Eat your veggies every day—lots of them.

• **Taking supplements.** It's difficult to study the specific effects of supplements over 80 to 100 years when so many other variables affect longevity. But both animal and human studies demonstrate the many health benefits of supplements.

Recommendation: In addition to taking a multivitamin, there's convincing evidence that a combination of the antioxidant alpha-lipoic acid (300 mg to 400 mg daily) and the amino acid acetyl-L-carnitine (800 mg to 1,200 mg daily) has a rejuvenating effect, making people feel more energetic. These two nutrients are involved in the body's production of energy, which powers every cell in the body. They are safe for everyone, although people with diabetes or seizure disorders should take them under a doctor's supervision. A recent study published in *American Journal of Clinical Nutrition* found that a related supplement, L-carnitine (2 grams daily), which helps transport fatty acids into the mitochondria (cell structures that convert nutrients into energy to power the cells), reduced mental and physical fatigue in centenarians. This supplement is safe for everyone. Magnesium (400 mg daily) helps maintain the length of telomeres, the protective tips of chromosomes. Resveratrol (100 mg twice daily) activates the SIRT1 gene, which is involved in longevity. And vitamin C (1,000 mg daily) enhances immunity and reduces inflammation, both of which can contribute to longevity. It is safe to take all of these supplements.

• **Eating less.** Animal studies dating back to the 1930s have shown that nutritionally complete but calorie-restricted diets (generally with 30% fewer calories than national recommendations) often increase life expectancy by up to 30%. In human terms, that's roughly an extra 22 years, which can bring people very close to the century mark. Studies of people growing up in Okinawa, Japan, during the 1940s and 1950s found that they consumed about 11% fewer calories than their estimated calorie requirements (about 2,000 calories daily for men and 1,600 for women) until middle age, which contributed to greater longevity.

Guaranteed benefit: Eating less will help you maintain a normal weight and lower the odds of developing diabetes and heart disease.

Important: Only 30% of centenarians are overweight.

It takes great willpower to maintain a diet with 30% fewer calories than what feels "normal," but eating less than you do can be an important first step. Assuming that you aren't underweight, I recommend a calorie-reducing compromise—at each meal, eat until you feel 80% full. You may feel hungry initially, but you'll soon adjust to consuming less food.

• **Continuing to learn.** Even more than physical health, mental sharpness (such as memory and the ability to make decisions) is the most likely predictor of independence among people in their 90s and over 100 years of age, according to a *Journal of the American Medical Association* article. Researchers say that some deterioration in cognitive function is inevitable as we age but that building a brain "reserve," or extra brain power, can offset part of this decline.

Mental activity builds your brain's reserve. Be a lifelong learner by taking challenging classes…reading and discussing difficult material…and exposing yourself to new and provocative ideas. All of these activities increase connections among brain cells.

• **Exercising.** The more exercise you do, the better. A study conducted at King's College London in England found that physically active people have healthier cells than those who don't exercise. Researchers found that exercise lengthened telomeres, the tips of chromosomes, which, as I explained earlier, usually shorten with aging.

Recommendation: If you are not physically active, start by walking for 10 minutes daily. Gradually build up speed, time and distance over a few weeks or months.

• **Getting enough—but not too much—sleep.** Seven hours of sleep nightly is the amount most strongly associated with longevity. Getting less sleep—or more—is associated with shorter life spans. People who sleep less than five hours don't give their bodies enough time for physiological recovery, and that may lead to metabolic dysfunction. Metabolic dysfunction also can result from habitually sleeping for more than eight hours.

• **Maintaining a spiritual foundation.** Having a spiritual foundation is associated with longer life. I find that my own spiritual foundation relieves stress. You can develop your inner life through prayer and/or meditation.

• **Being optimistic.** Centenarians tend to be optimists who feel that they have control over major decisions in their lives.

• **Connecting with others.** Strong ties to family and friends play a big role in longevity. Studies show that married men tend to live longer than bachelors. Research also has shown that having friends is even more important than having family in terms of living longer.

My prescription: Take time to thoroughly enjoy the company of family and friends!

The Ultimate Stay-Young Workout

Joel Harper, New York City–based certified personal trainer who designs equipment-free workouts for Olympic athletes and business executives. His exercise DVDs are *YOU: Staying Young Workout, YOU: On a Diet Workout, FitPack Workout, FitPack Chair Workout* and *Dorm Room Diet*. The exercises described in this article are adapted from the program he created for *YOU: Staying Young* by Mehmet C. Oz, MD, and Michael F. Roizen, MD (Free Press).

If you would love to have strong, limber muscles but hate the idea of trudging off to the gym to lift weights or use exercise machines, there's a new no-equipment workout that uses your body to create strength-building resistance.

Muscle strength is key to staying robust as you age. In fact, research shows that building strong muscles is one of the best ways to stay out of a nursing home.

The following exercise plan should be performed three times a week, with at least one day of rest between workouts. The exercises, which take about 10 minutes to complete, are generally appropriate for people of any age or fitness level. Just be sure to check with your doctor before starting the program—especially if you have a chronic health problem. If the basic exercises seem too easy, try the advanced versions.

Important: If you catch yourself holding your breath during the workout, immediately start counting your repetitions out loud. This is a simple way to force yourself to breathe properly. Always count backward rather than forward—it tricks your mind into thinking that you're headed toward a finish line.

My stay-young workout…

TITANIC

Purpose: Stretches your chest, shoulders and arms.

Helps with: Maintaining good posture—especially for people who work at computers.

What to do: While standing with your feet slightly apart, hold your arms out to your sides, palms facing forward, two inches below your shoulders. Keeping your torso upright, stretch your hands back as far as you can reach. Hold for 20 seconds, while breathing deeply into your chest. This will expand your diaphragm, the large muscle that separates the chest and abdominal cavities.

Advanced version: Bend your wrists back and reach the backs of your hands toward each other.

DREAM OF JEANNIE

Purpose: Strengthens your quadricep muscles (in the fronts of the thighs), abdominals and shoulders.

Helps with: Walking up stairs.

What to do: While kneeling, cross your arms and hold them in front of your body like a genie, maintaining a straight line from the top of your head to your knees. Keeping this straight line, lean back slightly, pulling your navel in and squeezing your buttocks together. Hold for 30 seconds, while breathing deeply. If necessary, cushion your knees with a folded towel.

Advanced version: Lean back as far as possible while continuing to maintain the straight line from your head to your knees.

SUPERMAN
TOE TAPS

Purpose: Strengthens your lower back and buttocks.

Helps with: Gardening, making the bed or carrying luggage.

What to do: Lie on your stomach with your head turned to the side and resting on your interlaced fingers. Keeping your legs straight, lift them off the ground and raise your knees as high as you can. Tap your toes together 40 times.

Advanced version: Reach your arms (palm side down) as far as you can in front of you. While looking down, lift your elbows as far above the ground as possible, then press your thumbs together and apart 40 times, while tapping your toes together.

HAMMOCK
STRETCH

Purpose: Stretches your hips and hamstring muscles (in the backs of the thighs).

Helps with: Easing low-back tension—especially when caused by sitting for long periods, such as during an airplane flight.

What to do: Sit on the floor with your hands behind you and your palms on the floor. Keep your fingers pointing backward and your elbows slightly bent. Bend your knees and draw your heels in until they are two feet from your tailbone. Keeping the sole of your left foot flat on the ground, place your right ankle on top of your left knee and sit up as straight as possible. Focus on pressing your lower back forward toward your right calf. Resist raising your shoulders toward your ears. Hold for 15 seconds, then switch legs and repeat.

Advanced version: For a deeper stretch, gently press the knee of your crossed leg away from you while doing this exercise.

ABDOMINAL
BUTTERFLY

Purpose: Strengthens your abdominals.

Helps with: Building strength in the core muscles of the trunk, which, in turn, supports the back.

What to do: Lie on your back and bring your legs into the "butterfly position"—knees pointing out to the sides and the soles of your feet touching. Relax your legs and lace your hands behind your head, resting your thumbs on your neck to ensure that it stays relaxed. Using only your abdominals, lift your upper body two inches off the ground then lower it back down, pressing your belly button toward your lower back. Repeat 25 times. Next, hold your upper body off the ground and lift your legs two inches, then tap the sides of your feet on the ground 25 times.

Advanced version: Lift your legs as high as you can off the ground and simultaneously raise your upper body into a "crunch" 25 times, while tapping the sides of your feet on the ground after each crunch.

CROSS-LEGGED
TWIST

Purpose: Stretches your back, abdominals and hips.

Helps with: Releasing low-back tension and opening up the hips—good for those who sit at a desk all day and for activities such as tennis and skiing.

What to do: Sit on the floor with your legs crossed. Keeping your torso upright and the top of your head directly above your tailbone, place your left hand on your right knee and your right hand on the ground behind you. Slowly twist to the right. Take two deep breaths while holding the stretch. Switch sides and repeat, then do once more on each side.

Advanced version: Do this in the lotus position (legs crossed with ankles on top of your crossed legs).

The Power of Homeopathy

Mark A. Stengler, NMD, licensed naturopathic medical doctor in private practice, Stengler Center for Integrative Medicine, Encinitas, California...adjunct associate clinical professor at the National College of Natural Medicine, Portland, Oregon...author of many books, including *The Natural Physician's Healing Therapies* and coauthor of *Prescription for Natural Cures* (both from Bottom Line Books)...and author of the *Bottom Line/Natural Healing* newsletter. *www.drstengler.com*

In this country, homeopathy is a source of controversy for medical practitioners and confusion for health-care consumers. That's why I am providing readers with this guide to homeopathic medicine, a therapy that aims to stimulate the body's own healing responses by using extremely small amounts of specific substances.

In my professional practice, I use homeopathy for one reason—it works. Before I get into the science, however, I want to share a personal story about the power of this healing therapy.

My first child was born prematurely, more than three months before he was due. His underdeveloped lungs were not ready for life outside the womb, and he contracted life-threatening viral pneumonia. It was heart-breaking to see my baby boy with tubes down his tiny throat, as four pediatricians worked around the clock to save him. Though antibiotics do not work against viruses, the doctors administered intravenous antibiotics in case there also was a secondary bacterial infection. When my son's condition did not improve, the doctors seemed at a loss for what to do next.

At this point, I took matters into my own hands. I treated my son with homeopathic *Antimonium tartaricum*, a liquid solution derived from antimony (a metal) and potassium salts, which I rubbed onto his chest. Within one day, he had improved visibly. By the following day, my son was off the respirator and on his way to complete recovery.

THE HOMEOPATHY PRINCIPLE

Homeopathy was founded two centuries ago by the German physician Samuel Hahnemann, MD. It is based on the law of similars—the idea that "like cures like."

Underlying principle: The symptoms the body produces in response to illness, injury or stress are not extensions of the condition, but instead reflect the body's attempt to heal itself.

Homeopathy promotes healing by utilizing substances that mobilize the body's natural self-defense processes. For example, the same plant that causes an itchy rash also can cure that rash when given in very minute quantities. In conventional medicine, this principle underlies vaccination and allergy injections—which administer tiny amounts of a disease-causing or an allergy-provoking agent to stimulate the immune system to produce antibodies that protect against this same agent.

For uncomplicated health problems, such as occasional digestive upset or a cold, patients can be helped with simple, common homeopathic remedies sold in health-food stores. For more complex problems, practitioners depend on a deep understanding of the individual patient's health status, an array of potent remedies and careful monitoring of the patient's progress.

We spoke with Iris Bell, PhD, professor of family and community medicine at the University of Arizona School of Medicine in Tucson, whose research on the psychophysiological effectiveness of homeopathy has been granted funding from the National Institutes of Health. Dr. Bell explained, "The human body is a network. Changes to any one system can affect the entire network. Disease is a process that can activate any number of other problems that an individual person may be genetically prone to. That's why homeopathic practitioners look at the larger picture and treat the whole patient."

THE PREPARATIONS

Homeopathy uses thousands of substances derived from plant, mineral or animal sources. Over many years, homeopaths have catalogued the physical and mental symptoms these substances can cause and, from this information, have created substances that can cure these conditions.

Homeopathic remedies generally are safe for everyone, have no side effects when used properly, and are manufactured in accordance with standards set by the FDA.

The process: The particular substance is dissolved in a "mother tincture" of alcohol or alcohol plus water. It is vigorously shaken, then further diluted with alcohol and/or water and shaken again. This process is repeated multiple times, further diluting the substance each time. When the appropriate potency is achieved, the substance is converted into a form appropriate for use—powder, liquid, ointment or tiny tablets (called pellets) to dissolve in the mouth.

A remedy's potency depends on the degree of dilution it undergoes. Classifications include X (for 10, meaning a potency based on a ratio of one part substance to 10 parts dilution), C (100) and M (1,000). Products are formulated by multiples of these ratios. For example, a 6X remedy contains one part active substance to 10^6—which is 10 x 10 x 10 x 10 x 10 x 10, or one million—parts carrier substances.

Now, here's the seeming paradox of homeopathy—the more diluted the substance is, the more potent it becomes. No one knows why for sure, but experience shows this does happen. Products used for minor conditions, such as colds and headaches, are sold over the counter in health-food stores. A prescription from a licensed health-care practitioner is required for homeopathic drugs that treat more serious problems, such as severe strep infections, as well as for all M-potency products. These can be filled at compounding pharmacies.

Recently, a medical doctor expressed his skepticism regarding the dilution of homeopathic substances. I asked if he would treat a life-threatening allergic reaction by injecting *epinephrine* (adrenaline)—the standard medical treatment—and he said of course he would, because it works. I then pointed out that the epinephrine used for injection is far more diluted than many homeopathic remedies.

SCIENTIFIC EVIDENCE

Researchers have been studying homeopathy for decades. Overall, studies show mixed results. This does not mean that treatments are ineffective, but rather that they are used in a holistic way not easily measured in conventional studies.

Reason: Drugs and nutritional supplements can be matched to specific problems and studied accordingly. For example, the drug (Celebrex) and the natural supplement glucosamine (an amino sugar) both are used to treat osteoarthritis, so studies focus on their effectiveness against that particular disease. However, homeopathic treatment is highly individualized according to a patient's overall profile. If a patient has migraines, I select from among several dozen homeopathic remedies, taking into account the type and location of his/her migraines, how the weather affects him, his diet and exercise habits, etc. With so many variables influencing the choice of homeopathic remedy and the patient's response to it, I'm not surprised that study results sometimes are inconclusive.

Even so, more than 100 clinical trials have demonstrated homeopathy's benefits. For example, a study conducted at the University of Vienna involved 50 patients with chronic bronchitis and/or emphysema and a history of smoking. Compared with participants who received placebos, those who took homeopathic remedies had significantly reduced levels of the mucus secretions that impair breathing…and their average hospital stay was just 4.2 days, compared with 7.4 days for the placebo group. Researchers at the University of Glasgow analyzed data from four studies involving about 250 patients with allergic respiratory symptoms, such as asthma and rhinitis.

Findings: Participants who received a 30C potency homeopathic remedy for hay fever reported a 28% improvement in symptoms, compared with 3% in the placebo group.

Equally convincing, in my opinion, are the many reports I have received from patients who have been helped by homeopathic remedies—often after other treatments failed.

FINDING A HOMEOPATHIC PRACTITIONER

Homeopathy does not work for everyone. For best effect, try to be articulate and open in detailing your symptoms, as this will help practitioners to identify the most appropriate remedies. Also, some practitioners work with a limited number of substances that they have found especially effective—so if you do not get relief with a particular practitioner, try someone else.

In the US, homeopathy is practiced by many naturopathic physicians, chiropractors, nurses, dentists and some medical doctors. In most states, homeopaths are not licensed as such, and there are no national standards for training. However, the following organizations have stringent training requirements for members and offer online directories for finding practitioners in various areas.

•**American Institute of Homeopathy awards a diplomate of homeopathy (DHt) certification.** A practitioner must hold an MD or a DO license, accrue 150 hours of education credits in homeopathy, and pass various exams (888-445-9988, *www.homeopathyusa.org*).

•**All naturopathic physicians are educated in homeopathy.** Those with the most extensive training are eligible to join the Homeopathic Academy of Naturopathic Physicians.

Referrals: American Association of Naturopathic Physicians (866-538-2267, *www.naturopathic.org*).

For more information on homeopathy, contact the National Center for Homeopathy (703-548-7790, *www.nationalcenterforhomeopathy.org*).

LOOKING AHEAD

You may be surprised to learn that high-potency homeopathic remedies are diluted to the point where they do not contain any of the original substance—yet they continue to have powerful healing properties. This is an aspect of the emerging field of energetic medicine. Energetic medicine heals by affecting the electrical and electromagnetic activity of the body—the means by which cells communicate with one another. Magnet therapy and light therapy also are examples of energetic medicine.

In homeopathy, researchers now believe that the original electromagnetic frequency of the source materials imprints itself on the fluid used to produce the remedy. Because the human body is 70% to 80% water, a fluid medium is an effective way to transmit information throughout the body.

Does this sound far-fetched? Remember that practitioners of Western medicine used to claim that acupuncture and chiropractic were nonsense—yet now these alternative therapies generally are accepted as legitimate. Researchers at a number of major universities are now studying homeopathy's applications in energetic medicine. I believe we will be hearing much more about this therapy in the years to come.

Homeopathic Remedies

Mark A. Stengler, NMD, licensed naturopathic medical doctor in private practice, Stengler Center for Integrative Medicine, Encinitas, California…adjunct associate clinical professor at the National College of Natural Medicine, Portland, Oregon…author of many books, including *The Natural Physician's Healing Therapies* and coauthor of *Prescription for Natural Cures* (both from Bottom Line Books)…and author of the *Bottom Line/Natural Healing* newsletter. *www.drstengler.com*

Low-potency homeopathic remedies that are sold in health-food stores generally are safe for everyone. They can be used in combination with other homeopathic remedies. Follow instructions on labels. Consult a doctor trained in homeopathy before using remedies if you have a serious illness…take medication…are pregnant or nursing…or if symptoms do not improve after 48 hours of use.

For this condition…	The remedy is…
Allergies, hay fever	*Allium cepa*
Arthritis pain	*Rhus toxicodendron*
Back pain	*Rhus toxicodendron*
Bee stings, insect bites	*Apis*
Bruising, swelling, sprains	*Arnica*
Cold sores	*Rhus toxicodendron*
Coughs, colds	*Phosphorous*
Earache	*Chamomilla*
Emotional distress, anxiety	*Ignatia*
Fever	*Belladonna*

Flu	*Gelsemium*
Hangover, heartburn	*Nux vomica*
Migraine	*Belladonna*
Muscle cramps, muscle spasms	*Magnesia phosphorica*
Nerve injury	*Hypericum*
Poison ivy	*Rhus toxicodendron*
Sore throat	*Phosphorous*
Skin rash, eczema	*Sulphur*
Stomach cramps, nausea	*Nux vomica*
Toothache, teething pain	*Chamomilla*
Urinary tract infection	*Cantharis*

Your Genes Are Not Your Destiny

Mark A. Stengler, NMD, licensed naturopathic medical doctor in private practice, Stengler Center for Integrative Medicine, Encinitas, California...adjunct associate clinical professor at the National College of Natural Medicine, Portland, Oregon...author of many books, including *The Natural Physician's Healing Therapies* and coauthor of *Prescription for Natural Cures* (both from Bottom Line Books)...and author of the *Bottom Line/Natural Healing* newsletter. *www.drstengler.com*

Family history. It's something doctors always ask about, and for many of us, it's a source of worry. After all, our genes are our destiny, right? Heart disease runs in my family, you may say, or cancer, or diabetes. Adding to the concern are all those reports about scientists discovering a gene that may influence our risk for contracting a certain condition. So far, their discoveries include genes that make us more susceptible to heart disease, Alzheimer's disease, breast cancer, prostate cancer, arthritis, diabetes, obesity, depression, osteoporosis and more.

Some of the news stories also mention the good news on the flip side of the coin—that genetic research eventually may lay the groundwork for new medical treatments. But the big advances are, at best, many years away.

There is more good news that we can use right now—eating certain foods can help us fight disease-causing genes, thanks to something called *nutrigenomics*. Just like it sounds, this new field of science merges research on genes with nutrition. One of the most exciting concepts to come out of the labs is the recognition that our genes have a great amount of flexibility, good and bad. We may always have the genes that we were born with, but what we eat—or don't eat—affects how they behave. We can use nutrients as a form of safe, natural gene therapy that aims to help our genes work better and keep us in good health.

I'll give you an example. An acquaintance, Jim, underwent nutrigenomic testing and learned that he had a gene variation that greatly reduced his body's ability to use folic acid, a B vitamin. As a consequence, he had elevated levels of homocysteine, an amino acid that aids in cellular metabolism and, when present in high levels, becomes a risk factor for heart attack, stroke and Alzheimer's disease. Jim can't change the gene—it's hardwired—but he did start taking folic acid supplements, which normalized his homocysteine levels and helped offset his genetic risk.

WHY GENES MATTER

Here's a quick refresher on basic biology. Genes are microscopic biological programs that regulate how each of our trillions of cells functions. They work like computer software, programming the tens of thousands of biochemicals in our bodies. Most cells contain two sets of genes, one from each parent. We also inherit many mutations, or variations, that can alter gene activity. When genes don't function at their best, they can increase our risk for disease.

Nutrition affects our genes in three basic ways...

•**First, we need nutrients to make and repair genes.** We make new genes each time we need a new cell for growth, to heal injuries or to replace dead cells. By eating right and taking nutritional supplements, we help our bodies

333

make healthy new genes and do a better job of repairing those that get damaged.

• **Second, some nutrients, such as folic acid and *genistein* (an isoflavone found in soy), regulate gene activity.** For example, they help turn off cancer-promoting genes, so one of the benefits of these nutrients is a potential decrease in cancer risk.

• **Third, extra amounts of some nutrients can offset genetic weaknesses.** This was Jim's experience, and it is a major focus of nutrigenomic research.

Upping your intake of a few key nutrients can have big benefits when it comes to preventing disease and even slowing down the aging process. Here are the three powerhouse nutrients that you'll want to incorporate into your diet right away.

B VITAMINS SLOW THE CLOCK

Every living creature ages. On a microscropic level, aging occurs in large part due to the deterioration of our genes and their ability to provide accurate instructions to cells. This is like having genetic instructions increasingly filled with typos. A solid nutritional foundation protects our genes and slows this deterioration… and the accumulation of genetic typos.

For example, studies show that low levels of B vitamins, such as folic acid and B-12, actually increase gene damage…and that damage is reduced when people consume more of these vitamins. Bruce Ames, PhD, of the Children's Hospital Oakland Research Institute in Oakland, California, found that low intake of folic acid and magnesium interferes with gene-repair mechanisms, resulting in more mutations. More mutations translate into faster aging and greater risk for disease.

Dr. Ames has amassed a wealth of data showing that 50 inherited diseases can be improved by taking B vitamins and other supplements, such as vitamin C, magnesium, *indole-3-carbinol* (found in cruciferous vegetables, such as cauliflower) and *chlorophyllin* (a natural derivative of *chlorophyll*, the ingredient that makes plant leaves green). These diseases include cancer, cardiomyopathy (deterioration of the heart muscle), autism, Alzheimer's disease and coronary artery disease. I suspect that these

are just a fraction of the conditions that can be modified through nutritional therapies.

Smart strategy: Because B-complex vitamins are so important for gene function and overall health, I recommend that nearly every adult take a daily high-potency multivitamin or B-complex supplement with 800 micrograms (mcg) of folic acid and 50 mcg to 100 mcg of vitamin B-12. Exceptions include anyone who is taking *methotrexate* for rheumatoid arthritis and some chemotherapy patients, because high-dose B supplements may interfere with these treatments.

D IS FOR DEFENSE

Researchers and physicians are increasingly focusing on the health benefits of vitamin D in maintaining healthy bones and muscle as we age…preventing cancer…fighting infections… and lowering the risk for heart disease. Considerable evidence suggests that getting enough vitamin D—at least 1,000 international units (IU) daily—could substantially decrease the risk for breast, colon, lung and other cancers.

Genetics enter the equation when it comes to the amount of sun people need to make their own vitamin D. Those with fair skin can get enough by spending 10 to 15 minutes outdoors daily in the summer sun, while people with darker complexions usually need 30 to 40 minutes in the sun. Unfortunately, most people don't get nearly enough exposure to sunlight. Also, according to a study in the journal *Metabolism,* 35% of Americans have a genetic variation (known as *VDR bb*) that reduces their ability to benefit from vitamin D.

Low levels of vitamin D occur not just in northern states that are sun-starved during the winter. A new study found that one-quarter of adults in sunny southern Arizona were deficient in D. The deficit was higher in some people—38% of Hispanics and 55% of blacks.

Best dosages: Take a minimum of 1,000 IU of vitamin D3 (the form the body makes from sunlight) daily if you are fair-skinned… or 2,000 IU if you have a dark complexion. I would add that some fair-skinned people need 2,000 IU to 4,000 IU to achieve normal blood levels. There are no great natural food sources of vitamin D, and you won't find this much in most multivitamins, so you'll have to take an additional supplement.

SELENIUM STAVES OFF BREAST CANCER

Selenium, an essential dietary mineral, also helps maintain normal gene activity, and research indicates that it may protect against breast cancer. It is a component of *glutathione peroxidase*, a powerful antioxidant made by the body that works as a natural detoxifying agent.

Mutations in the BRCA1 genes are an established risk factor for breast cancer. Women of Jewish European heritage are at high risk for inheriting this gene, and it also is common in women of Hispanic descent. Men with BRCA1 mutations also have a higher-than-average risk for breast cancer (1,600 men are diagnosed with the disease annually in the US, compared with 200,000 women). But once again, your genes don't have to be your fate.

The BRCA family of genes is involved in repairing damaged genes. As we know, mutations can keep genes from functioning properly. If genes can't do a good job at repair, cell damage accumulates, increasing the risk for breast cancer.

Try this: Selenium is found in most multivitamin/multimineral supplements. If you are in generally good health, strive for 200 mcg to 300 mcg of selenium daily (most multis contain 200 mcg). Don't take more unless your physician recommends it, though, because high doses of this mineral are potentially toxic. Or you could eat a handful of Brazil nuts (about six) each day—they're the richest natural food source of selenium.

GENETIC TESTING FOR YOU

The best way to evaluate your genetic risk is to consult with a genetic counselor. To find a counselor in your area, visit the National Society of Genetic Counselors at their Web Site *www.nsgc.org*. Click the link "Find a Genetic Counselor." Genetic testing may be covered by your insurance (especially if you are in a high-risk group).

THE CARE AND FEEDING OF YOUR GENES

So how can you start putting some of this knowledge to use? I'll relate the experience of one of my associates who underwent nutrigenomic testing. The tests revealed that Joseph didn't have any single gene that could make or break his health—but he did have a cluster of gene variations that together might increase his risk for diabetes. In fact, he already had been diagnosed with prediabetes.

Through better eating habits, exercise and supplements (chromium, biotin, alpha-lipoic acid and others), Joseph normalized his blood sugar, cholesterol and triglycerides—and lost 20 pounds. He now is in better health than he had been for years. Knowing that he has a genetic risk for developing diabetes has motivated him to stick with a healthier lifestyle to improve his genes.

Is nutrigenomic testing right for you? If there is a strong pattern of illness in your family, it might be worthwhile to evaluate your genetic risk. And for anyone, test results can be a powerful motivator to make healthy dietary and lifestyle choices.

Why We Age

Over the course of a lifetime, our bodies face inevitable decline. Aging is characterized by an accumulation of cell damage. Some of this damage comes from destructive molecules called free radicals.

Another problem: Wear and tear erodes mitochondria, microscopic cell structures that provide us with energy and stamina. In addition, telomeres, the tips of chromosomes, shorten with age, which may accelerate the aging process.

Mark A. Stengler, NMD, licensed naturopathic medical doctor in private practice, Stengler Center for Integrative Medicine, Encinitas, California...adjunct associate clinical professor at the National College of Natural Medicine, Portland, Oregon...author of many books, including *The Natural Physician's Healing Therapies* and coauthor of *Prescription for Natural Cures* (both from Bottom Line Books)...and author of the *Bottom Line/Natural Healing* newsletter. *www.drstengler.com*

Drink Coffee...Eat Chocolate...and Other Surprising Ways to Live Longer

Michael F. Roizen, MD, chief wellness officer and chair of the Wellness Institute, Cleveland Clinic in Cleveland, Ohio. He is coauthor, with Mehmet C. Oz, MD, of several books, including *You: Staying Young* (Free Press).

Many of the proven strategies for living longer—such as restricting calories and exercising on a regular basis—can feel like punishment for some people. Fortunately, there are many enjoyable ways to stay healthy—but doctors don't recommend these strategies as often as they should. Research has shown that activities nearly everyone enjoys can literally add years to a person's life.

Fun-filled ways to live longer...

1. Get the Right Kind of Sleep.

Studies have found that people who get deep, restorative sleep typically live three years longer than those who don't. During deep sleep, the body normally produces higher levels of melatonin, a hormone that improves immunity and reduces the risk for infections as well as cancer. Deep sleep also increases levels of growth hormone, which improves energy and helps promote a healthy weight.

Good news: You don't have to sleep uninterrupted through the night to get the benefits of deep sleep, as long as you complete a series of at least 90-minute sleep cycles—each one beginning with light sleep (stages 1 and 2)...progressing through deeper sleep (stages 3 and 4) ...and then into the deepest stage, known as rapid eye movement (REM) sleep. As long as you complete this 90-minute cycle several times a night, it doesn't matter if you wake up a time or two.

2. Enjoy Your Coffee.

Many people assume that coffee—unlike green tea, for example—isn't a healthful beverage. But that's not true. Studies have found that caffeinated and decaffeinated coffee are a main source of antioxidants in the average American's diet.

Research has shown that caffeinated coffee decreases the risk for Parkinson's and Alzheimer's diseases by 30% to 40%—health benefits that are largely attributed to the beverage's caffeine. (Decaffeinated coffee does not offer these same benefits.) The caffeine in coffee also is good for cognitive health.

Important: Caffeinated coffee may cause several side effects, such as blood pressure spikes, abnormal heartbeat, anxiety and gastric upset.

My recommendation: If you do not experience any of these side effects, and you enjoy drinking coffee, have as many cups of caffeinated coffee as you like. If you do experience side effects, you may prefer to drink decaffeinated coffee. Even though it does not have the health benefits previously described, studies show that decaffeinated coffee may help fight off type 2 diabetes.

3. Go Dancing.

Men and women who get optimal amounts of physical activity—about 30 minutes a day, seven days a week—can make their "RealAges" (the "biological ages" of their bodies, based on lifestyle and behaviors) 6.4 years younger.

Many types of dancing give a superb physical workout. Ballroom and square dancing are particularly good for cognitive health. They involve both physical and mental stimulation (in order to execute the appropriate dance steps) and may help reduce the risk for dementia. Aim to dance at least 30 minutes a day.

4. Do Some Singing.

Whether you lend your voice to a choir or merely sing for pleasure in the shower, singing improves immunity and elevates levels of hormones known as endorphins and dopamine—both of which reduce stress and activate the brain's pleasure centers. Studies have shown that singing helps people with asthma...reduces stress hormones...and may temporarily help improve memory in patients with Alzheimer's disease.

5. Continue Learning.

People who take pleasure in expanding their minds—for example, by learning to paint, attending lectures or doing puzzles—

can make their RealAges about 2.5 years younger.

Studies have shown that people with higher levels of education, and those who continue learning throughout life, form more connections between brain cells, making them less likely to experience later-life memory loss.

6. Eat Some Chocolate.

The powerful antioxidants known as flavonoids in dark chocolate increase levels of the body's nitric oxide (NO), a gas that dilates arteries (to help prevent blockages) and can help reduce blood pressure in people with hypertension. This is particularly helpful for people over age 50, because age-related buildup of fatty deposits in the arteries (atherosclerosis) reduces natural levels of NO.

My recommendation: Eat one-half ounce of dark chocolate (at least 70% cocoa) twice daily. Don't overindulge in chocolate—it is high in calories. Other good flavonoid sources include brewed black or green tea...red wine...dark grape juice...strawberries, cranberries and apples...and brussels sprouts and onions.

7. Find Opportunities to Laugh.

People who laugh—and who make others laugh—tend to have better immunity than people who are humor-impaired. Telling a joke is also a good way to improve your memory. It requires the teller—as well as the listener—to pay attention, and we laugh when we expect one outcome but are surprised by a different one. Psychologists call this "conceptual blending." In addition, laughter is a well-known stress reducer. People who are calmer and more relaxed have lower levels of heart disease and cancer.

8. Have More Sex.

Men and women who have sex (that results in orgasm) an average of twice a week have arteries with greater elasticity (which helps prevent hardening of the arteries). Men and women who have sex daily, on average, are biologically eight years younger than those who have it once a week.

9. Rest More Often.

Everyone enjoys taking a break from life's stresses. Research shows that people who give themselves time to relax (thus minimizing the effects of stress) can live for up to eight years longer.

Stress reducers—such as meditating, taking long walks, watching the sunset—can add years to your life. Yoga is particularly good. It lowers blood pressure, heart rate and stress hormones, and increases levels of dopamine and the "feel good" hormone serotonin. Aim for about 10 minutes daily of a stress-reduction activity.

10. Get a Pet.

People who own pets can make themselves an average of one year younger. Studies show that taking care of and bonding with a pet reduces depression and blood pressure.

After a heart attack, people with pets have a one-year survival rate of 94%, compared with 72% for people who don't have pets. Studies show that dog owners, who live about three years longer, tend to be a little healthier than those with other pets—in part because they get regular exercise when they walk their dogs.

Drugs or Supplements?

Alan H. Pressman, DC, PhD, CCN, host of the daily radio show *Healthline with Dr. Pressman* on WWRL 1600 AM in New York City and syndicated nationally on Air America, *www.drpressman.com.* He is author of numerous books on nutrition and health, including, with coauthor Sheila Buff, *The Complete Idiot's Guide to Vitamins and Minerals* (Alpha).

For many conditions, dietary supplements, along with lifestyle changes, can be safe and effective alternatives to more powerful—and often more risky—drugs. Talk to your doctor before treating a medical condition with supplements instead of drugs.

Caution: When starting a new supplement, begin with the smallest dose and take it for several days to be sure that you don't have a bad reaction. Slowly increase the dose to a level that helps. With some supplements, such as glucosamine (for joint problems) and saw palmetto, you may have to take the pills for several weeks before you notice an improvement. Never go beyond the maximum indicated on the container or recommended by your doctor. Stop taking the supplement if at any time you notice any bad side effects.

Quality caution: Sometimes a supplement doesn't help because the quality is poor. Consider trying a different brand before you give up on it.

Note: Always keep a complete list of all the supplements and drugs you take and review it with your doctor at every visit.

Surprising Stress Protector

The live bacteria in probiotic supplements (and fermented foods such as yogurt) help reduce intestinal damage caused by chronic stress. Probiotics inhibit the ability of bacteria to penetrate the intestinal wall and to initiate tissue-damaging inflammation.

MedPage Today.

Alternative Treatment for Multiple Sclerosis

Mark A. Stengler, NMD, licensed naturopathic medical doctor in private practice, Stengler Center for Integrative Medicine, Encinitas, California...adjunct associate clinical professor at the National College of Natural Medicine, Portland, Oregon...author of many books, including *The Natural Physician's Healing Therapies* and coauthor of *Prescription for Natural Cures* (both from Bottom Line Books)...and author of the *Bottom Line/Natural Healing* newsletter. *www.drstengler.com*

Donna, 70, dragged herself into my office three years ago. Her complaints —muscle weakness and stiffness, fatigue, irritability and sensitivity to noise—were all due to *multiple sclerosis* (MS), a disease she had battled since age 21.

MS is a degenerative autoimmune disease in which immune cells attack the *myelin sheath* (fatty tissue that surrounds and protects nerve fibers), disrupting the flow of electrical impulses between the brain and the nerves. Symptoms may flare up when a patient is stressed or has a viral infection, such as a cold or the flu. Conventional treatment includes the immune-regulating drug *interferon* (Betaseron) or *glatiramer* (Copaxone), which suppresses immune activity against the myelin sheath...and steroids or chemotherapy to reduce inflammation. These therapies can have serious side effects, including depression and flulike symptoms.

Research suggests that a deficiency of vitamin B-12 may be associated with the development of MS. B-12 aids in repairing the myelin sheath, so B-12 injections may help to prevent and treat MS flare-ups. To relieve Donna's symptoms, I prescribed B-12 injections twice weekly, plus a daily sublingual (under the tongue) B-12 supplement. After a month, she had more energy, strength and flexibility... was less irritable...and was less bothered by noise.

I urged Donna to increase her intake of essential fatty acids (EFAs), found in fish, walnuts, almonds and pistachios. I also recommended a high-potency fish oil supplement and a *gamma linoleic acid* (GLA) supplement in the form of evening primrose oil. To encourage her, I showed Donna studies by Roy Swank, MD, a professor of neurology at the University of Oregon, which found that a diet limited in saturated fat (from meat and dairy foods) and hydrogenated oils (from margarines and baked goods made with vegetable oils) and rich in polyunsaturated fatty acids (from fish oil and vegetables) helps to halt the progression of MS.

I also tested Donna's blood level of vitamin D and found that it was low. Vitamin D is a critical nutrient for proper immune function, including prevention of auto-immune disorders. MS is more common in higher latitudes where sunlight—a key source of vitamin D— is limited. A study published in *The Journal of the American Medical Association* reported that higher levels of vitamin D in the body may reduce the risk of developing MS by up to 62%. For Donna, I prescribed 1,000 international units (IU) of vitamin D daily, taken in addition to the multivitamin/mineral formula she was already using.

Since she began this treatment three years ago, Donna has had only occasional minor flare-ups, for which she receives twice-weekly B-12 injections. In general, her condition is well controlled with just one monthly B-12 injection, plus the sublingual B-12 and the vitamin D supplements. She no longer requires steroid medication—and she says that despite having had MS for almost 50 years, she's now in better health overall than her septuagenarian friends.

27

Natural Cures from Your Kitchen

Handy, Money Saving Remedies

You don't need to go to the pharmacy to find powerful cures for everyday ailments. The answers could be in your kitchen. Joan and Lydia Wilen have been collecting, researching and testing folk remedies for more than two decades—and all their remedies have been reviewed for safety by medical doctors, naturopathic doctors and other experts.

Bonus: You might even save a few pennies in the process—having to turn no further than your own kitchen. If you have an existing health condition, check with your physician before trying any of these remedies.

BAD BREATH, GUM DISEASE AND TOOTHACHE

• **Coconut oil, baking soda.**

Coconut oil can soothe ailments of the mouth, such as bad breath, gum disease and toothache. For help with any of these conditions, brush your teeth with a mixture of one-eighth teaspoon of baking soda and one-half teaspoon of organic extra-virgin coconut oil (which you can find at a health-food store). Sore gums also are helped when you rub them with coconut oil.

BUMPS AND BRUISES

• **Lemon.**

Most bruises that turn black and blue go away on their own, but you can speed the healing process—and reduce both the swelling and the bruising—with this Mayan remedy. Cut a lemon in half, and rub the pulpy side over the bruise once an hour for several hours. Avoid any cuts or breaks in the skin.

Lydia Wilen and Joan Wilen, folk-remedy experts based in New York City. The sisters are coauthors of many books, including *Bottom Line's Healing Remedies: Over 1,000 Astounding Ways to Heal Arthritis, Asthma, High Blood Pressure, Varicose Veins, Warts and More!* (Bottom Line Books). *www.bottomlinepublications.com*

CONSTIPATION

• **Lemon, honey, prune juice, prunes, papaya, apples, dried figs.**

Drinking water on an empty stomach can stimulate bowel movements. Before breakfast, drink the juice of one-half a lemon in one cup of warm water. If it is too tart, sweeten it with honey. If that doesn't help move your bowels, try one of the following—prune juice (at room temperature, not chilled) or stewed prunes, papaya, two peeled apples or six to eight dried figs. (Soak the figs overnight in water. In the morning, drink the water, then eat the figs.)

DANDRUFF

• **Thyme.**

We all have dead cells that fall from our scalp as new cells come in. But some people have a greater number of cells falling that are bigger and easier to see. Dried thyme can help get rid of dandruff. Boil one cup of water, and add two heaping tablespoons of dried thyme to the cup. Let it simmer for seven to 10 minutes. Use a strainer to collect the thyme, and get rid of it. Let the tea cool. Wash your hair with a regular shampoo. While your hair is still damp, gently massage the cooled tea into your scalp. Do not rinse.

DIARRHEA

• **Milk, allspice, cinnamon and powdered cloves.**

There are several remedies from other countries that use milk. A West Indian remedy is one cup of milk (or warm water) with a pinch of allspice. The Pennsylvania Dutch recommend one cup of warm milk with two pinches of cinnamon. A Brazilian remedy includes two pinches of cinnamon and one pinch of powdered cloves in one cup of warm milk. (Do not drink milk if you are lactose intolerant. It may cause diarrhea.)

HEADACHE

• **Green tea, mint.**

Fatigue, anxiety and stress can trigger headaches. For fast relief, brew one cup of green tea and add sprigs of fresh mint. You can use either spearmint or peppermint. If you don't have fresh mint available, use a peppermint or spearmint tea bag. Combine a bag each of green tea and mint tea to make a powerful brew that will diminish your headache in about 15 minutes.

INDIGESTION

• **Grapefruit, potato.**

If you are prone to any of the unpleasant symptoms of indigestion, including stomachache or nausea, you can prepare this remedy in advance to have at the ready. Grate the peel of a grapefruit, and spread the pieces out on a paper towel to dry overnight. Store the dried peel in a lidded jar. When you feel the first signs of indigestion, eat one-half to one teaspoon of the grated peel. Chew thoroughly before swallowing.

Another remedy: Raw potato juice can neutralize stomach acid. Grate a potato, and squeeze the gratings through a piece of cheesecloth or a fine strainer to get the juice. Take one tablespoon of potato juice diluted with one-half cup of warm water. Drink slowly.

INSOMNIA

• **Whole nutmeg, grapefruit juice, yellow onion.**

Nutmeg can work as a sedative. Crush a whole nutmeg, and steep it in hot water for 10 minutes. Drink it 30 minutes before bedtime. Or drink a glass of pure, warmed grapefruit juice. If you prefer it sweetened, use a little bit of raw honey. Or cut a yellow onion and put it in a glass jar. Keep it near your bed. When you can't sleep, or if you wake up and can't fall back to sleep, open the jar and inhale deeply. Close the jar. Close your eyes, think lovely thoughts and you'll fall back to sleep.

MEMORY PROBLEMS

• **Carrot juice, milk, fresh ginger, sage tea, cloves.**

For mild memory problems, try this memory-improving drink. Mix one-half glass of carrot juice with one-half glass of milk—and drink daily. Or use daily doses of fresh ginger in cooking or in tea. Ginger is known to improve memory. Or brew one cup of sage tea, and add four cloves. Drink daily. Sage and cloves are believed to strengthen memory.

POISON IVY/OAK/SUMAC

• **Banana skin, lemon, garlic, tofu.**

These remedies can help ease the itching and redness of poison ivy. Rub the inside of a banana skin directly on the affected skin. Use a fresh banana skin every hour for a day. (Freeze the leftover banana pieces to use in smoothies or to eat on hot days.)

Or slice one or two lemons, and rub them on the area. This helps to stop the itching and clears the skin. Or chop up four cloves of garlic, and boil them in one cup of water. When the mixture is cool, apply it with a clean cloth to the area.

Another remedy: Mash up pieces of tofu directly on the itchy area—and hold them in place with a cloth or bandage. This should cool off the area and help any poison ivy flare-up.

SINUS PROBLEMS

• **Tomato juice, garlic, cayenne pepper, lemon juice.**

When your sinuses feel clogged and uncomfortable, this bracing drink can help. Combine one cup of tomato juice, one teaspoon of freshly chopped garlic, one-quarter to one-half teaspoon of cayenne pepper (according to your tolerance for spicy food) and one teaspoon of lemon juice. Heat the mixture until it is warm but not too hot to drink. Drink it slowly, and it should help clear up sinuses quickly.

Kitchen Spices Fight Deadly E. Coli

The food-borne bacterium *Escherichia coli O157* causes severe cramps, bloody diarrhea and kidney failure. Researchers studied the effects of extracts of 20 spices on the bacterium.

Results: Allspice significantly reduced E. coli O157 toxin growth...to a lesser degree, so did cloves.

Worth a try: Add ground allspice and/or cloves to burgers, vegetables and salads.

Kumio Yokoigawa, PhD, professor of food microbiology, University of Tokushima, Japan, and leader of a lab study.

Migraine Relief

Eliminate migraine pain with pepper. Capsaicin, an ingredient in cayenne pepper, cuts off neurotransmitters in the brain that cause headache pain.

Best: Dissolve one-quarter teaspoon of cayenne powder in four ounces of warm water. Dip a cotton swab into the solution, and apply the liquid inside your nostrils. It will burn—and by the time the burning stops, the headache pain will be reduced and sometimes gone altogether.

Eric Yarnell, ND, assistant professor, department of botanical medicine, Bastyr University, Kenmore, Washington. *www.dryarnell.com*

Natural Remedies For Nausea

Suzy Cohen, RPh, registered practicing pharmacist for nearly 20 years and author of *The 24-Hour Pharmacist* (Harper Paperbacks). Her syndicated newspaper column, "Dear Pharmacist," reaches more than 24 million readers. Based in Florida, she is a member of the Association of Natural Medicine Pharmacists and the American Holistic Health Association.

As a pharmacist for almost two decades, Suzy Cohen knows the importance of medication—but she also has learned to "think outside the pill" and recommend natural options that often are just as good or better at promoting health without the risk of dangerous side effects.

Here is the remedy she recommends most often for nausea.

GINGER FOR NAUSEA

Studies have shown that ginger can relieve nausea—due to pregnancy, seasickness, etc.—as well as or better than over-the-counter drugs.

How it works: Ginger increases the pH of stomach acid, reducing its acidity. In one study, published in *The Lancet,* volunteers were given either ginger or Dramamine (a nausea-preventing drug), then were seated in a chair designed to trigger motion sickness. Those given ginger were able to withstand the motion 57% longer than those given the drug.

How to use: Put one teaspoon of peeled, grated fresh gingerroot in a cup of boiling water. Let it steep for 10 minutes, then drink (you can filter out the ginger if you want). Or chew and swallow a piece of crystallized ginger, sold in health-food stores.

Caution: Ginger can increase the risk of bleeding when taken with blood-thinning drugs, such as *warfarin* (Coumadin).

Kitchen Cures... Shopping List

Lydia Wilen and Joan Wilen, folk-remedy experts based in New York City. The sisters are coauthors of many books, including *Bottom Line's Healing Remedies: Over 1,000 Astounding Ways to Heal Arthritis, Asthma, High Blood Pressure, Varicose Veins, Warts and More!* (Bottom Line Books). *www.bottomlinepublications.com*

Keep your kitchen stocked with these ingredients—and you'll have homemade remedies and cures at the ready!

- **Allspice**
- **Apples**
- **Baking soda**
- **Banana (skin)**
- **Carrot juice**
- **Cayenne pepper**
- **Cinnamon**
- **Cloves (whole)**
- **Cloves (powdered)**
- **Coconut oil**
- **Figs (dried)**
- **Garlic**
- **Ginger**
- **Grapefruit**
- **Grapefruit juice**

- **Green tea**
- **Honey**
- **Lemon**
- **Lemon juice**
- **Milk**
- **Nutmeg (whole)**
- **Onion (yellow)**
- **Papaya**
- **Potato**
- **Prune juice**
- **Prunes (stewed)**
- **Sage tea**
- **Spearmint or peppermint**
- **Thyme**
- **Tofu**
- **Tomato juice**

5-Cent Cure for Kidney Disease

Magdi Yaqoob, MD, professor of renal medicine, The Royal London Hospital, London, England.

Finally—some great news for the 26 million people with chronic kidney disease! Because the problem is progressive and incurable, it can seem hopeless, but new research shows that a natural remedy that is safe, effective and costs just a few pennies a day can dramatically slow down kidney decline. What is it? Baking soda, believe it or not—or, if you want to be technical, *sodium bicarbonate.*

Though it may well be the most medically important, this is hardly the first unconventional health-related use for this simple and inexpensive kitchen ingredient—some swear by it as a remedy for acid indigestion, while others use baking soda to brush their teeth or in lieu of antiperspirant or to soothe rashes and skin eruptions. For people with *chronic kidney disease* (CKD), however, it is important

343

to take this only under your doctor's close supervision—read on to learn why.

RATE OF DECLINE
SLOWED BY TWO-THIRDS

CKD affects one in nine adults. It runs the gamut from poor function and minor discomfort to end-stage renal disease that requires dialysis (getting hooked up to a machine to filter blood when your kidneys can no longer do so). The body naturally creates bicarbonate to help maintain the correct acid-alkaline balance (or pH), and insufficient levels can cause problems ranging from minor all the way to death. A low bicarbonate level (the condition is called *metabolic acidosis*) affects 30% to 50% of advanced CKD patients, and doctors have long speculated that baking soda might help boost kidney function by bringing up the level.

In a study of 134 people with advanced CKD and low bicarbonate levels, Magdi Yaqoob, MD, a professor of renal medicine at The Royal London Hospital in England and his colleagues put this theory to the test. They gave half the participants a small daily dose of sodium bicarbonate in tablet form at mealtime while also continuing their regular medical care.

Over a two-year period, investigators discovered that people who took the sodium bicarbonate experienced...

•**A two-thirds drop in kidney decline.** They lost kidney function at the rate of just 1% per year, compared with 3% in those who didn't take sodium bicarbonate. Though these percentages sound tiny, they are quite significant for people losing kidney function.

•**A dramatic decrease in the need for dialysis.** Only 6.5% in the bicarbonate group required dialysis, compared with 33% in the untreated group.

•**Better nutrient absorption.** Nutritional parameters, including the ability to metabolize protein effectively, improved in those who took bicarbonate tablets. While sodium levels rose, blood pressure did not.

Sodium bicarbonate seems to help people with CKD by suppressing production of ammonia and *endothelin* (proteins that constrict blood vessels and raise blood pressure), which in turn discourages scarring and dysfunction in the kidneys, Dr. Yaqoob explains. These

findings were published in the *Journal of the American Society of Nephrology* (JASN). They require further validation in a larger, multicenter study but are very significant and encouraging, Dr. Yaqoob said.

ASK YOUR DOCTOR

If you have CKD, Dr. Yaqoob recommends asking your doctor about incorporating sodium bicarbonate into your medical care—but stresses this should not be attempted on your own. Though easily available and very helpful for particular people, sodium bicarbonate is not an innocuous substance. Dosage must be carefully calibrated to keep blood levels within normal limits. Excess can lead to milk alkali syndrome (calcium deposits in kidneys and other tissue), especially for kidney patients—but also in otherwise healthy people who consume excessive amounts.

That said, sodium bicarbonate may be a simple and inexpensive treatment to add to our medical arsenal against CKD. Talk to your doctor about it.

Mother Nature's Cures For Outdoor Injuries

Mark Blumenthal, founder and executive director, American Botanical Council, Austin, Texas.

Ahh, summer—the delicious season when you can spend many pleasurable hours out of doors...and get bug bites, sunburn, blisters, rashes and, if you love picnics, maybe even food poisoning! Fortunately, for every minor hazard that nature brings, Mother Nature also provides safe, natural treatments that soothe and heal. You can put together an herbal arsenal that will serve you throughout the warm months. To find out what substances we should all have on hand, we called Mark Blumenthal, founder and executive director of the American Botanical Council in Austin, Texas. *His natural first-aid kit...*

OLBAS OIL

Blumenthal's first pick happens to be a product I use all the time—Swiss-made Olbas Oil, an extract of the essential oils of six medicinal herbs (among them eucalyptus, peppermint and wintergreen plus menthol). It is immensely popular in Europe and useful for so many things that Blumenthal, who always carries it with him when he travels and in his backpack for outdoor activities, jokingly refers to it as "20-in-one oil." Olbas Oil squelches a mosquito bite itch in three to five minutes and reduces the pain and swelling of bee stings almost as fast. When applied to a bruise, it minimizes both its size and discoloration (especially if applied soon after the bruising injury), and it soothes and helps heal blisters. Olbas can be delightful as a massage oil (added to a more neutral oil, such as almond oil) to limber up muscles before sports and afterward to relieve stiff and sore muscles. And that's not all...Blumenthal says you can put one drop (but no more) of Olbas into a glass of water and drink to ease an upset stomach...or place a drop or two on a tissue tucked in your pillow case to open stuffy nasal passages for a better sleep. This refreshing remedy is available in many health-food stores and online (*www.olbas.com*).

ACTIVATED CHARCOAL

Though food poisoning can strike at any time of year, there are some particular hazards during the warmer months when we eat so many salads and fresh produce (which has become the most common source of food-borne illness) and when higher temperatures bring on spoilage more quickly. Blumenthal said that a helpful treatment for nausea and minor vomiting from suspected food poisoning is pharmaceutical-grade activated charcoal. It neutralizes the toxins in your system by absorbing them so that they're able to pass through without causing further discomfort. Seek immediate medical attention if symptoms persist for more than several hours, worsen or you have frequent vomiting or diarrhea, or if you experience dizziness, fainting or violent cramping. Activated charcoal is sold in tablet or capsule form at health-food stores—there's also a cherry-flavored liquid version that can be a wise medicine cabinet staple for homes

with small children. Follow dosing directions on the manufacturer's label.

GINGER CAPSULES

For milder stomach symptoms, try ginger capsules. These may be especially helpful for quelling nausea from motion sickness—whether from riding in a car, on a boat or even on a roller coaster. To keep nausea at bay, take two ginger capsules (500 mg each) 30 minutes before you start your journey, and they might even help if motion sickness has already started. Unlike with the drugs *dimenhydrinate* (Dramamine) or *meclizine hydrochloride* (Bonine, Antivert), which are antihistamines and induce sleepiness, you will remain alert with ginger.

WITCH HAZEL

Poison ivy, a common summer problem, has been the subject of considerable research to establish which botanicals might successfully treat its itch, pain and blisters. One remedy from way back when is worth a try—witch hazel, a clear liquid made from the flowering tree of the same name. It can be dabbed on with a cotton pad to help dry and heal the blisters and reduce itch and redness. Blumenthal notes that many American commercial witch hazel preparations contain a small amount of alcohol, which may also help healing.

HIBISCUS TEA

Heat can leave you feeling drained and uncomfortable, and in the tropics, says Blumenthal, people often drink chilled hibiscus tea to help themselves feel better. People have long believed that the tea lowers blood pressure, and modern medicine has verified this with several successful clinical studies, the most recent from Tufts University. Many believe that the tea also reduces body temperature, although Blumenthal says this has not been scientifically substantiated—but given how pleasant it is to enjoy a tall, cold glass of iced hibiscus tea on a hot day, it's certainly worth a try. You can find hibiscus tea in health-food and gourmet stores.

MULLEIN FLOWER OIL

Known for its antimicrobial and anti-inflammatory properties, mullein flower oil is a traditional treatment for swimmer's ear (*otitis externa*), a painful bacterial infection of the outer ear canal, Blumenthal says. Just drip a few drops into each ear and cover with a cotton ball inserted into the outer ear.

Caution: Do not do this if there is any possibility you have a perforated eardrum, symptoms of which include discharge (clear, bloody or pus), ear noise or buzzing, increasing pain or a sudden decrease in pain followed by discharge or hearing loss.

In fact, it's best to check with a doctor before you use this oil or any other substance in the ear to determine if it is safe and will be effective for you.

ALOE VERA

Blumenthal recommends one more all-purpose natural remedy—aloe vera, the succulent houseplant that has long been valued for its medicinal properties.

You may be surprised at how much scientific evidence backs up its use, in particular for soothing and healing skin problems such as sunburn and minor kitchen burns.

While the gel inside the leaves of the aloe plant (just cut one across the middle and squeeze) is 95% water, it contains trace amounts of vitamins (A, C, E and B), enzymes and minerals.

These make aloe a moisturizer, an anti-inflammatory, an antimicrobial and an analgesic (pain killer) to boot. That's a lot of bang for your buck—and speaking of that, you don't need to purchase any of the many drugstore products that contain aloe vera unless you'll be traveling.

Keep a plant in a sunny spot in your house (plant in sandy, well-drained soil and water only when very dry) and pick the mature leaves on the bottom of the plant for instant first-aid gel.

Generally speaking, these natural soothers are safe for almost everyone—but, as always, it is smart to check with your doctor before adding these and other remedies, natural and otherwise, to your personal first-aid kit.

This precaution is even more important for people with any type of chronic medical condition.

Healing Spices: Surprising New Discoveries

David Winston, RH, Washington, New Jersey–based registered herbalist and professional member of the American Herbalist Guild. He is author of several books, including *Adaptogens: Herbs for Strength, Stamina and Stress Relief* (Healing Arts).

Researchers have now identified new health benefits for several popular spices. You may recognize the names of these spices, but the latest studies suggest uses that are not widely known. *Intriguing research…*

CAYENNE PEPPER

•**Cholesterol.** Artery-clogging fatty buildups are created or worsened when cholesterol oxidizes, a biochemical process similar to metal rusting. Cayenne pepper (also known as chili pepper) contains a plaque-fighting antioxidant (capsaicin), which is also available in supplement form.

Recent research: When researchers asked 27 people to eat a diet that included cayenne-spiced chili or the same diet with no chili for one month, the spicy-chili group had much lower harmful cholesterol than those who did not eat chili. In addition to protecting cholesterol from oxidation, cayenne pepper also stimulates digestion and improves circulation—an important benefit for people with chronically cold hands and feet.

Recommendation: Use a cayenne-based hot sauce, to taste. Add it to a variety of foods, including chicken dishes and sandwiches.

Caution: In some people, cayenne causes digestive problems. If you experience stomach upset or anal irritation, use a milder hot sauce, cut back the amount or stop using it.

SAGE

•**Alzheimer's disease.** Herbalists and many doctors report that sage may help patients with mild to moderate Alzheimer's disease.

Recent research: Neurons of lab animals exposed to *amyloid beta* (the main constituent of harmful plaques in Alzheimer's) and sage leaves or *rosmarinic acid* (an active ingredient in sage) were less damaged than when the cells were exposed to amyloid beta alone. However, you cannot achieve this potential health benefit from the amount of sage used in cooking.

Recommendation: Drink sage tea.

What to do: Pour eight ounces of boiling water over a tea strainer or tea ball that contains one-half teaspoon of ground sage. Let sit for 15 to 20 minutes. Drink four ounces twice a day. (Refrigerate any unused portion and gently reheat before drinking.)

Alternative: Use sage tea bags. Or add 20 to 30 drops of sage tincture to one ounce of water—drink this amount three times daily.

ROSEMARY

• **Cancer.** Laboratory studies of human cells show that rosemary may help prevent certain types of cancer.

Recent research: The rate at which human leukemia and breast cancer cells multiplied in a laboratory study was reduced when researchers exposed the cells to rosemary extract. More research is needed to confirm these benefits in human study subjects, but rosemary extract is safe to use in the meantime. Cooking with rosemary does not provide this potential health benefit.

Recommendation: Drink rosemary tea.

What to do: Pour 12 ounces of boiling water over a tea strainer or tea ball that contains one-half teaspoon of rosemary. Let sit for 15 to 20 minutes. Drink four ounces, three times a day. (Refrigerate unused tea.)

Alternative: Use rosemary tea bags. Or add 40 to 60 drops of rosemary tincture to one ounce of water—drink this amount three times daily.

HOW TO USE SPICES

The active ingredients in spices can eventually deteriorate after processing. For example, the levels of antioxidants, known as carotenoids, in paprika drop by 75% after three months of storage.

Recommendation: Buy no more than a one-year supply of any spice you plan to use—and replace it annually. Keep your spices away from light, moisture and heat—for example, not near the oven. Consider buying whole rather than powdered spices, and grind them right before using, with a mortar and pestle or spice grinder. To tell whether a spice is rich in health-promoting compounds, smell and/or taste it—the richer the odor and flavor, the better the spice.

My Favorite Natural Treatments for Itching

Jamison Starbuck, ND, naturopathic physician in family practice in Missoula, Montana. She is past president of the American Association of Naturopathic Physicians and a contributing editor to *The Alternative Advisor: The Complete Guide to Natural Therapies and Alternative Treatments* (Time-Life).

The causes of itching are so varied that there is at least one associated with nearly every letter of the alphabet—starting with allergies, bug bites, contact dermatitis (from such things as soap or chlorine), drug reactions (antibiotics and painkillers are common culprits), eczema, fungus, gallbladder disease and hives. Exposure to poison ivy, oak or sumac is another common cause. Unfortunately, the instinctive desire to scratch an itch can exacerbate the underlying problem. Many people scratch their skin raw in an effort to get relief. *Natural medicines that gently—yet effectively—treat the most common causes of itching are much better options...*

• **Chamomile tea.** For itching due to insect bites, eczema, hives or poison ivy, oak or sumac, use two tea bags per 12 ounces of water and let it steep for six minutes. Soak sterile gauze or clean cotton cloth in the tea, and apply compresses for 15 minutes to the itchy area several times per day.

*Pregnant or lactating women should consult their physicians before trying herb-based products.

• **Calendula and comfrey salve.** These plants are common ingredients in topical salves that often include vitamins A and E in an olive oil base. This salve works best for dry, scaly rashes that result from contact dermatitis, fungus or eczema. For a moist, itchy rash with oozing clear or yellow fluid (such as that caused by insect bites or poison ivy, oak or sumac), use a tea or tincture preparation of calendula only. Apply the tea in a compress or pour or spray it on the area.

• **Oatmeal.** It is best for itching caused by hives or insect bites.

What to do: Fill a muslin or cotton bag with one cup of raw, rolled oats. Attach the bag to the spout of your bathtub and let the water flow through the bag as you fill a tub with warm (not hot) water. Lie in the oatmeal water for 20 to 30 minutes several times a day until the itch is gone. An oatmeal bath product, such as Aveeno, also can be used. For poison ivy, oak or sumac, use a compress of the oatmeal water.

• ***Grindelia ssp*** (gumweed). This is my favorite remedy for itching caused by poison ivy, oak or sumac. Wash the plant oil from the skin with soap and water, then apply a lotion or tincture of grindelia three times daily for several days.

• **White vinegar.** Itching caused by sunburn, bug bites or yeast responds well to white vinegar. Dilute vinegar with an equal amount of water and test a small area first to make sure the vinegar solution does not sting. Dab it on the skin or apply it with a compress. If tolerated, the diluted vinegar can be applied to itchy areas several times a day.

• **Water.** It's surprising how often simply drinking one-half ounce of water per pound of body weight daily can heal troublesome dry, itchy skin, which can result from inadequate hydration.

If itching is accompanied by a fever or if you notice skin discoloration or red or purple streaking near a bite, or if you have confused your medications, are urinating frequently, are having shortness of breath or are in significant pain, see your doctor. These could be signs of an infection, a reaction to medication or a medication overdose

Home Remedy For Insomnia

The Wilen sisters have been using home remedies all their lives, and for the last quarter of a century, they've been researching and writing about them as well.

The Wilens share their remedy for insomnia.

INSOMNIA

Our new best friends are nuts—in this case, walnuts. They're rich in serotonin, the brain chemical that calms anxiety and allows us to turn off the pressures of the day to get a good night's sleep. Eat a palmful (one ounce) of raw walnuts before going to bed. It's important to chew each mouthful thoroughly, until the nut pieces are ground down.

Lydia Wilen and Joan Wilen, folk-remedy experts based in New York City. The sisters are coauthors of many books, including Bottom Line's Healing Remedies: Over 1,000 Astounding Ways to Heal Arthritis, Asthma, High Blood Pressure, Varicose Veins, Warts and More! *(Bottom Line Books).* www.bottomlinepublications.com

Nature's Remedies for Sunburn and Bug Bites

Jamison Starbuck, ND, naturopathic physician in family practice in Missoula, Montana. She is past president of the American Association of Naturopathic Physicians and a contributing editor to The Alternative Advisor: The Complete Guide to Natural Therapies and Alternative Treatments *(Time-Life).*

If you're tired of using the same old products to prevent or treat sunburn, bug bites and other summertime skin problems, there are a number of natural remedies that I've found to be effective in my clinical practice.

My favorite natural remedies for...

• **Sunburn protection.** Beta-carotene is a naturally occurring pigmented compound that helps guard against sunburn—perhaps due to its powerful antioxidant properties. To prevent sunburn, supplement your sunscreen use by loading up on beta-carotene–rich foods. (This nutrient also improves general immunity, so it makes sense to eat these foods year-round.)

Best food sources of beta-carotene: Most orange-colored vegetables and fruits (such as carrots, sweet potatoes, mangos, cantaloupe and apricots)…and green veggies (such as broccoli, spinach and kale). Adults with fair, sun-sensitive skin may also reduce sunburn risk by taking a beta-carotene supplement (50,000 international units daily) June through September in North America.

Note: Some research has suggested that this dose of beta-carotene may be harmful to smokers. If you smoke, consult your doctor before taking beta-carotene. Even though beta-carotene helps protect against sunburn, you still need to wear sunscreen (check a natural-foods grocery store for a chemical-free product). The combination provides even more protection than when either is used alone.

●**Sunburn relief.** If you do get a sunburn, calendula is an herb that may help soothe burned skin, reduce pain and speed healing. Calendula flowers (used to make a soothing tea) and calendula tincture and lotion are readily available wherever botanical medicines are sold. The flowers also can be easily grown in home gardens (most nurseries stock both plant starts and seeds). Use one tablespoon of fresh flowers or two teaspoons of dried flowers per cup of water for tea. Put calendula tea, tincture or lotion directly on sunburned skin three times daily until symptoms improve. You can splash the tea or tincture on your skin or dab it on with cotton balls.

Caution: Do not use calendula if you are allergic to plants in the daisy family.

●**Bee stings.** A homeopathic remedy made from the honeybee, Apis 30C reduces swelling and pain. Take two pellets (under the tongue) twice daily for one to three days.

Caution: Do not take Apis if you are allergic to bees. You can also use calendula tea, tincture or ointment topically for relief.

●**Insect bites.** Homeopathic Lachesis 30C relieves the pain of swollen, tender insect bites, such as those caused by green bottle flies and house flies. The typical dose is two pellets (under the tongue) twice daily for one to three days. Echinacea (a well-known cold and flu preventive) in tincture form can be applied directly on any insect bite, including one caused by a mosquito, to reduce inflammation and soothe irritation. Apply as needed.

Caution: Do not use echinacea if you are allergic to plants in the daisy family.

Anti-Wrinkle Foods

When dietary data for 4,025 women was analyzed in a recent study, those with high intakes of vitamin C and the essential fatty acid *linoleic acid* had fewer wrinkles than women with lower intakes.

Theory: Vitamin C is an important component in collagen synthesis (which keeps skin supple), and *linoleic acid* promotes normal skin structure.

For younger-looking skin: Eat vitamin Crich fruits and vegetables, such as oranges and broccoli, and foods high in linoleic acid, such as soybeans and sunflower oil.

Maeve C. Cosgrove, PhD, research scientist, Corporate Research, Unilever Colworth Science Park, Bedford, UK.

Spice Up Your Health With Everyday Seasonings

Jonny Bowden, certified nutrition specialist and author of *The 150 Healthiest Foods on Earth* (Fair Winds) and *The Most Effective Natural Cures in the World* (Fair Winds). His free audio course on 7 SuperFoods is available at *www.jonnybowden.com.*

Cinnamon is so good for you it can almost be considered a health food—simple, ordinary, pumpkin-pie flavoring cinnamon, the same stuff they now have in shakers at Starbucks. Its exciting to see the increasing focus of research on the health benefits of everyday spices like this—capsaicin for prostate cancer...turmeric to reduce inflammation...ginger for nausea, to name just a few. A recent *Wall Street Journal* article reported how several plants abundant in China are being studied as a potential source of medicines by drug company Novartis AG. Its no surprise. Herbs and spices, derived from various plants, have a long history of medicinal use in Chinese medicine. So what else is there in the spice rack that we can use to healthify our meals in a delicious way?

Everyday spices are an amazing source of phytochemicals, which are plant compounds with extraordinary healing properties, explained Jonny Bowden, author of *The 150 Healthiest Foods on Earth* (Fair Winds). Many of these spices have been used in traditional medicine for hundreds of years, and Western medicine is just beginning to realize their potential. *Here are a few of Bowden's top picks for powering up your foods...*

CINNAMON

Lets take another look at cinnamon, for example. There are anti-inflammatory compounds in cinnamon that can be helpful in alleviating pain, stiffness and even menstrual discomfort, said Bowden. Additionally, compounds in cinnamon increase the ability of the cells to take in sugar, which is how it effectively lowers blood sugar and reduces the need for higher levels of insulin. A study published in *Diabetes Care* showed that cinnamon lowered not only blood sugar, but also triglycerides, total cholesterol and LDL (bad) cholesterol in people with type 2 diabetes. Though its not always the case with our other plant-based remedies, with cinnamon the inexpensive supermarket variety is basically as good as any of the pricier oils and extracts sold in specialty stores.

GINGER

Then there is ginger, known as the "universal medicine" in Ayurvedic medicine. Ginger can be used to soothe an upset stomach and quell nausea. In fact, in one study on ginger root, it was shown to be as effective as Dramamine in holding seasickness at bay. Ginger also packs plenty of powerful antioxidants, Bowden told me. "And animal studies show that ginger has antimicrobial effects and helps boost the immune system as well."

TURMERIC

Turmeric—the spice Bowden was most enthusiastic about—is a member of the ginger family, and also a heavy hitter in health benefits. "It's as close to a magical substance as you're likely to find in the kitchen cupboard," he told me. He attributes this spice's anti-inflammatory properties to "curcumin," which is also responsible for making Indian food and curry dishes yellow. In India, turmeric is used to treat arthritis precisely because of its ability to lower inflammation, Bowden said, noting that research indicates that curcumin also may have an anti-tumor effect. If you're not an Indian food eater, you can try it in rice dishes or even on eggs. Do not use medicinal amounts of turmeric during pregnancy, though, because it stimulates contraction of the uterus.

OREGANO

Another spice touted for its health properties is oregano, which Bowden tells me "has been shown by research to have 42 times more antioxidant activity than apples and 12 times more than oranges." Oregano contains a powerful cancer-fighting compound called *rosmarinic acid* as well, and its anti-inflammatory properties make it useful in supporting joint function. Oregano is also a source of calcium, magnesium, zinc, iron and potassium.

GARLIC

Of course garlic is not always used as a spice, but it does have a well-deserved reputation for adding flavor and boosting health. One of the oldest medicinal foods we know of, it is recognized even by conservative mainstream medical professionals as being helpful in reducing cholesterol. Bowden cited a study that found garlic reduces triglycerides by up to 17%. It has a small but notably positive effect on blood pressure. "In places where the consumption of garlic is high, theres a decreased risk of stomach and colon cancer," Bowden added.

Some other spices that have health-promoting properties include...

350

• **Cardamom.** Another member of the ginger family, cardamom is in spiced chai tea and used to flavor Turkish coffee, and is added to baked goods in Scandinavia. It stimulates digestion and flow of bile.

• **Mustard seeds.** These are a source of magnesium and selenium, and can be taken orally to stimulate appetite and circulation, and to help neutralize inflammatory materials in the GI tract.

• **Parsley.** A good source of vitamin K and potassium, and also helpful for detoxification.

• **Rosemary.** Contains lots of antioxidants and anti-inflammatory compounds, plus substances that help prevent the premature breakdown of *acetylcholine*, a neurotransmitter thats vital for memory and healthy brain function.

• **Sage.** Contains rosmarinic acid (like oregano), which is both an antioxidant and an anti-inflammatory, along with *thujone*, which can be protective against salmonella and candida.

• **Thyme.** Helps relieve chest and respiratory problems, including coughs and bronchitis.

MORE THAN A PINCH?

Since many of the research studies on these items used high doses of them, we asked Bowden how much of each is needed to make a difference. The answer varies, he said, but usually more than is typically used for seasoning is required to achieve a notable benefit—though it seems logical that adding a variety of spices, more often and in plentiful amounts, would have a cumulative positive effect. Though some of the dried spices retain their healthful properties, usually fresh herbs are nutritionally superior—not to mention delicious, and fun and easy to grow.

One thing that is especially nice about Bowden's recommendations is the fact that all of these spices are common flavors you can add to all sorts of foods—they're easy to find and don't require a refined palate to enjoy. So go ahead and spice up your menu—your food will taste more interesting and you'll feel better, too.

28

'Slightly Crazy' Cures

Chewing Gum Makes You Smarter

We all know to eat a healthy diet, but some brain-boosting foods may very well surprise you...

BRAIN BOOSTERS

• **Chewing gum.** OK, it's not exactly a food, but it's more than just something to keep your mouth occupied. Researchers at Northwestern University found that people who chew gum have increased blood flow to the brain—and a corresponding increase in cognitive performance. People who chew gum also report a reduction in stress, which protects brain cells from stress-related hormones.

Recommended: Chew gum when you are stressed or have challenging mental work to do. Opt for sugarless.

• **Frozen berries.** Raspberries, blueberries and strawberries are among the best sources of brain-protecting antioxidants. Researchers at the USDA Jean Mayer Human Nutrition Research Center on Aging at Tufts University found that animals given blueberries showed virtually no evidence in the brain of the cell-damaging effects of free radicals—and they did better on cognitive tests.

Frozen berries typically contain more antioxidants than fresh berries because they're picked and processed at the peak of ripeness.

Recommended: One-and-a-half cups of frozen or fresh berries at least two to three times a week. Darker berries contain the most antioxidants.

• **Turmeric.** It's one of the most potent anti-inflammatory spices. People who eat turmeric several times a week can have significant drops in C-reactive protein, a substance that

---

David Grotto, RD, LDN, registered dietitian and founder and president of Nutrition Housecall, LLC, a consulting firm that provides nutrition communications, lecturing and consulting services along with personalized, at-home dietary services, Chicago. He is advisory board chair for the Produce for Kids and PBS Kids health initiatives and author of *101 Optimal Life Foods* (Bantam).

indicates inflammation in the brain and other tissues.

A study that looked at more than 1,000 participants (average age 68.9) found that those who often or occasionally ate turmeric performed better on mental-status evaluations than those who rarely or never ate it.

Recommended: Add at least one-quarter teaspoon of turmeric to recipes several times a week. (Turmeric is one of the spices in curry.)

•**Hazelnuts.** These contain the highest concentration of folate of all the tree nuts (including walnuts, almonds and pecans). Low levels of folate have been associated with poor cognition and depression. Other foods rich in folate include spinach, beans, oranges, avocados and wheat germ.

Recommended: A handful of hazelnuts several times a week.

•**Cilantro.** This herb, also known as coriander and Chinese parsley, has long been used in Iranian folk medicine for stress relief. Stress has been linked to a speeding up of the aging process of the brain. Modern research also has revealed the benefits of cilantro—an animal study demonstrated that cilantro eased stress.

Recommended: One tablespoon of fresh cilantro several times a week. It's often used in salsa and guacamole and to top tacos, chili, stews and soups.

THREE "GOOD" VICES

You may have heard that certain "bad foods," such as coffee, red wine and chocolate, are good for the heart. *They also are good for the brain...*

•**Coffee.** A Finnish study of more than 1,400 participants found that regular coffee drinkers were less likely to develop dementia than those who didn't drink coffee. Those who drank moderate amounts of coffee in midlife (three to five cups daily) had the lowest risk, probably because the antioxidants in coffee inhibit age-related brain damage.

The caffeine in coffee—a five-ounce serving of coffee typically contains 30 milligrams (mg) to 150 mg, depending on how it is prepared—also improves mental abilities. Studies of university students have shown that when students drink coffee before a test, they score higher than when they abstain.

Recommended: One to three cups daily. If coffee gives you the jitters, try green tea, which also is good for the brain but has slightly less caffeine.

•**Red wine.** Red wine contains resveratrol, a polyphenol, that helps prevent inflammation and oxidation of brain tissue. People who drink moderate amounts of red wine have lower risks for stroke and dementia. Laboratory studies indicate that red wine can reduce the accumulation of *beta-amyloid*, the substance found in the brains of Alzheimer's patients. (In a healthy brain, beta-amyloid is broken down and eliminated.) White wine also contains polyphenols but in lower concentrations than reds.

Recommended: Up to two glasses of wine daily for men and one glass daily for women. Moderation is important because too much alcohol has been linked to increased risk for dementia.

Alcohol-free option: Concord grape juice. Some studies suggest that it may be just as healthy as red wine when it comes to improvement in cognitive skills. Aim for one cup a day.

•**Chocolate.** The cocoa flavonols in chocolate inhibit free radicals. Flavonols also relax the linings of blood vessels. This helps reduce high blood pressure, a leading cause of dementia.

One study, conducted at Brigham and Women's Hospital in Boston, found that participants who drank one cup of high-flavonol cocoa daily had, after two weeks, an average increase in brain circulation of about one-third.

Chocolates with a high percentage of cocoa don't necessarily have a high concentration of flavonols—processing techniques can destroy the protective compounds.

Recommended: Look for products that advertise a high flavonol content on the label (60% to 85%). One ounce is enough to get the benefits without unnecessary sugar and calories.

DON'T FORGET FISH

You probably have heard that fish is "brain food," but we couldn't do a brain-boosting article without mentioning it. A study of 3,660

353

adults age 65 and older found that those who ate omega-3–rich fish three times a week or more were 25% less likely to have silent *infarcts*, blockages in blood vessels that can cause dementia.

Ancient Healing Secrets From Tibet

Phuntsog Wangmo, TMD, director of the Shang Shung Institute's Traditional Tibetan Medicine Program, Conway, Massachusetts.

Global medical traditions offer different perspectives for understanding health —such as the importance of the seasonal cycle in Ayurvedic Medicine from India or the Traditional Chinese Medicine emphasis on balance. An ancient healing tradition that is not as widely known as those is Tibetan Medicine, which is very "of the moment" with its connection to the five elements—earth, water, fire, wind and space.

To find out more about this ancient form of healing, we called Phuntsog Wangmo, TMD, president of the American Tibetan Medical Association and director of the Shang Shung Institute's Traditional Tibetan Medicine Program in Conway, Massachusetts. She explains that at the core of Tibetan Medicine is the concept that the body, spirit and mind are interconnected and that illness results from an imbalance among them. Also relevant is their interaction with the external environment.

ELEMENTS & HUMORS

The central concept is that there are five elements that exist in the world and our bodies, which directly affect health—earth, water, fire, wind and space. Each corresponds to a body system, for instance, water relates to the body's fluids...fire is expressed in its metabolic functions...wind is involved in all types of circulation...earth corresponds to the stable body parts, including bones and muscle...while space has to do with the body's cavities.

Additionally, there are three systems, called *humors* that control body processes:

• **Wind**—circulation and nervous system impulses. Balance is characterized by mental focus, ease of movement and efficient elimination of impurities. An imbalance can cause symptoms such as anxiety, insomnia and mental instability.

• **Bile**—energy and digestion. In balance, bile brings determination and proper digestion as evidenced by a glowing complexion. Fevers, sharp pain and headaches can indicate an imbalance of bile, which ultimately may lead to anger, aggression and hatred.

• **Phlegm**—or the body's fluids, bring good judgment and a sense of calm. Symptoms of imbalance can include loss of appetite, nausea, depression and laziness.

No single element or humor is more important than another, notes Wangmo, emphasizing that it is the totality of the elements and humors, how they come together and how they are balanced or imbalanced in an individual that is the essence of understanding Tibetan Medicine. Imbalance is usually caused by disruptions, internally and externally.

WHAT HAPPENS AT A VISIT?

The initial visit always begins with an in-depth interview to help the practitioner find what your imbalances and disturbances may be. Usually these are rooted in incorrect diet, unsuitable behavior and/or general unhealthy lifestyle. Next, a Tibetan medical practitioner looks at the interplay between environmental factors, your body and mind, and where illness and mental distress may result. If you have headaches, for example, the practitioner may ask you to describe the nature of your pain...then will ask about a host of possible contributing factors such as time of onset... when, what and how much you ate before it, and also how your body responded to the meal...your mood...and the emotional tenor of the day. Gathering these details helps in understanding and treating the unique "whole" of you, Wangmo explained.

Next comes a simple in-office urinalysis, with the practitioner observing the color, odor and, after vigorously shaking the sample, the sediments and number, size and persistence of

354

bubbles in the urine. He or she then evaluates the 12 organ positions of the pulse. The purpose is to measure pulse strength, speed and quality, all of which helps define and locate the illness. The exam concludes with a check of the color and coating on your tongue and eyes.

TREATING THE ILLS

The first step in treatment is addressing diet and behavior factors. Due to our overscheduled lives, Wangmo says that many Westerners have imbalances in the wind (often resulting in mental imbalance) and fire (leading to lots of digestive issues). To help correct mind issues, she might suggest adding ginger, garlic, leafy greens and pomegranate to the diet, as well as warm, heavier foods such as lamb. For digestive problems, her suggestions would tend toward light foods. She tempers her dietary advice according to the season, the patient's personality and age and where the patient lives —people in cold climates might be advised to use warming spices, for example.

With regard to lifestyle, she observes that our Western tendency to worry and overcommit causes yet more imbalances in, once again, the wind humor. And so in addition to dietary changes, Wangmo teaches relaxation methods—for instance, a variety of breathing techniques. To balance the elements, she guides patients with specific suggestions about breathing such as to picture certain colors while inhaling and others while exhaling. Other techniques include meditations geared to the specific nature of problems, counseling, and working with patients to restructure daily habits, including exercise, sleeping schedules, food selection and timing of meals.

Often the combination of changing diet and lifestyle is sufficient to resolve patients' problems. When it is not, though, practitioners of Tibetan Medicine next turn to some of the huge number of herbs, minerals and animal substances available to them, and again individualize a combination to your needs. They may also add a variety of physical techniques as well—acupuncture, massage, cupping (applying a container with heat inside to create a vacuum effect to draw out harmful fluids) and moxibustion (applying a heated herb to certain points in the body).

HOW TO FIND A TIBETAN MEDICAL PRACTITIONER

At this time there are only a few people practicing Tibetan Medicine in this country—Wangmo estimates around 50.

However the Institute that she heads has a four-year medical school and is graduating its first class—of seven mostly American students—in 2009. The only other major schools are in India and Tibet.

No licensing yet exists, but the American Tibetan Medical Association (ATMA) is working toward that goal.

In the meantime, if you want to consult with a practitioner trained in Tibetan Medicine, visit the Shang Shung Institute

Web site: *www.shangshung.org/home/school.html*. There are a number of other Web sites that also list practitioners in the US, including *www.dharma-haven.org/tibetan/medicine-clinics.htm*.

Treatment under Tibetan Medicine may be highly individualized, but the practice has a message for everyone.

Balancing our bodies, our minds and our spirits with the environment helps to maintain excellent emotional, mental and physical health.

Chuckle for Cardio

Laughter yoga combines traditional yoga stretches and poses with exercise designed to make people laugh.

In terms of cardiovascular benefits, one minute of laughter (about 100 giggles) is the equivalent of six to 10 minutes on a rowing machine.

Laughter has aerobic benefits and can help lower blood pressure, lift mood and boost immunity.

For more information, call 212-956-5920 or go to *www.laughteryoga.org*.

Alex M. Eingorn, DC, laughter-yoga instructor and director, Better Health Chiropractic, New York City.

10 Surprising Ways To Stay Healthy and Control Your Weight

Mehmet C. Oz, MD, medical director of the Integrative Medicine Program and former director of the Cardiovascular Institute at New York–Presbyterian Medical Center and professor and former vice chairman of surgery at Columbia University, both in New York City. He is coauthor, with Michael F. Roizen, MD, of *You on a Diet: The Owner's Manual for Waist Management* (Free Press).

Whether you're trying to lose weight or simply find a healthful eating plan you can stick with, you are bound to fail if you try to stay on a diet. Invariably, people on diets end up depriving themselves of certain foods and/or scrupulously counting calories.

Problem: Virtually no one can maintain long-term deprivation because our bodies are programmed to avoid this type of ongoing discomfort. And calorie restriction causes your metabolism to slow down in order to preserve energy, often resulting in more stored fat.

The secret is to work with your body's chemistry rather than against it, so healthful eating becomes automatic, not forced.

Recent development: Body weight used to be considered one of the best indicators of overall health.

Now: Research has shown that your waist measurement (at or just below your navel) may be more reliable. That's because abdominal fat is especially harmful due to its proximity to your vital organs, where it can lead to harmful increases in cholesterol and triglyceride levels. Fat in this area has been linked to heart disease, cancer and diabetes. Studies have found that men should strive for a waist measurement of 35 inches or less, while women should aim for 32½ inches or less. When these measurements are exceeded, health risks increase. For example, risk for metabolic syndrome (a group of conditions, including hypertension and abdominal obesity, that raises diabetes and cardiovascular disease risk) increases by

40% at 40 inches for men and 37 inches for women.

Important: Even if your weight is ideal, you still can benefit from some of the strategies described below because they promote healthy cholesterol and blood pressure levels. *My recommendations…*

1. Spice up your morning eggs. Cayenne and other forms of red pepper contain capsaicin, a substance that suppresses appetite signals, increases metabolism and decreases the desire for food later in the day. In addition, eggs are high in protein, which tends to induce feelings of fullness.

2. Consume fiber early in the day. Fiber increases levels of appetite-suppressing signals in the small intestine. Eating fiber early in the day makes people less hungry in the afternoon—the time when most of us tend to eat snacks and other calorie-dense foods. Consume about 30 g of fiber daily in the form of high-fiber cereals, fruits and vegetables, and 100% whole grains.

3. Eat nuts. The monounsaturated fat in nuts stimulates the production of *cholecystokinin* (CCK), a chemical messenger that slows the rate at which the stomach empties and reduces appetite without putting your body into starvation mode—that is, the point at which it starts conserving calories, rather than burning them. Before lunch and/or dinner, have about six walnuts, 12 almonds or 12 hazelnuts.

4. Drink coffee instead of soft drinks. Coffee (caffeinated and decaffeinated) is a rich source of antioxidants, and Americans consume more of it than any other antioxidant-rich food. Coffee is much lower in calories (if you don't add a lot of sugar and/or creamer) than sugary soft drinks.

Bonus: Caffeine stimulates the release of *norepinephrine*, a hormone that suppresses appetite and promotes calorie burning by increasing heart rate and metabolism. Green tea also is a rich source of antioxidants as well as caffeine.

5. Supplement with *5-hydroxytryptophan* (5-HTP). Related to the amino acid tryptophan and sold as a weight-loss supplement, 5-HTP increases brain levels of serotonin, a neurotransmitter that controls appetite. In one study, people taking 5-HTP for six weeks lost an average of 12 pounds, compared with only four pounds in a control group. Recommended dose: 300 mg daily. Bonus: 5-HTP has mood-enhancing benefits.

6. Turn up the thermostat. One reason that people tend to eat more during the cold months is that cold temperatures stimulate appetite. Also, people with naturally low body temperatures tend to have a slower metabolism and are more prone to weight gain. Staying warm may be a natural form of appetite control, particularly if you increase body temperature with exercise. Every one degree increase in body temperature increases metabolism by 14%.

7. Ask your doctor about Tagamet. The active ingredient (*cimetidine*) in this heartburn drug is thought to activate appetite-suppressing CCK. One 12-week study found that people taking a prescription form of Tagamet (400 mg, three times daily) had about a 5% decrease in waist size.

Important: Tagamet is unlikely to cause significant side effects, but should be taken to aid weight loss only if you have heartburn symptoms.

8. Consider using nicotine. It's common for people who quit smoking to gain weight, probably because the nicotine in tobacco suppresses appetite, increases metabolism and damages taste buds, which makes food less appealing. Studies have shown that nicotine—in the form of patches and gum, not from cigarettes—when combined with small amounts of caffeine, can help some people lose weight.

If you've hit a weight plateau: Talk to your doctor about combining a nicotine patch with two cups of coffee daily. Even for non-smokers, this approach can be used temporarily (to avoid possible addiction risk) to jump-start weight-loss efforts.

9. Smell grapefruit. Grapefruit oil, available from aromatherapy shops, emits an aroma that is thought to affect liver enzymes and help promote weight loss. In preliminary research, animals exposed to grapefruit scent for 15 minutes, three times weekly, had a reduction in appetite and body weight.

10. Control emotional stress. People who live with chronic stress (due to family pressures, a fast-paced job, etc.) produce high levels of *cortisol*, a stress hormone that increases the propensity for the omentum—a structure located near the stomach—to store fat. Excessive fat in the omentum can significantly increase waist size.

Important: Exercise is among the best ways to lower stress—and curb accumulations of omentum fat.

Recommended: A 30-minute walk and five minutes' worth of stretching daily...and three weekly sessions that include basic exercises, such as push-ups, shoulder shrugs, abdominal crunches, etc.

Enjoy Life, Live Longer

Michael F. Roizen, MD, chief wellness officer and chairman of the Wellness Institute, both at Cleveland Clinic in Cleveland, Ohio. He is coauthor, with Mehmet C. Oz, MD, of several books, including *You: Staying Young* (Free Press).

Many of the proven strategies for living longer—such as restricting calories and exercising on a regular basis—can feel like punishment for some people. Fortunately, there are many enjoyable ways to stay healthy—but doctors don't recommend these strategies as often as they should. Research has shown that activities nearly everyone enjoys can literally add years to a person's life.

FUN-FILLED WAYS TO LIVE LONGER

1. Enjoy Your Coffee. Many people assume that coffee—unlike green tea, for example—isn't a healthful beverage. But that's not true. Studies have found that caffeinated and decaffeinated coffee are a main source of antioxidants in the average American's diet.

Research has shown that caffeinated coffee decreases the risk for Parkinson's and

Alzheimer's diseases by 30% to 40%—health benefits that are largely attributed to the beverage's caffeine. (Decaffeinated coffee does not offer these same benefits.) The caffeine in coffee also is good for cognitive health.

Important: Caffeinated coffee may cause several side effects, such as blood pressure spikes, abnormal heartbeat, anxiety and gastric upset.

My recommendation: If you do not experience any of these side effects, and you enjoy drinking coffee, have as many cups of caffeinated coffee as you like. If you do experience side effects, you may prefer to drink decaffeinated coffee. Even though it does not have the health benefits previously described, studies show that decaffeinated coffee may help fight off type 2 diabetes.

2. Go Dancing. Men and women who get optimal amounts of physical activity—about 30 minutes a day, seven days a week—can make their "RealAges" (the "biological ages" of their bodies, based on lifestyle and behaviors) 6.4 years younger.

Many types of dancing give a superb physical workout. Ballroom and square dancing are particularly good for cognitive health. They involve both physical and mental stimulation (in order to execute the appropriate dance steps) and may help reduce the risk for dementia. Aim to dance at least 30 minutes a day.

Photos for Pain Relief?

Naomi Eisenberger, PhD, assistant professor of psychology, director of the Social and Affective Neuroscience Laboratory, as well as co-director of the Social Cognitive Neuroscience Laboratory, University of California at Los Angeles.

We all take comfort from the presence of a loved one during tough times—and here is a way to tap into those feelings even if that person isn't able to be physically present. Researchers have found that bringing a picture of a loved one to a medical procedure can help make it less painful—literally.

Naomi Eisenberger, PhD, assistant professor of psychology, director of the Social and Affective Neuroscience Laboratory, at University of California, Los Angeles, led a team exploring how social support can help people cope with physical pain.

Twenty-five female undergraduate students were recently recruited to participate in a study that they were told would "explore how people respond to comforting and uncomfortable stimuli."

The study required participants to bring a loved one to the one-hour session.

To produce the "uncomfortable stimuli," researchers placed a probe onto each participant's forearm. It could be heated to a temperature high enough to cause pain but not high enough to create a burn.

As the probe heated up, each subject was asked to rate the level of pain on a scale of 0 to 20. There were six different scenarios tested for each participant: holding the hand of her loved one...holding a stranger's hand...holding a "stress ball" to squeeze to release tension... gazing at a computer screen on which was displayed a photo of the loved one...a photo of a stranger...or a photo of a chair.

Predictably enough, participants felt less pain while holding the hands of their loved ones compared with when they held either a stranger's hand or the stress ball.

But it also turned out that simply looking at a loved one's photo greatly reduced pain—in fact, more effectively even than holding the loved one's hand.

So this is easy advice you can put to use right away—carry a photo of your partner, family or a friend (or all of them!) with you to look at when something hurts.

You can do this for others, too—if you can't be with someone you love who is sick or having a medical procedure, send a photo and explain why you think it will help—chances are, it will.

Intestinal Worms May Help Your Health

Joel V. Weinstock, MD, professor, immunology, Tufts University School of Medicine, and chief, division of Gastroenterology/Hepatology at Tufts New England Medical Center, Boston, Massachusetts.

Are we too clean for our health? That's the theory behind a surprising (and growing) area of research. Doctors and scientists are exploring the use of *helminths*—more typically known as parasitic intestinal worms—to treat a range of ailments, from inflammatory bowel diseases like Crohn's disease and ulcerative colitis to severe seasonal allergies and asthma to neurological disorders, including multiple sclerosis and even autism.

The thinking is this: Throughout history and in the normal course of our lives, humans have had lots of contact with creepy critters like helminths—in fact, to the point that some helminths are exclusive to humans, meaning that they grow and reproduce only in our systems. However, we've gotten much cleaner these days—with our indoor plumbing, antimicrobial cleansers, frequent laundering and bathing and, in many areas, less exposure to farm animals. This means we now share our homes (and bodies) with far fewer of these tiny, unseen creatures. Meanwhile the same time line has brought an increase in the incidence of inflammatory bowel diseases, asthma, seasonal allergies and the like—problems related to an overreactive immune system. Interestingly, these diseases are still uncommon in countries that don't have hygiene standards similar to ours.

THE HIDDEN CONNECTION

Could there be a connection? Scientists are exploring the possibility that helminths play a role in the healthy human immune system—and it appears that there may be some merit to this odd (and frankly unpalatable) theory.

We asked Joel Weinstock, MD, a professor of immunology at Tufts University School of Medicine in Boston and a leading expert on this topic, to tell us about the latest research. He told us that we should all be aware that there are two major functions of the immune system, noting that most people are familiar with just one—the "fight and kill" response. "But what would happen if you got an infection in your arm and your immune system didn't know when to turn off? That generally doesn't happen because the immune system's regulatory aspect kicks in," he explained. According to Dr. Weinstock, this self-regulating aspect is what gets out of whack in people with conditions like inflammatory bowel disease, in which the mucosal immune system perceives organisms in the gut as much more dangerous than they are—and then attacks them. This same premise also applies to other immune system-related problems, such as asthma, allergies and the like.

Where do the worms come in? Helminths can help regulate an overreactive immune system, Dr. Weinstock explained. Some of his group's early research appears to support this theory, at least in the case of inflammatory bowel diseases: A randomized controlled trial using *Trichuris suis* (pig whipworm) therapy for ulcerative colitis found an improvement in symptoms in 43.3% of those receiving the whipworm treatment, as opposed to 16.7% given the placebo. A similar study for the treatment of Crohn's disease showed similar results. In fact, Dr. Weinstock told us that those studies showed so much promise that helminth therapy is now being studied for other conditions—including a clinical trial that's going to explore using helminths in patients with multiple sclerosis. (Meanwhile, another recently completed trial found that whipworm was ineffective as a treatment for pollen-induced allergic rhinitis, so don't be surmising that this particular organism works for everything!)

WHAT'S NOT SO GREAT

Apart from the "ick factor," there are valid concerns about the growing interest in helminth therapy—most particularly that some unscrupulous human opportunists are worming their way onto the market to peddle parasites that could, in fact, turn out to be quite dangerous. Though he is optimistic about the potential of helminth therapy, Dr. Weinstock points out that an FDA-approved helminth-based treatment is still years away at best… but, because these parasites occur naturally in the wild, some enterprising individuals are already selling them to the public. This could bring more harm to patients who are already vulnerable and suffering, not to mention to the reputation of this promising therapy.

"These products are not monitored or approved by the FDA," Dr. Weinstock says. Many parasites look enough like each other that only a scientist can distinguish among different strains and species, so there is no way for a consumer looking at a Web site hawking parasites to know what is actually delivered. "It could be salt or sugar—or worse, you could end up with a treatment that is worse than the disease—because some parasites (unlike pig whipworm, which is relatively harmless) can be very harmful," he points out. With no oversight and no certification or standards, there is no way to know that what you're buying is safe, let alone effective against a particular complaint.

If you are a person who does happen to have inflammatory bowel disease or another of the immune-related diseases for which this therapy might be helpful, is there any safe, reliable way to try parasite therapy? *Dr. Weinstock offered these important cautions…*

•**Don't go it alone.** "This applies to any alternative approach," he says. "You want to have an expert in the disease work with you to make sure that you don't do any harm." This is a situation where it is a good idea to enlist a physician who specializes in your disease and can help guide the therapy.

Try established, proven therapies first. Before trying helminths, make sure that you and your physician have considered all the conventional therapies, since these less controversial treatments have been proven beneficial for many and are far more straightforward, at least at this point in time.

•**Look for clinical trials.** If you are interested in going forward, the best place to find opportunities to do so safely is to explore clinical trials and studies, most of which are announced through the nonprofit societies that support disease research, such as the National

Multiple Sclerosis Society. You can also find them at *www.clinicaltrials.gov*. Another resource for information and research is the site of the manufacturer of the whipworm used in the earlier studies, *www.ovamed.org*.

This ancient "medicine" may someday become conventional again, but it's not to be undertaken casually—stick with resources you know to be clean and safe, "above ground" in every sense of the term.

3-Second Energy Boost

Patt Lind-Kyle, MA, PhD, psychotherapist and executive coach based in Nevada City, California, and author of *Heal Your Mind, Rewire Your Brain* (Energy Psychology Press).

Yawning is something we mostly stifle—after all, it's embarrassing to yawn in the face of another as if to announce that you didn't get enough sleep or, worse, that you're bored. That's a shame—because researchers have discovered that the humble yawn is a major contributor to mental alertness…keeps our brains properly cooled (literally)…and helps us to shift from one activity to another, even to adjust from one time zone to another. They recommend using yawning consciously as a tool to make life better. For example, yawn soon after awakening to rev up your brain for the day or at night to help calm yourself and promote sleep.

THE SCIENCE OF THE YAWN

Most people believe that we yawn to bring oxygen from the air into the body, but that's wrong, says psychotherapist Patt Lind-Kyle, MA, the author of *Heal Your Mind, Rewire Your Brain*. She calls yawning an "exercise for the brain" based on the growing number of studies that have found that it facilitates mental efficiency. Yawning does its magic by literally forcing extra blood directly to the brain. When you yawn, your facial muscles broadly contract and then relax, and this action pushes oxygen-rich blood into the brain's prefrontal cortex, the location of the "executive function" that covers planning, organization, decision-making, personality expression and many other crucial activities.

The yawn also sends blood to stimulate an area called the *precuneus*, which is involved in consciousness along with memory and motor coordination. As far as serving to cool the brain, a study at State University of New York-Albany found that performing difficult mental tasks, such as processing lots of information, actually increases brain temperature. Though we're all familiar with the way ongoing mental labor can trigger yawning, it's not because it is tiring. Again, the yawn sends blood to the brain to curtail its rising temperature, which is how it helps to maintain mental efficiency. Interestingly, both yawning and body thermo-regulation seem to be controlled by the same area of the brain, the hypothalamus.

PUTTING YOUR YAWNS TO WORK

Okay, so now we know that yawning can increase our efficiency in a number of areas... how can we take better advantage of this? Just decide to yawn and then do it—and I mean do a real face-stretcher! *I'll tell you how in a moment, but first here are some situations in which Lind-Kyle suggests adding a yawn...*

•**To stimulate better thinking.** When you are preparing for an exam, a presentation or an important conversation, you can enhance your performance by yawning several times first. During an exam, don't be shy about yawning when you find yourself losing focus or starting to stumble in your thoughts—it will help.

•**To reduce jet lag and reset energy levels.** At 20 weeks gestation, fetuses start to develop a wake/sleep pattern and as part of the process, they yawn...a lot. Lind-Kyle says that we can consciously use yawning to help reset our wake/sleep patterns, including when suffering jet lag. To start, yawn five times or so as soon as you get off the airplane. When you've experienced how well this refreshes you, Lind-Kyle says you may soon begin to do it intuitively—you'll find yourself yawning whenever you feel yourself starting to drag. She says that yawn-ing can be used in this manner to help you acclimate to high altitudes and to reset your energy level as you switch from one activity to another, such as from sleep to wakefulness.

•**To improve your mood...and, possibly even your relationships.** Yawning is associated with increased levels of *dopamine*, the neurotransmitter released from the hypothalamus that is associated with pleasure, motivation and sociability. Lind-Kyle says that when two people yawn together, it can help diminish tension in the relationship...and fortunately, yawning is highly contagious, so it's easy for both of you to get in on the act. If nothing else, a shared yawning session should make for a few ice-breaking laughs.

•**For relaxation.** Curiously, although yawning serves to stimulate the brain, a deep yawn and wide stretch also relax the body. Lind-Kyle, who leads meditation classes, always starts with a healthy yawn, which she says gets people relaxed quickly. She said that bringing on a few deep yawns at bedtime may help you get to sleep.

HOW TO BRING ON A YAWN

We think of yawns as automatic, but it's surprisingly easy to make yourself yawn...

•**Focus thoughts on yawning.** Yawns are not only contagious from person to person—even thinking about a yawn can help trigger one, says Lind-Kyle. Close your eyes and picture a yawn, or say the word "yawn" repeatedly to encourage one.

•**Fake a yawn...**or two...or three until a real one sets in. Lind-Kyle says she generally gets a real yawn after one or two fakes, but however long it takes, stick with it—it will happen.

•**Consciously slow your breathing.** The decreased oxygen may help trigger a yawn—flaring your nostrils as you breathe in may make this happen faster.

And finally, the best yawn is one you fully experience, Lind-Kyle says. So go all the way—open your mouth wide, scrunch your face fully, and take a deep, full breath. Just be ready to explain yourself if you're in company!

Index